FOUNDATIONS OF COMPLEMENTARY THERAPIES AND ALTERNATIVE MEDICINE

Also by Robert Adams:

A Measure of Diversion? Case Studies in Intermediate Treatment (co-author)
Problem-solving Through Self-help Groups (co-author)
Self-help, Social Work and Empowerment *
Protests by Pupils: Empowerment, Schooling and the State
Prison Riots in Britain and the US *
Skilled Work with People
Working with and within Groups
The Personal Social Services: Clients, Consumers or Citizens?
Quality Social Work *
The Abuses of Punishment *
Social Work: Themes, Issues and Critical Debates * (co-editor)
Critical Practice in Social Work * (co-editor)
Social Policy for Social Work *
Social Work and Empowerment *
Practising Social Work in a Complex World * (co-editor)
Foundations of Health and Social Care *
A Short Guide to Social Work
Foundations of Childhood and Early Years Work *
Empowerment, Participation and Social Work *

* Published by Palgrave Macmillan

Foundations of Complementary Therapies and Alternative Medicine

Edited by
ROBERT ADAMS

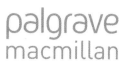
palgrave
macmillan

First published 2010 by
PALGRAVE MACMILLAN

Palgrave Macmillan in the UK is an imprint of Macmillan Publishers Limited, registered in England, company number 785998, of Houndmills, Basingstoke, Hampshire RG21 6XS.

Palgrave Macmillan in the US is a division of St Martin's Press LLC, 175 Fifth Avenue, New York, NY 10010.

Palgrave Macmillan is the global academic imprint of the above companies and has companies and representatives throughout the world.

Palgrave® and Macmillan® are registered trademarks in the United States, the United Kingdom, Europe and other countries.

ISBN-13: 978–0–230–21143–8

This book is printed on paper suitable for recycling and made from fully managed and sustained forest sources. Logging, pulping and manufacturing processes are expected to conform to the environmental regulations of the country of origin.

A catalogue record for this book is available from the British Library.

10 9 8 7 6 5 4 3 2 1
19 18 17 16 15 14 13 12 11 10

Printed in China

To my late father-in-law
Nasser Cassim Athraby 1922–2005

Brief Contents

Full Contents

List of Resource Files

List of Figures

List of Tables

Acknowledgements

Chapter 3 – Table 3.2 is used with the permission of Family Doctor Publications, Poole.

Chapter 9 – The authors and publishers would like to thank the Nursing and Midwifery Council, the College of Occupational Therapists and the General Osteopathic Council for their permission to reproduce their codes of practice.

Chapter 14 – The photographs are by David Mitchell and were taken with permission at the AECC Chiropractic College, UK.

Chapter 28 – The authors and publishers would like to thank GIA publications for the use of the two images in Figure 28.1 © 2000 by Barbara H. Conable and Benjamin J. Conable. Distributed by GIA Publications, Inc., 7404 S. Mason Ave., Chicago, IL 60638, www.giamusic.com, 800.442.1358. All rights reserved. Used by permission.

Chapter 29 – The authors would like to acknowledge the following, who have brought invaluable information to the West from Japan: Robert Jefford, who in 1954 started working with a number of students and friends of Usui in Japan, and in particular with the hands-on techniques known as reiki; and Chris Marsh, who in 2000 started working with a student of Usui's, known as Suzuki, focusing on the meditations and techniques 'to achieve personal perfection'.

Chapter 31 – The author would like to say thank you to the arts and play therapists who were willing to be interviewed for this chapter.

Every effort has been made to trace copyright holders but, if any have inadvertently been missed, the publishers will be pleased to make the necessary arrangements at the first opportunity.

Notes on Contributors

Robert Adams is Professor of Social Work in the School of Health and Social Care, University of Teesside and visiting Professor in the University of the West of Scotland. He has edited and written more than 100 publications, including more than 20 books, with translations into Chinese, Japanese and Korean. He has researched, written and lectured in the UK and abroad on empowering people in health, social work and other human services.

Sue Armstrong is a lay homeopath (RSHom) for human patients and a qualified veterinary surgeon (MRCVS) and veterinary member of the Faculty of Homeopathy (VetMFHom) for her animal patients. Having been in full-time practice since 1984, she set up her current practice Balanced Being in Wetherby in 2003, which has homeopathy as its core philosophy. At this clinic, Sue offers treatment to the whole family regardless of the species. Sue is a partner of the Homeopathic Professionals Teaching Group, which provides professional homeopathic training for doctors, veterinary surgeons, physiotherapists, chiropractors, dentists and nurses. Sue is the President of the British Association of Homeopathic Veterinary Surgeons and President of the Canadian College of Animal Homeopathy. She lectures extensively internationally and has written numerous journal articles. In 2008, Sue set up the Balanced Being Foundation, dedicated in part to clinical research into homeopathy and integrated medicine. Sue can be contacted at www.balanced-being.com.

Sally Canning taught an introduction to complementary therapies and now works in the field of meridian energy therapies, energy psychology and holistic health. She is an international trainer at Inner Solutions, an organization offering complementary therapies, and works with, among others, Phoenix Aid, a charity working with individuals and groups in Bosnia and Herzegovina. She is an advanced practitioner of emotional freedom technique, and also practises EmoTrance and Tapas Acupressure Technique. Sally can be contacted at www.innersolutions-uk.com.

R Mike Chan is a practitioner of traditional Chinese medicine who is registered with the British Medical Acupuncture Society in England, and since 1997 he has been a member of the Association of Hong Kong and Kowloon Practitioners of Traditional Chinese Medicine and is listed with the Chinese Medicine Council of Hong Kong. He was taught by his uncle, one of a family line of TCM practitioners extending back seven generations. He spent eight years in the Royal Navy as a medic in Hong Kong. He holds the Member of International Acupuncture Society

(China), is a member of the British Medical Acupuncture Society (UK) and is a UK registered mental nurse. He practises at clinics in Hull and East Yorkshire. Mike can be contacted at www.jqt-chinesemedicine.com.

Hugh Gemmell is a qualified chiropractor as well as holding a doctoral degree in health promotion. He is Principal Lecturer at the Anglo-European Chiropractic College and has practised chiropractic for 30 years. His main interests are teaching and research in myofascial pain medicine. Hugh is also active in postgraduate teaching and seminars.

Nicola Hall is Director of The Bayly School of Reflexology, which holds training courses in London, Edinburgh, Birmingham and overseas. She is the author of eight books on reflexology, which have been translated into many languages, and has also contributed to a number of complementary therapy texts. She is Chairman of The British Reflexology Association and has been a reflexology practitioner in Worcestershire for over 30 years.

Sue Jennings is a state registered dramatherapist, play therapist, supervisor and author, with over 30 books published in many languages. *Neuro-Dramatic-Play and Attachment* will be published in February 2010, by Jessica Kingsley. She has pioneered dramatherapy and 'arts become healing' in many countries and lives in the UK and Romania with her partner Peter. In Glastonbury, Somerset, they have their own art gallery and studio The Rowan Centre, which has become the hub of artistic activity of all kinds. Sue can be contacted on suejphd@gmail.com.

Andrew Maddick trained at the British College of Osteopathic Medicine (BCOM) and graduated in 1999. His first job was at the Osteopathic Centre for Children where he gained a Diploma in Paediatric Osteopathy and a Masters in Research. Andrew has a specialist interest in paediatrics and research, and he works as a consultant osteopath at the Foundation for Paediatric Osteopathy, a Senior Lecturer at BCOM, and in private practice in Norfolk. He has taught across the UK and Europe, and is involved with research into osteopathy for preterm infants and children with cerebral palsy. Andrew lives and practises in Norfolk and London.

Fanyi Meng was educated in Beijing Chinese Medicine University and qualified as a medical doctor and Chinese medicine doctor in 1983, holding a research degree the equivalent of a PhD in medicine. He was an Associate Professor in Beijing before moving to the UK. He has been Course Leader and Clinical Director of Acupuncture at the University of Lincoln for four years. He has written three books, contributed eight chapters in books and written more than 20 research reports. He is also an elected council member of the Association of Traditional Chinese Medicine (UK), the professional body of TCM practitioners, and a council member of the Sub-Health Society of the World Federation of Chinese Medicine.

Rosemary Pharo has been practising reiki since 1998, predominantly in Western styles and latterly Eastern. She is a qualified childbirth educator and complementary therapist and has a background in writing. She is a member of Reiki Healers and Teachers Society and the Complementary Therapists Association. She has been involved in developing practitioner standards for reiki in the UK since 2003.

Lama Rabsang was born in 1971 and brought up in Tibet. He became a monk aged 11 and studied and worked in Buddhist monasteries, first in Tibet and later in India. He has practised meditation for many years. He lives in Brynmawr, Wales, where he teaches Buddhism and meditation at the Buddhist centre, Palpung Changchub Dargyeling (www.palpung.org.uk).

Jacqueline Richards is Lecturer in Adjustive Technique, as well as an Assistant Lecturer in Neuro-Orthopaedics, in the faculty of Chiropractic Sciences at the Anglo-European College of Chiropractic, Bournemouth. She has an interest in research, specifically in the area of psychomotor skill training.

Doreen Sawyer has practised reiki for 10 years and has experience in both Eastern and Western styles. She is a qualified teacher, trainer, assessor and complementary therapist and is involved with the UK Reiki Federation. Having worked for a number of awarding bodies during her career, she has lectured at both Swindon and Newbury College in a range of business subjects and teaches both NVQs and complementary therapies from her own training centre in Ludgershall near Andover. She has worked with National Occupational Standards since their inception and was involved with the 2008/09 revision of NOS in complementary therapies.

Lena Schibel-Mason has practised the Alexander technique full time for 18 years. She founded the York Alexander Technique School (yats@thorpestreet.org) and has been the director since 2003, has taught dancers at Scarborough University, actors at acting schools and music students at the Music Department of York University. In her private practice, she teaches a wide range of ages (from 6 to over 80) and people from all walks of life and with all manner of activities or ailments they want to improve, including back, neck, shoulder pain and a wish for a more wholesome posture and for diminishing tiredness. She has taught the Alexander technique as part of a module of alternative medicine to medical students in Leeds.

Andrew Stableford is Senior Lecturer in Herbal Medicine at the University of Lincoln, where he is the Programme Leader for the course. His academic and research interests are to develop an integration of contemporary herbal medicine therapeutics with mainstream biomedical knowledge to expand the understanding of how herbal medicine can intercede in the complexities of body, mind and spirit dynamics and be truly holistic. He is currently working on a book on this 'energetic' approach to herbal medicine therapeutics.

Karen Tinker practises aromatherapy in Barnsley, Yorkshire, and has been heavily involved in charity work in Bosnia for five years, treating war victims with physical and emotional trauma, congenitally disabled children and vulnerable adults with aromatherapy and various other holistic therapies. Karen began her holistic therapies in 1999 and teaches and practises various forms of energy healing – reiki/ seichem, quantum touch and Egyptian cartouche – and her own channelled work along with some metaphysical emotional release work. Karen has just completed a qualification in lomi lomi (Hawaiian massage) and Ayurvedic massage. Her book on channelled work is due for publication.

Jason J.W. Tsai holds degrees in pharmacy and traditional Chinese medicine and received his training in conventional medical and Chinese medical sciences in Taiwan and China. He received a PhD in Biological Sciences from the University of Warwick and undertook a number of years of research in Biochemistry and Molecular Biology at Imperial College London. He teaches on the Complementary Medicine Programme of the University of Lincoln and sits on the editorial board of the *Global Journal of Health Science*.

Introduction

My purpose in this book is to equip those who wish to use complementary and alternative approaches, as practitioners and/or self-carers, with the knowledge and understanding to be critical and self-critical in their practice. This is not a negative goal, but it means questioning rather than simply providing information. The topic of this book is of growing importance in the modern world, as we turn increasingly from high-tech, high carbon input products and services towards traditional, more environmentally sound ways of living, as individuals and in groups and communities.

The use of the somewhat cumbersome term 'complementary therapies and alternative medicine' indicates the problematic territory of the subject of this book. It is not that the subject is unknown so much as the terminology reflects the differing status of a huge number and range of different approaches. As is apparent below, some of the approaches considered here form the mainstream of traditional medicine in many non-Western countries, while others are regarded by many people as already part of, or moving into, the mainstream of conventional Western medicine.

Purpose of this Book

It would be easy, but mistaken, to begin this book by reflecting on some of the rhetoric of advocates of complementary therapies and alternative medicine, rather than questioning it. What do I mean by this? Well, let us take the example of Frawley's (2003: 1) authoritative handbook on the Indian subcontinent's ancient 'Ayurvedic' system of medicine, which is practised widely nowadays in Western as well as Eastern countries. This begins:

> We are in the midst of a global paradigm shift in health care. At the center of this change is Ayurvedic medicine, a healing system which promotes health using natural nontoxic substances and which recognizes the important role of the mind and emotions.

I do not say that Frawley is necessarily wrong in putting Ayurvedic medicine at the centre of a revolution in healthcare throughout the world. However, rather than simply reflecting his view, along with the views of other advocates of complementary and alternative approaches, the purpose of this book is to become engaged in reflecting critically on them. Is there a revolution? Is it worldwide? Is the (historically) ancient Indian system at the core of the revolution?

My thoughts about this are that there are many traditions of healthcare that we inherit from ancient history. Ayurvedic medicine is one of them and it is true that, like other traditions, it has made the transition from nonindustrialized countries, which we (in a somewhat condescending way) often call 'developing', to largely Western industrialized countries, those we often call 'developed'. Alongside this trend, there are many approaches that have developed within the past two centuries and these also have become popular in Western countries, among others. Some have remained 'alternative' to conventional medicine, while others have become 'complementary' to them. Surely it is questionable to regard these traditional approaches, which are all that approximately half the people in the world will ever know of health services in their lifetime, as alternative? Quite simply, many people have no alternative.

We need to adopt a questioning approach to the dominant attitude of Western medicine implicit both in the title of this book and in the above discussion – that the approaches considered in this book are marginal, that is, complementary and alternative, while Western medicine is mainstream. In most countries of the world, traditional medicine is mainstream.

Linked with the above point, we can ask: is the book solely about 'medicine'? The answer is a definite 'no'. Some of the approaches discussed in this book would resist being medicalized at all – the educational Alexander technique, for example. Others would reject a Western biomedical model – reiki, for example, which is a spiritual approach often used in healing, one of many holistic approaches.

Let us return to my previous point, that there is rapid growth in complementary and alternative approaches, which may or may not amount to a revolution. This is a matter of opinion. Your view may depend on whether you are a complementary practitioner yourself or a doctor. It may depend on whether your relative was cured by conventional surgery or helped by a complementary practitioner, or indeed whether your relative may not have been cured or helped. The picture is complex. At the start of this book, it is important to be aware of the relative positions of different systems of health and wellbeing theory and practice, because this point is neither made clearly from within conventional medicine, nor is it accepted by many of its practitioners. This book will be mapping complementary and alternative approaches, exploring their richness, but at the same time examining the evidence base for their uses complementary with, as an alternative to, or as an integrated part of, conventional healthcare and medicine.

Aim of this Book

The aim of this book is to provide an authoritative base for students, self-carers and practitioners across the entire field of complementary therapies and alternative medicine. These approaches are growing in prominence yet many of them remain somewhat controversial. This book sets out the basis for a professional approach to critical practice in this field. This entails practitioners practising with due regard both to the evidence base for their particular approach and also to the bedrock of values and ethics in which their principled approach is based. I argue that practitioners in complementary therapies and alternative medicine need to develop an evidence-based, ethical and principled practice. The ethical basis for practice is as important as evidence-based practice, because both are equally concerned with the professional actions of the practitioner, the latter with what is done and the former with how it is done.

The bookshelves on complementary and alternative approaches are laden with three types of books:

1. There are hundreds, probably thousands, of informative guides to particular approaches to complementary therapy or alternative medicine. Also, there is a growing number of encyclopedic general guides across numbers of complementary approaches (Hulke, 1978; BMA, 1993; Woodham, 1994; Fulder, 1997; Shealy, 2000; Lewith, 2002; Bratman, 2007). These form the bulk of what we may call the 'popular' literature.
2. There are also many books of the 'how to practise' variety, which claim to cover what the potential practitioner needs to know.
3. Finally, there is, by comparison, a tiny number of evaluative books focusing on research studies into complementary and alternative approaches. This heightens the need for a text that opens up and lays out the main areas of this complex field, provides a well-evidenced source of key areas of knowledge and understanding and discusses the main areas of debate.

This burgeoning literature is one sign that the industry of complementary therapies and alternative medicine is growing rapidly in the UK and other Western countries and is still widespread in some of the largest and most populous and economically powerful territories such as China, the Indian subcontinent, Japan, Malaysia and Indonesia. By 1998, sales of complementary medicinal products in the UK totalled £93m, of which £50m was sales of herbal medicines, £23m homeopathic medicines and £20m aromatherapy essential oils. This was a 50% increase in the £63m total in 1994, with evidence of a continued further increase (House of Lords, 2000). The increasing popularity of complementary and alternative healthcare and self-care accompanies the growing acceptance by more people of the principles and practices inherent in a diversity of approaches to wellbeing.

Despite the widespread use of complementary and alternative routes to wellbeing, they remain controversial and debates over their efficacy continue. Official, that is, professional, antagonism from within the health services in Western countries has persisted since the nineteenth century. At the same time, various estimates indicate their use by between a quarter and a third of people in the West, while it is likely that usage in developing countries is far higher. Estimates vary, but research indicates that by the late 1980s, more than 90% of GPs in the Netherlands were referring patients to alternative practitioners such as homeopaths and acupuncturists (Visser and Peters, 1990). Research also shows that more than two-thirds of people in the USA have tried at least one form of alternative medicine (InterSurvey, 2000). This represents an increase from 33.8% in

1990 (Eisenberg et al., 1993) and 42% in 1997 (Eisenberg et al., 1998), these figures being based on use of at least one of 16 alternative therapies during the previous year.

Structure of this Book

This book is structured so as to take the reader through the main aspects that are required in study and practice development.

Part I deals with the skills needed for learning and studying (Chapter 1) and the knowledge and understanding required to grasp the main aspects of professional development (Chapter 2).

Part II introduces some important contextual themes that form the basis for knowing about, and critical understanding of, complementary approaches, notably their social, policy and legal bases (Chapters 3–5).

Part III sets out the main ethical, multiprofessional, business, health and safety and hygiene aspects of managing your practice, whether employed in the health service or working independently (Chapters 6–8).

Part IV deals with the areas of knowledge, understanding and skills required for working with patients and clients (Chapters 9–12).

Part V deals with the historical, philosophical and scientific knowledge of the main areas of practice and of anatomy, physiology, pathology and the differential diagnosis of different conditions and illnesses (Chapters 13–18).

Part VI deals with the main different areas of practice (Chapters 19–31). These areas of practice have been selected because individually they represent the character of their particular approach and collectively they represent the huge variety of the field.

The process of selection means that some important areas have not been given a chapter. To have allocated a chapter to each area would have required several volumes of the size of this one. For example, the ancient status of Ayurveda as a traditional Indian medicine that predates most other systems is recognized. While we devote a chapter to the associated beliefs of traditional Chinese medicine and then a chapter to its practice, Ayurvedic practice is not dealt with here in a separate chapter. This is because it was deemed that both Ayurvedic and traditional Chinese systems of medicine have in common, among their own bases for practice, the major elements of earth, water, fire, metal and wood, the practices of pulse and tongue diagnosis that contribute to assessment, and use holistic treatments (such as massage, herbs and aromatherapy) based on the notion of restoring physiological harmony and balance between the elements. However, Ayurvedic principles and practice have not been adopted in Western countries to the extent of traditional Chinese medicine.

Part VII deals with the important topic of maintaining your continuing professional development throughout your career (Chapter 32).

Features of the Book

The book contains an array of features to engage and enhance the reader's experience.

At the start of the chapter:

■ *Learning Outcomes:* Statements that summarize what you can expect to learn by reading it.

Throughout the chapter:

■ *Key Concepts:* Important ideas that are referred to in bold in the text and listed in Appendix 2.
■ *Practice Examples:* Short illustrations drawn from practice, which highlight relevant points.
■ *Activities:* Suggested things to do that may enable you to focus on a key message in part of a chapter.

At the end of the chapter:

■ *Review Questions:* Questions that encourage you to check back and see whether you have gained a particular piece of knowledge or understood a key idea.
■ *Chapter Links:* Suggestions about other chapters in which you will find other material of relevance to the chapter you have just read.
■ *Further Resources:* Relevant readings and websites.

At the end of Parts I–V, immediately following Chapters 21, 22, 24, 28, 30, 31 and at the end of Part VII:

■ *Resource Files:* Particular topics of importance, relating to the preceding part or chapter(s).

Abbreviations

AAA	abdominal aorta aneurysm	GH	growth hormone
ACTH	adrenocorticotrophic hormone	GHRH	growth hormone-releasing hormone
ADH	antidiuretic hormone (also called vasopressin)	GnRH	gonadotrophin-releasing hormone
A&E	accident and emergency	GP	general practitioner
ANS	autonomic nervous system	GRCCT	General Regulatory Council for Complementary Therapies
AOC	Aromatherapy Organisations Council	HDL	high-density lipoproteins
ATC	Aromatherapy Trades Council	HRT	hormone replacement therapy
BCA	British Chiropractic Association	HVT	high velocity thrust
BCMA	British Complementary Medicine Association	IBS	irritable bowel syndrome
		IHD	ischaemic heart disease
BCTCVSR	British Complementary Therapies Council for Voluntary Self Regulation	LBP	low/lower back pain
		LDL	low-density lipoproteins
BMA	British Medical Association	LH	luteinizing hormone
CAM	complementary and alternative medicine	MI	myocardial infarction
		MRI	magnetic resonance imaging
CBT	cognitive behavioural therapy	MRSA	methicillin resistant *Staphylococcus aureus*
CHD	coronary heart disease		
CNHC	Complementary and Natural Healthcare Council	MS	multiple sclerosis
		NASW	National Association of Social Workers (USA)
CNS	central nervous system		
COT	College of Occupational Therapists	NCAHF	National Council Against Health Fraud
CRH	corticotrophin-releasing hormone	NIMH	National Institute of Medical Herbalists
CT	computed tomography	NSAID	non-steroidal anti-inflammatory drug
DM	diabetes mellitus		
EBP	evidence-based practice	OA	osteoarthritis
ECG	electrocardiogram	OTC	over the counter
EFT	emotional freedom technique	PCOS	polycystic ovarian syndrome
EU	European Union	PCT	primary care trust
FIH	Foundation for Integrated Health	PD	Parkinson's disease
FSH	follicle-stimulating hormone	PFIH	Prince's Foundation for Integrated Health
GCC	General Chiropractic Council		
GOsC	General Osteopathic Council	PNS	peripheral nervous system

RA	rheumatoid arthritis	UK	United Kingdom
RCT	randomized controlled trial	UKCC	United Kingdom Central Council for Nursing, Midwifery and Health Visiting
SMT	spinal manipulative therapy		
TB	tuberculosis		
TCM	traditional Chinese medicine	VBA	vertebrobasilar artery
TIM	traditional Indian medicine	WHCCAMP	White House Commission on Complementary and Alternative Medicine Policy
TM	traditional medicine		
TRH	thyrotrophin-releasing hormone		
TSH	thyroid-stimulating hormone (also known as thyrotrophin)	WHO	World Health Organization

Learning, Studying and Professional Practice

Part I
Learning, Studying and Professional Practice

Introduction

Part I is written in the expectation that many readers of this book will be from a nontraditional educational background and new to further or higher education and may therefore welcome the opportunity for some additional learning support at the start of the programme. Indeed, English may not be your first language, or you may have enrolled on a course which takes for granted that you are already 'up to speed' in the practicalities of being a student. With this in mind, Part I is a preliminary to the main content, aiming to orient new students to learning and equip them with the confidence, skills and learning resources necessary to tackle the subject matter.

Chapter 1 deals with the skills required in order to engage in college, university and work-based learning. Chapter 2 deals with the important matters of personal awareness and professional development, which are threaded through all the chapters. You need to read and think carefully about the material in Chapter 2, so that you can engage in the process of critical reflection throughout the rest of this book.

Skills for College and Work-based Learning

ROBERT ADAMS

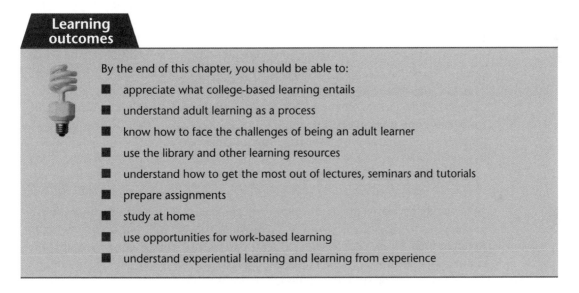

By the end of this chapter, you should be able to:

- appreciate what college-based learning entails
- understand adult learning as a process
- know how to face the challenges of being an adult learner
- use the library and other learning resources
- understand how to get the most out of lectures, seminars and tutorials
- prepare assignments
- study at home
- use opportunities for work-based learning
- understand experiential learning and learning from experience

This book begins with material in this chapter intended to help you to learn more effectively. But this is only to help build your confidence and, perhaps, give you a quick start with books, learning, studying for assignments and writing essays. The heart of learning and working as a practitioner lies in how we reflect on experience and use this in our subsequent actions. These first two chapters in this book start this process.

I do not intend this to be a mechanical primer; it does not focus merely on your study skills; it does not present the journey to becoming proficient as a complementary practitioner as though it consists merely of acquiring knowledge and learning techniques. It is much more exciting than that. It is about becoming a critical and reflective practitioner – a journey which, when you embark on it, should engage you for the rest of your life. This book puts forward complementary practice as a lifelong process. When we reach Part VI of the book, you will gain some sense of this, as the different practitioners in our writing team each share with you important aspects of their own development as practitioners. They write from this direct experience. If you want to understand what the book is all about, you can dip into these chapters now, selecting an area of practice in which you want to specialize. But you will need to return to the earlier parts of the book as well, in order to develop a fuller understanding of this area of practice.

This first chapter moves towards understanding learning as much more than study skills alone, but as an approach to reflecting on, and bringing together in an integrated way, three very different sources of experience:

- experience at work
- experience as a student
- previous life experience.

This chapter is written on the assumption that you will probably be learning, working and studying simultaneously for much of the time that you are reading this book. This will be the case whether you are on a course, or not. It is likely that in the field of complementary practice, you are doing some form of related work, even if you are also taking a course, such as a foundation degree. We shall spend much of the chapter considering these two major areas of learning opportunities: college-based learning (by which I include sixth form, further education and university) and work-based learning.

College-based Learning

Not everybody learns at, or through, college. Half my undergraduate and post-graduate university degrees were gained when working full time and studying in my own time. Many people spend at least part of their college course juggling the competing demands of work. Foundation degrees are designed on the assumption that learners will be studying alongside relevant work.

However, college is where most people go to acquire qualifications beyond school and studying complementary therapies and alternative medicine is likely to entail being based, whether full time or not, in a college or university. Some programmes of study are distance based, which means the student does not attend college, or they may be flexible, involving some short blocks of full-time study and the use of work-books, study guides or other learning resources to support learning at a distance.

People take up college or university courses at different stages of their lives. In some ways, a student moving straight from school to college may find the transition easier than someone who has been away from the classroom for years. However, the more experienced adult learner brings a wealth of experience on return to college and invariably is highly motivated to use the time positively. So while the adult learner finds it challenging, there should be no doubt that the college benefits from the diversity of adult learners' experiences and their high motivation to learn and do well.

Becoming an Adult Learner

Adult learning does not happen to us simply by paying our fees and registering for the course. It is a process we take part in, which involves us developing new areas of knowledge and understanding, engaging in discussion of ideas and practice and being challenged by viewpoints that are different from our existing ones. All in all, we may find this rewarding, but there are bound to be some times when we find it tiring, even exhausting. Some parts of learning may involve us discarding our existing ideas and assumptions and this can be painful.

Meeting the challenge of learning

Many would-be complementary practitioners have been away from education for many years when they are studying for their qualification. It is possible to meet the demands of becoming a student by being organized, but first of all it may be somewhat daunting to find oneself back in the classroom as an adult student, faced with a pile of handouts, course outlines and reading lists. It is important to realize that the key to success at this point is being well organized. Do the following:

- Do not panic.
- Develop the habit of organizing all the material as it accumulates, in folders separately labelled with each subject, with lecture notes and topics indexed within them.
- Carry an appointments diary and jot down the date and time of every meeting and other event that matters, day by day, as you find out about it.
- Keep phone numbers, addresses, the names of people and places all together where you can easily find them. Keep a copy at home in case you lose your diary.

Using the Library

The library, or learning resources centre, is the hub of learning. These days, students can often access university libraries from home, using Athens or a similar scheme. If you register at college or university, you will be able to find out about these opportunities by asking the library staff. Some courses use Blackboard as a means of communicating with students off campus. Tutors may put information, including reading lists, about their courses on Blackboard, for the benefit of off-campus students.

Library staff will give guided tours to many college libraries, which usually take place at the beginning of the term when new courses begin. These are an invaluable source of tips on how to search for material. There is no substitute, however, for browsing and becoming familiar with the books in particular sections. Often libraries differ in how the material is laid out.

While books and journals are the mainstay of libraries, the modern library gives access to many other sources of learning, including learning packages deposited with particular courses in mind, archived material, DVDs and tapes and, of course, online sources.

Reading

It is easy to be intimidated by the wealth of material available on a particular topic. Everybody studies in their own way, but the following hints are worth bearing in mind:

- Clarify the task.
- Choose a manageable number of appropriate books and/or journal articles.
- Be realistic about how much you attempt to read in a limited period.
- Select the most up-to-date edition of a book.
- Take notes while reading.
- Think critically while reading.
- Write out key quotes 'verbatim', that is, using the exact words and punctuation of the original. Record the page number, book title, author, publisher and place; or journal title, volume, issue and page numbers.

Taking notes

The key skill of taking notes is to learn how to summarize. When reading a page, practise the art – and it is an art, it takes practice – of making a list of bullet points comprising the main points the author is making. Try this after reading the entire page, rather than making notes line by line. If it proves difficult, be tough and decide that the entire page has to be summarized in no more than three bullet points.

Lectures, Seminars and Tutorials

College and university courses usually are built around a core of activities that bring groups of students together with tutors and lecturers in various programmed events:

- *Lectures* tend to take the form of largely one-way communication from the lecturer to the students.
- *Seminars* are more of an open discussion. Some students are more forthcoming in seminars, while others find them intimidating and do not make a contribution. It is important to use seminars in the way the college intends. They may follow particular sequences of lectures and each may be intended as opportunities to clarify ideas raised in the preceding lecture. They may be built around required reading and it will be important to do this in advance.
- *Tutorials* are relatively rare opportunities for students to meet with tutors, either individually or in small groups. Again, it is important to ensure that the best use is made of these.

Throughout, it is important to assume that only one opportunity exists to learn about any particular topic, so even if other students say a lecture, seminar or tutorial is not important, invariably it is. Realizing this afterwards is too late.

Doing Assignments

Assignments are assessment tasks that need to be completed as a course proceeds. It is realistic to think of an assignment as an iceberg. Experts tell us that approximately six-sevenths of an iceberg lies below the surface of the water and only one-seventh is visible. Similarly, most of the work of doing an assignment – reading, taking notes, thinking and writing drafts – is not visible in the end product. However, a marker can tell from the quality of the writing how much work has gone into an assignment, so it is important not to neglect this.

Some basic tasks are entailed in any learning task. The secret of studying for a particular assignment is to focus clearly on the topic and work through a prescribed sequence.

Once the studying for an assignment is well under way, it is best to begin to draft it, which means sketching it out and writing as much as you can, in rough rather than in best, instead of waiting until you have completed all the preparation. The process of actually drafting the assignment reveals what gaps there are and the questions that remain unanswered.

Developing Study Skills and Planning Study Time

People study in different ways and everybody has particular preferences when it comes to settling down to concentrate on thinking about and studying for a particular assignment. A good deal of published guidance is available on study skills and many of the short texts in local bookshops are clearly written and very good value.

We live busy lives and even the act of reading this book takes time that we may feel we cannot afford. However, without setting aside time to study, it will not be possible to move forward in learning about complementary approaches. It is important to make quality time to study. The competing demands on time mean that making time to study reduces the time spent on other activities.

Planning study time entails making a weekly plan in the diary and slotting into it realistic chunks of time when study can take place. The plan should cover all seven days and not be limited to college days. The competing pressures of work and home may mean that study time will be limited to college days. However, a detailed look at home time may suggest spaces – half an hour here or there – where study could take place. It is important to have a book placed strategically, with a notepad to take notes, so that these half-hour slots can be used effectively.

Work-based Learning

Put simply, work-based learning is learning at work, or while engaged in a particular task. However, work-based learning is a challenging activity and in order to tackle the challenge, we need to understand its basis and what it entails. Some foundation degrees, vocational and professional courses in complementary approaches will include a work-based learning component. This is where you as the student can learn about practice settings, exercise appropriate skills and understand the relevance and relationship between theory and practice.

Work-based learning components can either take place as part of an organized placement (found by the student or the university/college) or, if you are on a work-based route, by using your current places of work as a learning resource for practice. In either case, it is important to establish the boundaries of the work-based learning and the knowledge, skills and values you are expected to demonstrate. It is also important to recognize and understand the partnership that will be established between the student, practice placement and tutor and what the roles of the respective participants will be. This should be established within a practice agreement prior to the commencement of the practice period. The role of the placement and the partners may include elements of the following:

- Identifying your needs as a student in relation to practice and reviewing and adapting these as the practice period progresses
- Identifying the sequence of learning opportunities to be provided
- Identifying and establishing links between the academic and practice elements of the programme
- Enabling you as a student to recognize and transfer existing knowledge, skills and values to the current practice and academic settings
- Assessing the knowledge, skills and values that the placement aims to enable the student to develop and demonstrate
- Giving feedback to you as a student – when and in what format
- Supervising you, the student – who will do this and what it will focus on.

Experiencing and Learning from Experience

The idea of experiential learning can help with work-based learning. It has some limitations, as we shall see, but it provides a good starting point, which we can use critically to develop a useful model for work-based learning.

Experiential learning is the term often used on courses to refer to different ways in which people draw on their previous and current learning from experience. The literature on experiential learning is rooted in cognitive psychology. The word **cognition** refers to those processes by which we are aware of, experience and know the world around us. These two forms of learning have a lot in common, but in reality are quite different from each other. Kolb has written about experiential learning and brief reference to his work enables us to introduce two different ideas – learning styles and the process of experiential learning.

Learning styles: Kolb

Kolb (1984) developed a four-stage model of the process of learning through experience (Figure 1.1).

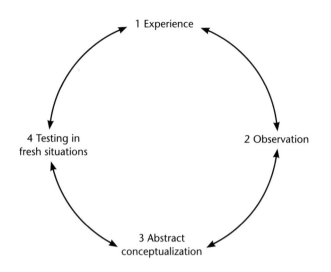

Figure 1.1 Kolb's experiential learning cycle

The cycle begins with (stage 1) the concrete experience of the person, moves on to (stage 2) observation and reflection on this, continues with (stage 3) abstract conceptualization, when the learner develops ideas that provide a model of what has been observed and continues again (stage 4) when the learner sets out to test what has been learned.

Kolb linked a key process with each stage, which he identified as a role performed by the learner (Figure 1.2).

Concrete Active	Concrete Reflective
Active learner: **'learning through doing'**	**Reflective learner:** **'learning through thinking** **about'**
Abstract Active	Abstract Reflective
Pragmatic learner: **'learning through applying in** **practice'**	**Theorist learner:** **'learning through theorizing** **about practice'**

Figure 1.2 Learning styles adopted in the process of experiential learning

Kolb's ideas have the advantage of focusing attention on how we learn and enabling us to understand how different people approach their experience differently. However, beyond this, it is a mistake to do what many lecturers do, which is to present students with the diagram and invite them to explore which kind of learner they are. The four types are very much models or ideal types, rather than an attempt to impose on a particular person a single learning style. Most of us learn in different ways in different situations and probably change our style in the process. The strengths of Kolb's approach are that he:

- highlights for tutors the message that people learn differently from each other
- emphasizes the important contribution that a person's experience makes to their learning
- confronts us with the reality that knowledge in the form of college lectures is meaningless unless we can relate it to our own thoughts and feelings, ideas and experiences.

Some weaknesses of Kolb's approach are that:

- it concentrates on primary learning from experience
- it does not emphasize the value of secondary, formally structured work-based learning.

Let us recognize these two equivalent but very different major sources of experiential learning:

1. *Primary learning from experience*, which involves you learning from previous experience and work experience, independently of any formal courses. Some people refer to this as 'life' experience.
2. *Secondary learning from experience*, which refers to formally acquired learning from planned placements, for example those set up by the college or university as part of your present course of study. The purpose of this placement normally will be to enable you to build on existing, and develop new, areas of knowledge, understanding and skills. The main benefit of work-based experiential learning is that it takes place in a 'real practice' setting, one which approximates to the conditions encountered in everyday practice.

Putting these two forms of experiential learning together, these are some of the different ways in which people learn from experience:

- in cognitive ways – through thinking about and reflecting on what happens to them. Cognitive learning involves acquiring new knowledge, understanding and expertise through the process of conscious thought and reasoning
- through gathering information – by reading books and so on
- in diverse ways in different cultures – according to background and habits
- in socially situated ways – in one way at college and in other ways at work and at home.

We can use these different approaches as the basis for developing our own useful model for running work-based learning projects. The student benefits by being able to use all the different sources and methods of learning mentioned above, so that they all enable us to reflect critically and improve our knowledge, understanding and skills. When these combine, we call the product 'expertise'. This is quick to write, but actually is complex, involving us continuing to develop in personal and professional terms, as the different forms of experience and learning combine (Figure 1.3).

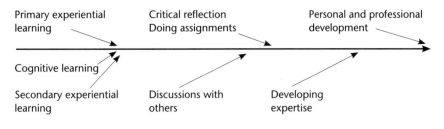

Figure 1.3 Process of college, home and work-based learning

Chapter Summary

This chapter has dealt with how to become equipped to meet the demands of learning about complementary approaches to practice. This requires a combination of learning and study skills as well as an understanding of what is entailed in learning as an adult.

REVIEW QUESTIONS

1   What are the main points you need to consider when preparing to write an assignment?

2   What key tasks will you face when carrying out a work-based learning placement?

3   What preparation will help you to gain the most from lectures and seminars?

CHAPTER LINKS

For further discussion of what developing as a reflective and critical practitioner entails, see Chapter 2.

For details of further opportunities for professional and personal development, see Chapter 32.

FURTHER RESOURCES

Burns, T. and Sinfield, S. (2003) *Essential Study Skills: The Complete Guide to Success at University*, London, Sage. A useful practice guide to studying.

Collins, S.C. and Kneale, P.E. (2003) *Study Skills for Psychology Students: A Practical Guide*, London, Arnold. Despite its title, a helpful source of tips on study skills for students of complementary practice.

---

2 Personal Awareness, Critically Reflective Practice and Professional Development

ROBERT ADAMS

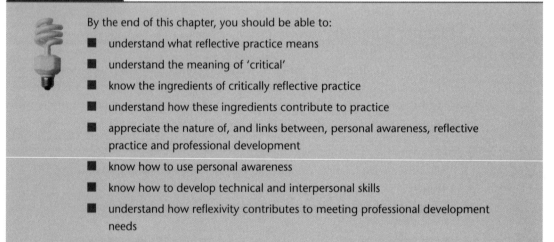

Learning outcomes

By the end of this chapter, you should be able to:

- understand what reflective practice means
- understand the meaning of 'critical'
- know the ingredients of critically reflective practice
- understand how these ingredients contribute to practice
- appreciate the nature of, and links between, personal awareness, reflective practice and professional development

- know how to use personal awareness
- know how to develop technical and interpersonal skills
- understand how reflexivity contributes to meeting professional development needs

I begin this chapter by linking it with what I said at the start of Chapter 1. Our college and work-based learning and professional development are intimately bound up with how we make sense of our experiences and this interacts with our personal development.

This chapter introduces the notion of critically reflective practice and shows how it contributes to personal and professional development. It is important to appreciate how interwoven these different topics are and how they relate to other aspects of professional practice. Your personal values, knowledge and understanding will be important contributors to the process of you becoming a critically reflective practitioner.

Becoming Critically Reflective in Practice

The meaning of reflection

Reflection is a simple word that carries a lot of meanings. We use the word 'reflection' in everyday life to refer to our image, thrown back at us when we look into a mirror. Another meaning of reflection is more sophisticated than this, when we examine our practice, as though we were a mirror, reflecting its reality back to ourselves. It is the professional meaning of reflection – as the core of the learning process.

This reflective process helps us to decide what to do next. If you can imagine us going through this process continually, this is the unending learning process that makes up reflective practice.

What is Reflective Practice?

Reflection brings together the actions involved in the continuous process of analysing, interpreting and evaluating. These are what we do when we reflect on our practice, that is, engage in **reflective practice**. Schön (1983) wrote extensively about reflective practice. Using his work, we can distinguish between reflective and unreflective practice (Figure 2.1).

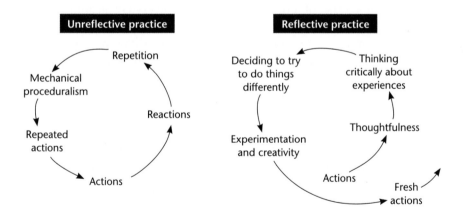

Figure 2.1 Contrasting processes of unreflective and reflective practice

In unreflective practice, the practitioner is trapped in an endless cycle of not learning from experience and repeating the same old problem-laden practice endlessly. There are dangers in this of harming clients or patients by not identifying new situations they bring to the consulting or treatment room and not treating them appropriately.

In reflective practice, the practitioner uses the initial stimulus of the first meetings and subsequent practice as the starting point for an endless process of questioning and self-critical thoughtfulness. This leads to evaluating previous practice and deciding to try something different next time, not for the sake of being different, but because there are always fresh problems demanding a questioning approach. This defines practice as a process of experimentation offering opportunities for creative work with patients and clients. They appreciate this, as the practitioner is always bringing freshness and vigour to the next appointment. The practitioner's reputation is enhanced as clients, patients and colleagues all gain from proximity to this reflective practice.

While discussing being reflective, it is important to distinguish this from the process of being reflexive. Reflection extends practice beyond your comfort zone by encouraging the habit of trying new ways of understanding and developing your practice. **Reflexivity** refers to the way you bring to bear on your reflections on another person's situation your emotions and thoughts in relation to your own experience and learning. There are two aspects to reflexivity: awareness of yourself and critical awareness of your practice and its context. Let us examine this word 'critical'.

The Meaning of Critical

What I have just described is what some people refer to as 'critical practice'. 'Critical' is another of those words that has an everyday meaning and a meaning in our professional practice. In everyday life, critical can be used when we want to say something negative about somebody or something. We say 'you are very critical of me', when somebody has criticized our speech or actions. Critical can also mean crucial or important, as when we say: 'the money you lent me was critical to my professional development because it enabled me to pay for my degree.' Closer to the meaning of 'critical' in our professional practice is the activity of the music, drama or book critic, who reacts to a particular work by writing a review. As we know, critics are meant to provide balanced reviews but sometimes are regarded as being too negative or 'critical'.

In our professional practice, we should be striving to give the patient or client the best possible service, based on the available evidence. We use our critical powers to appraise this evidence continually as we practise and we incorporate our critical appraisal of the latest evidence into our practice.

Ingredients of Critically Reflective Practice

What makes us critically reflective in practice? We do not acquire a simple set of skills that will one day enable us to wake up in the morning and say: 'yesterday, I wasn't a critically reflective practitioner, but now I have read that book and completed that course I am one.' For a start, reflection is as much about the kind of person you are becoming as what techniques you use. It is about being as much as doing. The best way to think of reflectiveness and reflexivity is that these are attitudes of mind, or ways of being. You become a critically reflective practitioner by developing this attitude. It is similar with critical reflectiveness. It is as much an attitude as it is a technique.

Let us try to identify the components of critically reflective practice. I shall do this by looking at the practitioner and asking: 'what aspects contribute to critically reflective practice?' The answer to this is 'qualities', knowledge or what I prefer to call 'understanding', commitment to 'values' and skills or what I prefer to call 'expertise'. Let us briefly examine each of these.

Qualities

It is important to recognize that practitioners use themselves – their own personal qualities and attributes, which some people refer to as 'gifts' – in their practice. Another term often used is 'personality', which in everyday speech does not mean what the psychologist means when administering a test of 'personality types'. It refers more to qualities such as warmth, empathy (the ability to understand and to an extent feel the emotions and share the experience the client or patient is undergoing), and the capacity to make the patient or client feel reassured and relaxed.

The word 'quality' draws attention to some aspects of our practice that depend more on aspects of ourselves which are partly inherent in the kind of person we are. This is not to say absolutely that we cannot develop or change them, but this certainly cannot be done as simply as learning to touch-type, for example. We are not talking about technical skills.

Activity

Make a list of no more than six key qualities you would regard as essential in a complementary therapy practitioner you visited as a client or patient.

My list includes the following:

- warmth
- empathy
- capacity to relax and reassure
- capacity to make professional relationship
- sensitivity
- self-awareness.

Understanding

Our second component is knowledge, or as I prefer to call it, understanding. The word understanding is helpful as a reminder that learning a fact is not the same as appreciating the meaning of something.

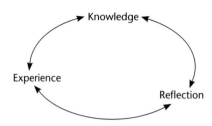

Figure 2.2 Components of understanding

In the first place, we have experience. We build our experience continually and, while this entails us learning new knowledge, when on our course of study, we are likely to acquire new knowledge through formal means. Whether this is greater in quantity or superior in quality depends on many factors, such as the standard of the course, how stimulating our teachers are, the books we read from the library and so on.

While on our course of study, we have the opportunity to reflect on this knowledge and experience (Figure 2.2). These three components – experience, knowledge and reflection – are bound together and interact with each other continually, as we turn over different ideas and topics. In complementary practice, is it important to understand the meanings of the terms, concepts, remedies, treatments and prescriptions applied and not just to know the technicalities.

Values

The third component is the values expressed in your practice. A value is something we believe is good and desirable. Sometimes people attach the word 'morality' to their beliefs. Values are a personal matter and they can be expressed as absolutes. For example, I have an absolute value concerning my opposition to capital punishment. This exists irrespective of any arguments about its effectiveness. I regard it as 'morally wrong'. It is helpful to think of our professional values as not segregated from our personal values. There is a hierarchy of values and principles that guide our practice. Values are the most abstract expression of what we believe is good, while principles tend to be the active expression of values in practice. Often professions produce codes of practice or ethical guidelines, which act as lists of principles to guide practice.

Expertise

Last but not least, there are skills, or as I prefer to say, expertise. Expertise covers those aspects of skills and techniques which, as a practitioner, you incorporate so thoroughly into your practice that they become part of your professional approach. There is a difference between this and a technique you acquire that does not become part of your distinctive practice.

I have indicated above that personal and professional aspects overlap and interact. Let us try to bring these different components together.

Personal Awareness, Practice and Professional Development

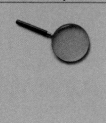

Practice example

Gemma is a complementary therapist – I shall not specify her particular specialism. Her background was in administrative work before she changed professions and her main priority is bringing efficiency to her practice. Unfortunately, her clients complain behind her back that she has absolutely no personal skills at all and seems capable only of asking a series of questions and delivering very straight advice, with no attempt to engage with them as people. As a result, most people visit her once, or at most twice.

I have begun with this example because it highlights key characteristics of great relevance to the linked topics in this section. Let us work through these as we consider the shortcomings in Gemma's performance and how these may be tackled:

1. Gemma needs to learn how to reflect on her practice, be self-critical and feed what she learns from this into her future practice.
2. Gemma lacks personal awareness, or is not using such personal awareness as she possesses. She needs to learn from people's failure to return.
3. Gemma is not making a connection between the different aspects of professional skills she needs to acquire and develop – in her technical competence and her interpersonal understanding and skills in communication and interaction with people.
4. Gemma needs to use the interplay between her personal and professional development to improve the latter.

Let us work through these in turn.

Learning how to Reflect on Practice

Reflection on practice is a continual process, not a task to be completed first so that we can move onto other things. Gemma is going to find this difficult at first. She will have to adjust to a state of being rather than doing. I once heard reflectiveness described as a state of becoming, which captures very well the task facing Gemma.

Developing and Using Personal Awareness

Gemma needs to develop her qualities of sensitivity and self-awareness. I think of these two aspects as on the border between qualities and skills. That is, they are akin to artistic talent – they are more part of the culture of some people's lives and consequently are built into their everyday way of acting, rather than being techniques they have learned. Let us assume that Gemma already possesses a modicum of sensitivity and self-awareness and just needs to strengthen them in her practice. What do we mean by sensitivity? In this context, we mean trying to tune into what her client or patient is saying. More than that, it may mean reading between the lines and appreciating the body language of the person, that is, what the person is not saying, but what comes across in other ways (see Chapter 10 for discussion of using body language in interacting with people). What do we mean by self-awareness? We are concerned here with the ability of Gemma to seek inside herself some of the emotions and thoughts that will help her to work with the person. Gemma needs to know herself. She needs to understand her own responses and appreciate how they can influence her work with people.

Developing a Repertoire of Technical and Interpersonal Skills

We are building now on the previous two points. Gemma needs to work hard at building on her reflectiveness and develop her repertoire of skills alongside and integrated with her self-understanding and understanding of other people. It is important for Gemma not to forget her grasp of technical and administrative skills. These are useful attributes and many sensitive and self-aware professionals working with people do not possess them. For Gemma, however, the balance is the other way. She needs to strengthen her interpersonal skills and ensure there is a balance between them and her efficient office manager manner, when she is working with people.

Developing Reflective Practice through Reflexivity

In this final point, we build on the previous three points. Reflexiveness involves using your abilities, qualities and experiences, thoughts and feelings, and bringing them to bear on what you do, how you practise. Gemma needs to be reflexive in her reflective practice, so as to further her professional development.

The word 'reflection' has many different aspects because it conjures up many meanings, in the dictionary and in everyday usage. This makes it necessary for us to be precise about how we are using it. So, to summarize, reflective practice is the systematic process of describing practice, identifying its main features, highlighting its significance, exploring its complexity, evaluating its strengths and weaknesses and clarifying what would be done differently next time. What does this mean in practice?

Activity

Focus for a few minutes on the task of reflecting on your own practice. Here is a set of tasks to help you do this:

1. Identify a piece of your practice.
2. Make brief notes about what it entailed.

3.   Give brief details of the agency, its location, 'clients' and main working methods.
4.   Describe your practice briefly.
5.   Write a reflective review of your practice, by answering these three questions:
   ■ What did I do well?
   ■ What did I do less well?
   ■ How would I do things differently next time?

This activity should have helped you to fill out the process of reflecting on your own practice. This reflection is critical, because you are asking yourself evaluative questions. Schön (1983) distinguishes between two aspects of reflection:

1.   *Reflection-in-action*, which takes place in practice, at the time, as the practice happens. It enables the practitioner to consider and immediately apply in practice what is learned from the present situation.
2.   *Reflection-on-action*, which takes place afterwards and draws on previous experience. It enhances knowledge and understanding of previous practice and, in the process, links this with previous learning, including learning through study as well as through experience.

Chapter Summary

This chapter has examined the nature and importance of reflection and criticality and how to apply them in practice. This is a vital ingredient of professionalism in complementary practice, to counter the criticism that the practitioner seems not to be sensitive and self-aware and the practice is not self-critical. Criticality in practice is necessary in order to base the development of expertise on the continually expanding evidence base. For practitioners to maintain their criticality, they need to be confident in appraising the worth of research and applying it to practice.

REVIEW QUESTIONS

1   What does the term 'reflection' mean in work with patients and clients?

2   What is the main difference between unreflective and reflective practice?

3   How would you distinguish between your 'expertise' and the 'techniques' you use in your practice?

CHAPTER LINKS

For more discussion of ethical aspects of practice, see Chapter 9.

For more discussion of important aspects of evidence-based and research-aware practice, see Chapter 12.

FURTHER RESOURCES

Brechin, A. (2000) Introducing critical practice, in A. Brechin, H. Brown and M.A. Eby (eds) *Critical Practice in Health and Social Care*, London, Sage. Helpful discussion of ideas and practicalities involved in developing critical practice.

Bulman, C. and Schutz, S. (2004) *Reflective Practice in Nursing*, Oxford, Blackwell. Detailed discussion of theories and practice in reflective practice within the healthcare sector.

Resource file

Collecting and Organizing Information

A qualified and experienced practitioner needs to become confident in locating and handling information. A major contribution to this is practising while a student – using the tasks of researching for an essay, presentation or for practice.

Sources of Information

You will find information about complementary approaches in many places, because they are important to so many people. The main sources are listed below. You can probably add one or two more of your own:

- Government departments' websites and publications, such as official reports
- Professional bodies
- Research and conference reports
- Reports by research bodies, voluntary agencies and, for example, organizations for different complementary approaches, many with their own websites
- Academic textbooks
- Journals
- Newspaper articles.

Searching Books, Journals, Reports and Other Publications

1. Choose a subject for your search
2. Limit the scope – too wide and it will be unmanageable
3. Clarify the broad category of information, for example academic, fiction, biographies
4. Narrow down the types of information, for example statistics, official reports, books, journal articles based on research
5. Arrive at keywords to use, for example reiki, meditation, aromatherapy
6. Identify where to find the information, for example on databases in the library
7. Leave enough time, for example spend a regular amount of time each day for a week, allowing extra time because searching generally takes longer than you anticipate
8. Do the search
9. Write down a summary of each item and take a full note of the reference to it (see details on creating references below)
10. Evaluate your search, that is, look back at the search and ask four questions:
    - How adequate were my sources?
    - How well did I carry out the search?
    - Am I very pleased, pleased, displeased or very displeased with the result?
    - Why is this?

Searching on the Internet

Go to your nearest library – usually the college or university library is best – and ask for help with search engines at the IT or learning resources desk. The best way of searching the internet is to go straight to one of the websites listed below, or another website you already know about. If you use Windows Internet Explorer, you can use the search box to type in your favourite search provider, or access a 'drop down' menu or list. You may have a favourite 'search engine'. A search engine does a lot of the work of searching for you. You could try out several search engines. These are some of the most commonly used search engines:

- Google   www.google.co.uk
- Excite   www.excite.com
- Yahoo   www.yahoo.com
- Altavista   www.altavista.digital.com
- Jeeves   http://uk.ask.com

You can type in keywords to one of these. The disadvantage is it often produces a huge number of results and you will need to learn to narrow down the choice by using very specific terms. Try the search engine Google first. You could use Google Scholar, which targets academic sources. Or you could search for general information by trying sources such as the

British Complementary Medicine Association at Info@ bcma.co.uk, www.bcma.co.uk; the Internet Health Library at www.internethealthlibrary.com; *British Medical Journal* articles since January 1998 on complementary medicine at http://bmj.com/cgi/collection/complementary_medicine.

Subject Gateways

You can narrow down your search by using a subject gateway. Subject gateways are internet-based, searchable sources of information about specific, usually academic, subject areas. For example, there is a large gateway to health and social sciences information that was under the banner heading of Biome but is now called Intute. You can access the health and life sciences category of this by typing in www.intute.ac.uk/healthandlifesciences/ and then typing complementary medicine into the search box. This produces over 80 items, which you can browse through. Typing in alternative medicine produces around 90 items.

University and College Libraries

You may be a student at a college or university. In this case, you will gain most benefit by asking in person, emailing or phoning library and learning resources staff in the library or learning resources centre and asking for details of relevant databases. A database is a list of information and knowing the names of relevant ones will save you a lot of time.

For example, the library at the Robert Gordon University in Aberdeen has a useful internet resource. If you go to www.rgu.ac.uk/library/resources/, you can access the nursing and midwifery section and within this look down the list and click on complementary therapy. This gives a useful list of web links. Web links are extremely helpful because they can start you off on more detailed and focused searches within your specialist area.

If you are researching a particular topic, try to jot down a short list of keywords before you start. Your aim now is to gather as full a list as you can of articles and publications – books and reports – relevant to the topic:

- Remember to try to focus your search and not become sidetracked
- List the main words you think are useful, for example for healing, your keywords might be healing, reiki, energy
- Type your topic in the search box in lower case
- If you think a particular word is especially important, type a plus (+) before it
- Enclose a whole phrase in double inverted commas, for example "transcendental meditation"
- Use NOT to exclude a word from the search, for example meditation, NOT transcendental
- Use OR to broaden the search, for example – of massage – sports OR therapeutic
- Use AND to link two ideas, for example Chinese AND Ayurvedic.

Here are two important points at the outset:

1. Clarify the topic.
2. Don't be afraid to narrow the topic down. Most people start with too broad and ambitious a topic and can find the number of results overwhelming.

Use keywords from your topic. If your topic is uses of acupuncture in the NHS, try using the main nouns from your topic as keywords, on their own at first and then together, as in acupuncture and NHS.

For example, rather than traditional medicine, focus on traditional Chinese medicine. Linking two subjects narrows down the topic. Linking three narrows it down still further, as in traditional Chinese herbal medicine. I tried these topics, using Google. I typed in 'traditional medicine' and received 14,700,000 hits. This is far too many for your search. I then added 'Chinese', making it 'traditional Chinese medicine', which reduced the hits to 9,740,000. Adding 'herbal', as in 'traditional Chinese herbal medicine', massively reduced the hits to 620,000. Adding the word 'research', making it 'research traditional Chinese herbal medicine', reduced it further to 284,000.

Organizing Information

When you have identified an item you want to include, follow up the reference and open it. Print it out if possible. Read through the item and file it in a clip folder, using a system of indexing so that you can find it again.

Taking Notes

Don't rely on your memory alone when you come across interesting or relevant information. You should try to take notes on information you gather, whether from a book or article or in class. Bear in mind the following when taking notes:

- Don't leave writing something until later. You may have forgotten it then. Write it down now.
- Carry a small memo pad or notebook with you all the time, night and day, in your bag or pocket.
- Transfer information at home onto A4 sheets in folders or ring binders.
- Label these separate holders with subjects such as 'Law' or 'Essays' and divide each into sections, labelled with the different topics in a subject, such as 'Material for case study on ... '.
- Summarize the information in note form.
- Use bullet points or lists of numbers to help you summarize points.
- Try to summarize arguments in a word or phrase that strikes you as easy to remember. Have confidence in your ability to recall a point from that single word or phrase.

Using Information

Writing an Essay

Preparing for the Essay

- Check you understand the title or question set.
- Confirm the deadline and what you have to hand in.

Collecting information for the essay

- Set a timetable for yourself with a deadline well before the hand-in date.
- Decide what kind of information you need.
- Gather the information, avoiding being diverted from your topic.
- Modify the topic and your information if necessary:
  - Don't stick with a topic you become convinced is unworkable.
  - Renegotiate an unworkable topic or change it if you can.
  - Don't collect too much information.
  - Don't gather information you feel is irrelevant but interesting.

Planning the Essay

Plan the main headings of the essay. Most essays have three sections – introduction, main body of the essay and conclusion – plus, at the very end, a list of the work referred to (for how to refer to other people's work, see below).

Introduction: The most important first job is to try to come up with a sentence in the introduction, summarizing your approach – which we call here the argument – in your essay. Here are some common ways of starting your essay as an argument:

- 'This essay discusses the pros and cons of ...'
- 'In this essay, we examine the evidence for the statement that ...'
- 'This essay critically reviews the statement that ...'
- 'I have chosen to study ... for my special topic and I am tackling the question of whether ... or ...'.

Main body of the essay: Jot down the topic for each paragraph. Try to map out the whole essay in paragraphs or sections, based on the chunks of information you've collected. Put your plan to one side for a while and come back to it after a gap of several hours or preferably a day or two.

Conclusion or *Conclusions* (whichever you prefer): This is a few sentences bringing your essay to an end, perhaps by rounding off the argument or saying what you've found or shown. Your conclusion should not introduce any new ideas, particularly those quoted as references from things you've read.

Writing the Essay

- Now have another look at your essay plan. Alter anything which looks wrong.
- Confirm the sequence of your main paragraphs. Say, for example, your word limit is 2,000 words. Have no more than 10 long paragraphs or 20 short ones.
- Write a simple sentence summarizing the main point of each paragraph. Each single sentence should be no more than 30 words long (three lines). Any longer and you should try to split it into two sentences.
- Each single sentence now becomes the first sentence in each paragraph. Add four or five more sentences to it explaining its key point in that paragraph. Repeat for every paragraph in the essay. Your essay should be near its final length.
- You may be able to add a paragraph at the end under the heading 'Conclusions'. This brings together all the points you've made in a few sentences summarizing your argument.

Making References and a Bibliography

If you copy or paraphrase (that is, summarize) the words or ideas of an author or web-based source and do not acknowledge this in your writing, you will be guilty of plagiarism. Plagiarism is a serious offence and is treated as dishonesty. Plagiarism can be direct, as in quoting other people's words without putting quotation marks round your extract, or indirect, as in summarizing their ideas without acknowledging the source, so always make written acknowledgement of other people's work, as indicated below.

There are two common ways to quote or refer to other people's writing in our own work:

1. *Listing references:* You can go through your written

work putting a number in brackets after each item you refer to or quote from. Then, at the end of the written work, you list the numbers and after each give a full statement of the source of the reference: author or editor, initials, date, title, edition (if later than the first), place of publisher, name of publisher.
2. *Bibliography – Harvard system:* This is an easier system for you to use. You put a main name, date and, if necessary, page number in brackets at the point where you refer to a person's work. Then, at the end of your written work, you list in alphabetical order all the items you have referred to. We shall use the Harvard bibliography system below and throughout this book.

The Harvard System

Quoting From or Referring to Books

In the main part of your written work, put a bracket like this: (Webb and Jones, 2003: 94). Or, if you mention Webb and Jones: As Webb and Jones (2003: 94) say, 'blackberries are sweet'. If there are more than two authors, in the text this is written as: (Webb et al., 2008). At the end of your written work, list all the books you've quoted from or referred to, like this:

> Webb, J.H. and Jones, K.D. (eds) (2003) *Fruits of the Forest*, 3rd edn, London, Best Books.

So the formula is: author(s)' or editor(s)' surname (if there are more than three authors, use et al. after the first three names), initials of forenames, (ed.) if edited, if it not, omit, date using all four numbers (2003), title in italics and edition, if later than the first edition, place of publication and name of publisher.

Quoting From or Referring to Journal Articles

Journal articles are similar. In your written work, put a bracket as for books: (Brown, 2004: 274). At the end, in the bibliography, put the author(s)' surname, initials, the date, the title of the article inside single quotation marks, the title of the journal in italics, volume number, issue number in brackets and finally the page numbers of the entire article. For example:

Brown, L. (2004) 'Complementary practice', *Journal of xxxxx*, **88**(2): 270–87.

Quoting From or Referring to Websites

Follow the same sequence as above for authors and their works. Then put the website followed by the date you referred to it. For example:

www.west.ac.uk/central (accessed 4 May 2001).

Note: This resource file is adapted from similar resource files in Adams, A. (2007) *Foundations of Health and Social Care*, Basingstoke, Palgrave Macmillan.

Contexts for Practice

Part II
Contexts for Practice

Introduction

This book argues that we need to review the relative importance of different conventional and traditional health systems and remedies to the health and wellbeing of the world's population, in the light of the significant contribution made by therapies and medicines deemed complementary and alternative by those who practise conventional medicine.

We need to distinguish between health services based on conventional medicine and the full span of health systems, remedies and practitioners in developed as well as developing countries. When we view global traditional medicine, we see that it extends far beyond the Western view of medical services. Beyond people's relatively formal relationships with doctors, hospitals and 'national' health services lies a rich array of learning and experience of health and wellbeing.

Part II is contextual and intended as a basis for the major areas of knowledge and skills covered in Parts III to VI. Chapter 3 provides a general introduction to complementary approaches. Chapter 4 discusses different models of the promotion of health and wellbeing. Chapter 5 deals with the policy and legal basis of complementary approaches.

Introduction to Complementary Therapies and Alternative Medicine

ROBERT ADAMS

Learning outcomes

By the end of this chapter, you should be able to:

- refer to the changing use of terms used to refer to complementary approaches
- discuss the main features of complementary approaches
- compare categorizations of complementary approaches
- recognize the categorization of complementary approaches used in this book

At the start, let us acknowledge the basic irony inherent in the subject of this book. Over the last couple of centuries, Western industrialized countries have adopted new medical approaches based on scientific research, in the Enlightenment tradition, that is, what many positivist scientists (who assume that inherent in physical and social phenomena is a core of essential truth waiting to be discovered) regard as making progress in the search for knowledge. This medicine is not regarded as new, however, so much as conventional or established. In contrast, traditional medicine and natural therapies, which over thousands of years have become conventional and established in many Eastern, developing and nonindustrial countries, have, over the past century, spread and become increasingly popular in developed countries, where they are labelled variously as 'complementary', 'alternative', 'unconventional' and are regarded as 'new'. In this novel setting, policy makers, health professionals, practitioners, patients, clients and members of the public increasingly turn to these approaches, while many simultaneously struggle with questions of their reliability, safety and effectiveness, and debate whether to ignore them, covertly or overtly recognize them or even ensure that the state registers their further development.

This chapter begins the task, undertaken in this book as a whole, of making sense and presenting a critical yet balanced view of this complicated and on occasions contradictory situation. In the process, we delve into the principles and practice of some of the most common and established areas of complementary practice.

Changing Use of Terms

Complementary approaches to health and wellbeing have enjoyed a revival in Western countries, which has accelerated since the 1960s when many people rebelled against their conventional lifestyle and experimented with alternatives (Table 3.1).

Table 3.1 Terms used to refer to complementary approaches

Pre-1970s	1970s–80s	1990s onwards
Non-conventional and fringe treatments	Alternative treatments	Complementary and alternative treatments

Since the 1990s, the spread of new technologies for sharing information globally has empowered more people to question the authority of their treatment by professionals in healthcare and medicine in particular and to seek alternatives to conventional approaches. The growing popularity of complementary and alternative approaches has led to the USA and European countries reviewing their policies towards them and making more flexible and inclusive arrangements than hitherto for people to have access to them. Although some of these approaches remain controversial, there are indications that some of them are being incorporated as legitimate complements and respectable alternatives to conventional healthcare. In subsequent chapters, we consider different issues raised by these developments.

Activity

Consider how the terms 'conventional', 'complementary' and 'alternative' relate to each other, in the fields of therapy and medicine.

The term 'complementary' indicates that the approach overlaps and to some extent integrates with conventional medicine rather than replacing it (Figure 3.1). Complementary approaches may integrate with medical and social practice across the health and social work professions, particularly where a person's full assessment points to multiple needs. Some techniques of practice appear in widely different therapeutic and medical systems. For example, generic methods such as massage are found in a wide range of Eastern and Western approaches, ranging from traditional Chinese medicine (TCM) to remedial massage therapy in sports injury and physiotherapy (Cash and Ylinen, 1992; Cash, 1996) and the use of facial massage in cosmetology (the study, theory and practice of beautifying the face, hair and skin) – used, for example, where cosmetic practice contributes to the rehabilitation of accident victims.

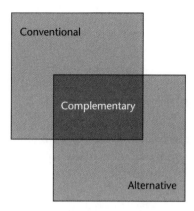

Figure 3.1 Conventional, complementary and alternative approaches

The term 'alternative' indicates that the approach replaces conventional medicine. The British Medical Association (BMA, 1993: 6–7) specifies complementary approaches as 'those which can work alongside and in conjunction with orthodox medical treatment'. This includes self-help (for example yoga), educational (for example Alexander technique), relatively noninvasive (for example healing and massage) and interventionist (for example acupuncture and chiropractic) approaches. In contrast, alternative approaches are used 'in place of orthodox medical treatment' (BMA, 1993: 6), although these authors acknowledge that in certain circumstances, any nonconventional therapy could be used as an alternative treatment. They give the example of herbal medicines given instead of orthodox medication (BMA, 1993: 7).

Conventional and Nonconventional Medicine

The term 'nonconventional medicine' is sometimes used to refer to different approaches, yet this raises the question as to what we mean by conventional medicine. The BMA (1993: 7) defines conventional medicine as 'that treatment which is delivered by a registered medical practitioner'. Yet this is confusing, because some registered medical practitioners undergo training in complementary and alternative approaches, such as homeopathy. Does this mean that homeopathy delivered by a registered medical practitioner becomes conventional medicine? This is unlikely to be generally recognized by the medical professions. The BMA (1993: 7–8) negotiates this hurdle by defining nonconventional therapies as:

> those forms of treatment which are not widely used by the orthodox health-care professions, and the skills of which are not taught as part of the undergraduate curriculum of orthodox medical and paramedical health-care courses.

There is a tendency for some approaches to be grouped under medicine, while others are broadly therapeutic. This does not cover all approaches. For example, the Alexander technique is set out by its originator as broadly educational rather than therapeutic. Other holistic approaches are not specifically therapeutic, in the sense that they aim to bring about wellbeing rather than tackling specific illnesses or conditions.

Main Features of the Field of Practice

Complementary therapies and **alternative medicine**, or traditional medicine (TM) as these approaches are commonly described in many countries, cover a vast array of practices, which fall into two groups:

1.   those that overlap with or are closely related to specific areas of conventional medical practice
2.   those that share little or nothing with conventional medical practice.

The word 'traditional' in traditional medicine, as used by the World Health Organization (WHO), has a precise meaning. It either means medical prescriptions (often herbal) passed by word of mouth from generation to generation, with families specializing in their own prescriptions, or a system of medicine practised in its country of origin (WHO, 2001: 2). Traditional medicine is:

> a comprehensive term used to refer both to TM systems such as traditional Chinese medicine, Indian Ayurveda and Arabic unani medicine and to various forms of indigenous medicine. TM therapies include medication therapies – if they involve use of herbal medicines, animal parts and/or minerals – and non-medication therapies – if they're carried out primarily without the use of medication, as in the case of acupuncture, manual therapies and spiritual therapies. In countries where the dominant health care system is based on allopathic medicine, or where TM has not been incorporated into the national health care system, TM is often termed 'complementary', 'alternative' or 'non-conventional' medicine. (WHO, 2002: 1)

Traditional medicine is defined by the World Health Organization (2001: 1–2) as:

> a diversity of health practices, approaches, knowledge and beliefs incorporating plant, animal and/or mineral-based medicines, spiritual therapies, manual techniques and exercises, applied singly or in combination to maintain well-being, as well as to treat, diagnose, or prevent illness.

Complementary and alternative approaches involve:

- a practitioner and a client or patient
- a process involving the practitioner suggesting to the client or patient some treatment or activity that could be beneficial in some way.

Beyond that, there is no common set of beliefs that underlies them all. Sometimes they are rooted in traditional practices that are centuries old. Others are linked with religious or spiritual beliefs. Others again have a basis in philosophies or metaphysical systems. Yet others are linked with, or have grown out of, various experiences of conventional approaches and developed into systems for promoting health and wellbeing. The seven categories of complementary and alternative therapies identified by the National Institutes of Health's Office of Alternative Medicine (1994) are:

1. alternative systems of medical practice
2. mind-body therapies
3. bioelectromagnetic therapies
4. manual healing therapies
5. herbal therapy
6. diet and nutrition therapies
7. pharmacologic and biological therapies.

A Growing Field of Practice

Whether or not we advocate, are indifferent to, or are hostile towards complementary and alternative approaches to conventional health and medical services, we are living in the era of their rapid growth. In the UK, the NHS spends £50m per year on complementary therapies and alternative medicine, and the total annual spending is upwards of £4.5bn and increasing.

The number of complementary and alternative approaches is growing fast also and rivals conventional approaches in size and scope. Typical directories of these approaches (Albright, 1997; Credit et al., 2003; Bratman, 2007) are likely to go into detail about dozens of those whose clinics are commonly encountered, or can be found attached to beauty parlours, hairdressers shops, health centres and hospitals, indeed, almost everywhere. There are hundreds, even thousands, of therapies and treatments and the most common of them are available as walk-in services in most communities. In the UK, there may be as many as 50,000 practitioners, spread across many different aspects of practice.

A growing proportion of people use complementary approaches, perhaps between a quarter and a third, at some point in their lives. In the USA (www. intersurvey.com), more than two-thirds of people have tried at least one form of alternative medicine. The use of at least one of 16 alternative therapies during the previous year increased from an estimated 33.8% of the population in 1990 (Eisenberg et al., 1993) to 42% in 1997 (Eisenberg et al., 1998). This is reflected in the expanding number of self-help guides, enabling people to understand, manage and in some cases self-administer their own complementary treatments (BMA, 1993; Woodham, 1994; Fulder, 1997; Austin et al., 1998; Young, 2002; Credit et al., 2003). If we add the developing countries, the worldwide use of complementary and alternative approaches is huge – an estimated four-fifths of the world's population being reliant on what we can call traditional remedies for primary healthcare (WHO, 2001).

A Field of Practice that is Difficult to Name

There is some difficulty in arriving at a convenient label to use for this area, which is acceptable to different interests. Although we may refer to it as traditional in developing countries, in developed countries it is often regarded as unconventional. In so being, is it also complementary or alternative? Is it medicine or therapy, or education or a developed form of traditional self-help remedies? Is it unconventional or simply part of the diversity of therapies and medicine?

It is important that we understand the different emphases implied in these different labels. We should also bear in mind that the use of some titles such as a medical 'doctor' is governed by law. It is also necessary that we appreciate that the situation is changing and what applied 10 years ago may not apply nowadays. Terms such as 'complementary health', 'complementary therapy', 'complementary medicine', 'integrated medicine' and 'alternative medicine' are used in different contexts and in different countries. A common term is complementary and alternative medicine (CAM). Sometimes the word 'unconventional' is used, in contrast with conventional medicine. Also, more flatteringly perhaps, the term 'holistic' is used in some approaches, which, rather than tackling a single illness or symptom, aim to improve the whole person's wellbeing. The notion of integrated approaches to health and wellbeing has gained momentum in the twenty-first century (see Chapter 4).

There is no ready consensus about what to call complementary approaches. The WHO definition of alternative medicine is 'health care which usually is outside the official health sector' (Bannerman et al., 1993). The emphasis on 'medicine' is interesting as it is a more restrictive term than 'therapies', which in turn is more restrictive than 'approaches'. The term 'complementary and alternative medicine' is widely used in some Western countries, notably the USA. However, this does not take account of a huge range of approaches that do not regard themselves as medical. The BMA report (1993) distinguishes between 'complementary medicine', which tends to be used by the general public, and 'non-conventional medicine' and 'non-conventional therapies', which are also used in the report. This label of 'nonconventional' should be used with caution. It could imply a degree of marginality and even eccentricity. In fact, between 1993 and 1997, the two research studies published by Eisenberg and colleagues shifted from using the term 'unconventional medicine' to 'alternative medicine' (Eisenberg et al., 1993, 1998).

The BMA (1993: 5) notes that the use of the WHO definition would lead to the inclusion of more than 160 approaches:

> including physical therapies such as osteopathy, psychological therapies such as hypnotherapy, and paranormal therapies such as healing. Indeed, Lord Skelmersdale, the Under-Secretary of Health, informed Parliament during a debate on complementary medicine in November 1987 that he had identified no fewer than 160 therapies, or variations of them.

Much of the richness of the complementary field is characterized by this diversity. In order to accommodate this, I have adopted the dual heading of complementary therapies and alternative medicine for this book. Even this does not take account of those approaches, such as the Alexander technique and many holistic approaches, which do not define themselves as therapies or medicines. In the interests of brevity and to avoid the tedium of repeating the long title, I use the term 'complementary approaches' in many places, where it does not detract from the meaning. Sometimes the sense of the context demands a different term.

We need to specify what the term 'complementary therapies and alternative medicine' covers. Although in theory this label covers every approach to treating the whole person as well as illnesses and conditions of parts of the body, we follow the decision of Fulder's research survey and exclude the purely psychological and psychotherapeutic therapies such as psychosynthesis, encounter groups, Gestalt therapy and what Fulder (1997: 5) refers to as 'about 140 other psychotherapies listed by President Carter's commission on mental health'.

The field we know as conventional or orthodox medical practice is known as **allopathic medicine**, a general label for conventional medicine, based on the Greek word 'allopathy' meaning 'other suffering'. The 'other' are the external agents – viruses, bacteria or chemicals – which attack the body and cause illnesses and conditions. Over the past two centuries, in Western countries, orthodox medicine has gained ground and now dominates health and medical practice. Orthodox medicine grows from a relatively unified and homogeneous stock of knowledge about the body, its health and the conditions and illnesses that attack or under-mine it. In contrast, complementary therapies and alternative medicine are extremely diverse, reflecting the different knowledge bases of many different countries and cultures, with their associated belief systems about the human body, the mind and the spirit. Among the many different forms of complementary and alternative approaches are those which focus 'holistically' on the whole person, in contrast with orthodox medicine, which typically focuses on tackling particular symptoms, or the affliction of one part of the body.

Different Ways of Categorizing Complementary Approaches

Activity

Spend a few minutes listing all the different complementary approaches that occur to you. Now try to group them into no more than six categories.

The rest of this chapter explores different ways of tackling the difficult and demanding task of categorizing complementary approaches. Some groupings of complementary approaches are based partly on territorial origins and partly on conceptual and philosophical associations. Lewith (2002: 3), for example, lists six categories, with homeopathy placed, bizarrely, alone under the 'unique' heading (Table 3.2). Shealy (2000) classifies what he terms 'complementary therapies' into nine categories (Table 3.3), with yoga in a category on its own, rather than in the 'Eastern' category, and a section on arts therapies – interestingly, omitting drama-therapy – which is not shared by any other commentator. The inclusion of aroma-therapy in the 'touch' category is mystifying. The category 'feelgood' hardly warrants a distinctive place since all therapies might be assumed to have this as an aim. The category 'natural' also seems insubstantial, with many therapies potentially likely to claim this. Finally, there seems to be little logic in meditation being classified as a 'lifestyle' rather than a 'mind' therapy.

Table 3.2 Categories of complementary therapies

Connected with Chinese medicine	Acupuncture Acupressure Reiki Shiatsu Herbal medicine
Connected with Ayurvedic (traditional Hindu) medicine	Yoga Aromatherapy Herbal medicine
Massage and manipulative based	Chiropractic Osteopathy Reflexology Cranial osteopathy Massage
Mind-body	Autogenic training Biofeedback Healing Meditation Relaxation and visualization Therapeutic touch Hypnosis
Naturopathy related	Environmental medicine Naturopathy Nutritional medicine
Unique	Homeopathy

Source: Lewith, 2002

Table 3.3 Classification of complementary therapies

Lifestyle	Naturopathy Relaxation Visualization Meditation
Feelgood	Alexander technique Tai chi Chi kung
Natural	Homeopathy Herbalism
Touch	Massage Shiatsu Aromatherapy Reflexology
Yoga	Yoga

Arts	Dance therapy
	Colour therapy
	Art therapy
	Music therapy
Mind	Healing
	Psychotherapy
	Hypnotherapy
Eastern	Ayurveda
	Traditional Chinese medicine
	Acupuncture
Manipulative	Chiropractic
	Osteopathy

Source: Adapted from Shealy, 2000

Pietroni (1991: 180–1) developed a fourfold classification of different complementary treatments (Table 3.4).

Table 3.4 Classification of complementary treatments

Complete healing systems	Homeopathy, acupuncture (and TCM), herbal medicine, osteopathy, chiropractic
Methods of diagnosis	Hair analysis, kinesiology, iridology, aura diagnosis
Therapeutic modes	Aromatherapy, spiritual healing, hydrotherapy, massage, reflexology
Self-help approaches	Yoga, breathing and relaxation, meditation, visualization, fasting and dieting

Source: Adapted from Pietroni, 1991

This is simple, but not ideal, since it does not distinguish approaches in terms of their basic assumptions and purposes. In contrast, Gascoigne's (1997) book on Chinese complementary therapies conceives these as forms of self-help. Interestingly, the BMA report (1993: 61) identifies the four treatments mentioned under the first heading above – homeopathy, acupuncture, herbal medicine and osteopathy – as the most common and having the greatest potential for doing harm.

The nurse's handbook (Andrews et al., 1999: v) lists seven major categories of 'common alternative therapies' (Table 3.5).

Table 3.5 Classification of 'common alternative therapies'

Alternative systems of medical practice	Traditional Chinese medicine, Ayurvedic medicine, homeopathy, naturopathy, osteopathy, environmental medicine

Mind-body therapies	Art therapy, biofeedback, dance therapy, hypnosis, imagery, meditation, music therapy, prayer and mental healing, psychotherapy, sound therapy, tai chi, yoga
Bioelectromagnetic therapies	Electromagnetic therapy, magnetic field therapy, cell-specific cancer therapy, static electromagnetic field therapy
Manual healing therapies	Acupuncture, Alexander technique, applied kinesiology, chiropractic, craniosacral therapy, Feldenkrais method, hydrotherapy, qigong, reflexology, rolfing, therapeutic massage, therapeutic touch, Trager approach
Herbal therapy	Different herbal prescriptions
Diet and nutrition therapies	Orthomolecular therapy, anti-cancer diets, macrobiotic diet, fasting, juice therapy, enzyme therapy
Pharmacological and biological therapies	Apitherapy, aromatherapy, chelation therapy, light therapies, neural therapy, biological cancer therapies

Source: Adapted from Andrews et al., 1999

We can put the above classifications together and arrive at the classification that is used to categorize the approaches referred to in this book (Table 3.6).

Table 3.6 Categorization of approaches used in this book

Alternative medical systems	Homeopathic medicine (see Ch. 19) Traditional Chinese medicine (see Ch. 21) Tai chi, Ayurvedic medicine
Mind-body interventions	Meditation (see Ch. 22) Kinesiology, yoga
Biologically based therapies	Herbal medicine (see Ch. 23) Aromatherapy (see Ch. 24) Dietary approaches
Manipulative and body-based approaches	Chiropractic (see Ch. 25) Osteopathy (see Ch. 26) Reflexology (see Ch. 27) Alexander technique (see Ch. 28) Iridology Massage
Energy therapies	Reiki (see Ch. 29) Healing (see Ch. 30) Therapeutic touch Electromagnetic field therapies Sahaj Marg Shiatsu
Expressive therapies	Art therapy (see Ch. 31) Music therapy (see Ch. 31) Dramatherapy (see Ch. 31) Play therapy (see Ch. 31)

Controversies Associated with Practice

Two main sets of controversies are associated with the practice of complementary approaches:

1. questions over their intrinsic validity, reliability (safety) and effectiveness
2. debates about the credibility of the education and training, qualifications, expertise and regulation of their practitioners.

These are large areas, to which we return repeatedly in this book. They present complexities that are beyond a brief, simplistic conclusion here. However, the following is a summary of the general direction this book takes:

1. *intrinsic nature of practice* – there is a growing body of evidence that draws attention to the value that many patients and clients attach to the different approaches, irrespective of whether specific treatment outcomes are proven more effective than conventional treatments.
2. *credibility of practitioners* – education and training for practitioners in some areas of practice is leading to registration in some countries, notably the UK.

Chapter Summary

This chapter has examined some of the major ways in which complementary therapies and alternative medicine have been classified in the literature and by policy makers and practitioners themselves. Important shared features of these as well as a significant diversity of approaches have emerged through this discussion. The chapter has concluded with the classification adopted in this book.

REVIEW QUESTIONS

1 What is cosmetology?
2 What do the initials WHO, TM and TCM refer to?
3 What is Ayurvedic medicine?

CHAPTER LINKS

For further examination of the major categories of complementary approaches, see Part VI chapters and the related resource files.

FURTHER RESOURCES

Shapiro, R. (2008) *Suckers: How Alternative Medicine Makes Fools of Us All*, London, Harvill Secker. Critical study of the complementary therapy and alternative medicine industry.

4

Approaches to Illness, Treatment, Health Promotion and Wellbeing

ROBERT ADAMS

Learning outcomes

By the end of this chapter, you should be able to:

- locate changing views of illness and health promotion in their wider context
- understand the assumptions and focus of different models of illness, treatment and health promotion
- appreciate the distinctive nature of complementary and alternative approaches

Since Reich (1971) wrote *The Greening of America* – an argument for a holistic approach to people and the natural environment – perspectives on illness, health and wellbeing have been incorporated into the mainstream of environmental and preventive approaches to people's health and wellbeing. These lie outside the traditional preoccupations of healthcare and medicine with using conventional medicine to treat illness. Complementary therapies and alternative medicines remain an intrinsically contested area. They can be viewed either as occupying a somewhat contested territory on the fringe of medicine, or at the foreground of what Dr Pietroni (1991) calls the 'greening of medicine' in his book of this title, which advocates holistic policies of health and wellbeing, based on principles of the connectedness and interdependence of people, societies and the processes of nature.

In this chapter, we set out a framework that makes it possible to understand how perspectives on illness, healthcare and health promotion relate to approaches, models and methods, and highlights some of the issues of particular importance.

Changing Ideas about Illness and Health Promotion

The notion of what constitutes a healthy person is not an objective reality but is socially constructed. In this sense, it can change through time, as society changes.

Activity

Spend a few minutes thinking of an example of an aspect of people's everyday life and habits that has changed over the past half-century, as far as what we regard as healthy and unhealthy is concerned.

Practice example

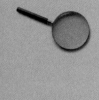

Smoking

Smoking was taken for granted as a social habit until the 1970s, as can be seen from its prominence in films and other media until that date. Gradually, as research proving the correlation of smoking with ill health and premature death has become more widely known, a consensus has arisen in many Western countries, including the UK, that smoking in public places should be banned and advertising should be restricted. This ban on smoking took effect in Scotland and France in 2006, Ireland and England in 2007 and Spain in 2008.

This example illustrates much wider shifts in views of illness and health that have taken place and are still occurring. Complementary therapies and alternatives to medically based interventions, such as those based on drugs and surgery, occupy a somewhat ambiguous territory, increasingly sought by the general public and yet ignored or criticized by the medical establishment. However, it remains undeniable that their position in relation to conventional health and medical services has shifted from being more alternative to being more complementary. In some countries, as the WHO worldwide review of TM suggests, it is misleading to use the terms 'complementary' and 'alternative' because they imply that these approaches are no more than supplementary to conventional healthcare. In reality:

> in some countries, the legal standing of complementary/alternative medicine is equivalent to that of allopathic medicine, many practitioners are certified in both complementary/alternative and allopathic medicine and the primary care provider for many patients is a complementary/alternative practitioner. (WHO, 2001: 1)

By the beginning of the twenty-first century, the situation of complementary and alternative approaches in the USA was sufficiently secure for a major publisher to publish a *Nurse's Handbook of Alternative and Complementary Therapies* (Andrews et al., 1999).

The health services of many Western countries have taken major strides since the latter half of the twentieth century away from a total adherence to **biomedical approaches** to health and towards social and **holistic approaches**. There is widespread and growing recognition of the social origins, not only of mental illnesses such as depression (Brown and Harris, 1978), but also a range of physical illnesses that can be made worse by social conditions (Totman, 1979). The growing cost of conventional 'illness-based' health services is one major factor encouraging the development of more preventive approaches to health and wellbeing. Many health services now engage in health education as part of health promotion and health development policy initiatives. Health promotion is not regarded as the exclusive preserve of health service organizations. Responsibility for it is split between social, collective and individual, private responsibility. It has become part of the debate about which public health services should be provided through the NHS and local authorities, and which should be privatized commodities available to people as part of their freedom to make lifestyle choices, through choosing what they eat and whether they exercise, for example, by becoming members of a private leisure centre.

Ideas, critical commentaries and research that have driven health policies since the 1990s in the UK have been given additional impetus by evidence of persistent links between poorer health and other negative consequences for people in society. Health is unequally distributed. The significant Black Report (1980) found that the worse off a person is, the worse their health is likely to be and the greater their chances of becoming ill (morbidity rates) and dying younger (mortality rates). Better off people suffer less from chronic conditions such as heart disease and chest complaints than poorer people. People's health and ill health are distributed unequally, not just in social class terms, but also geographically. Ill health costs the nation significantly in terms of healthcare resources – notably its financial burden – and there are continuing costs, in terms of people's loss of achievement and earning potential, associated with social and health inequalities in society.

These inequalities in the delivery of core health services have proved worryingly persistent in the quarter century since the Black Report. Sir Donald Acheson's government-sponsored review of these health inequalities concluded that they are still present and often are rooted in people's poverty, the quality of their housing and the extent to which they are able to access the services they need (Acheson, 1998).

In 2004, the White Paper *Choosing Health* (DH, 2004) placed health promotion as a high priority for central and local government. It set out the government's strategy to:

- encourage people to live healthier lives
- persuade people to make better informed and healthier decisions about diet and lifestyle
- take a broad approach to encouraging individuals and also sharing responsibility for health promotion with the commercial and cultural environment.

Health promotion in a locality involves adopting a coordinated approach, based on a mixture of prevention and early intervention, with the NHS leading local authorities and other partners in a multi-agency Healthy Care Partnership. The National Healthy Care Standard for looked after children and young people is intended to meet the five objectives outlined in the government publication *Every Child Matters*: to be healthy, stay safe, enjoy and achieve, make a positive contribution and achieve economic wellbeing (HM Treasury, 2003: 14). Areas of health promotion include healthy eating and physical activity, mental health, sexual health, substance and alcohol use, smoking, and play and creativity. The *National Service Framework for Children, Young People and Maternity Services* (DH/DfES, 2004):

- sets out standards for promoting children's and young people's health and wellbeing
- builds on previous government initiatives for children with particular needs, such as implementing the recommendations of the Healthy Care Programme for looked after children (NCB, 2005).

Many of these initiatives are debated, since ideas about the ingredients of a healthy life are matters of opinion rather than fact. We say they are 'socially constructed', which means they are the product of the interaction between people's individual views and collective views which develop for and against certain arguments in society. Debates about what constitutes a healthy lifestyle continue. The government's 2004 White Paper (DH, 2004) recommended healthier public areas and workplaces through improving people's diets and banning smoking in public places. Often the term **wellbeing** is used to refer to how a person feels rather than relating to objective measures of health or illness. Wellbeing is also associated with holistic approaches to health. The Foundation for Holistic Spirituality (www.f4hs. org/) is an example of an initiative that endeavours to cross disciplinary and professional boundaries and acts as a resource to encourage education and research.

Perspectives on Illness, Treatment and Health Promotion

We saw in Chapter 3 how terms such as 'nonconventional', 'alternative' and 'complementary' have been used in the fields of healthcare and health promotion and how this usage changes over time, depending on the relationship between the complementary and conventional professions and organizations. It is the case that whereas once complementary approaches were relegated to the margins by established professionals, since the 1960s in Western countries, they have moved from the margins and have begun to be taken more seriously by conventional medical practitioners. Complementary approaches play a more useful and practical role than hitherto in the growing field of health promotion. This is because while some therapies and treatments lie closer to conventional practice in their focus on particular conditions – such as the role of osteopathy and chiropractic in relation to a specific set of muscles or a joint – other treatments are rooted in holistic principles and may be preventive rather than remedial in character. This emphasis is much more in harmony with the contemporary direction of health policies, towards prevention and health promotion and development.

We can appreciate the broad span of perspectives on illness, treatment and health promotion by presenting them in tabular form, which highlights their different emphases. Table 4.1 presents a greatly simplified view of the major perspectives. It is simplified in the sense that some approaches cross between and draw on more than perspective.

Table 4.1 Perspectives on illness, treatment and health promotion

Perspective	Focus	Key ideas
Biomedical	Treating the illness and/or condition of the patient	Treatment model
Holistic	Treating the whole person to promote wellbeing	Holism
Social	Working with the person in the wider environment to maximize the quality of life	Social factors
Community action	Empowering people to take action to secure environmental improvements to prevent factors contributing to illness and promote health development	Empowerment, social action
Integrated	Drawing together biomedical, holistic, social and community models to empower people and improve health and wellbeing	Connectedness, interdependence

The different models and approaches that fall into, and between, the major perspectives referred to in Table 4.1, concerning promoting health, highlight the particular contrasts between medical and social perspectives on health. Whereas medical perspectives concentrate on treating the illnesses and conditions of the patient, social perspectives work with the person in relation to the influence of factors in their social environment on their sickness and health. Beyond this, as we also indicate in Table 4.1, there are holistic perspectives that even lie beyond the threefold division of health promotion strategies identified by Tones and Tilford (2001: 30), in terms of educational, preventive and empowerment approaches.

Biomedical Perspectives

The biomedical perspective on health asserts that good health is simply the absence of illness or abnormality. There are some medically based approaches to health promotion based on biomedical assumptions, including preventive schemes of immunization, or approaches based on a behavioural approach to health education – changing people's behaviour – such as the knowledge-attitude-behaviour model (Kemm and Close, 1995: 29). This is quite a restricted and discredited approach, which relies on the assumption that if professionals give information to people, this will change their attitudes and behaviour and lead to a reduced incidence of certain diseases and conditions.

The foundation of good practice from the biomedical perspective is assumed to be the evidence base, preferably in traditional, experimental research based on randomized controlled trials.

Holistic Perspectives

Holistic perspectives on health promotion are rooted in very similar holistic approaches to health and wellbeing encountered in many complementary and alternative approaches.

Activity

Spend a few minutes reflecting on what we mean by 'holism' in relation to our health and wellbeing.

Pietroni (1991: 25) has some helpful insights. **Holism** is a word derived from the Greek *holos* meaning a whole or complete. This is not the same as the so-called Gestalt view that the whole is greater in some ways than the sum of its parts. It is simply the parts arranged in a particular way so that they form the whole. It is also similar to the Gaia principle, which is the idea that the Earth, and its myriad systems of living organisms and inanimate substances, comprises an organic whole that functions as though it is a single organism. This relates closely to ecological ideas. 'Ecology' refers to the study of how organisms and non-living things relate to and interact with each other and their physical and biological environment. Pietroni (1991: 26) argues that it makes more sense to take a holistic view, outside the medical model of disease. It is worth quoting him at some length:

> We have surveyed some of the major conceptual ideas that underpin the 'greening process'; and seen how central the shift from causality to connectedness is. Rather than focus on and search for the causes as to why the universe is as it is, the greening process privileges a perspective which looks for the connections that make the universe as it is. The first necessitates a reductionist 'take the clock to bits' approach, the second observes the nature of the clock and how events and people will relate to its function – that of keeping the time.

So, the practices based on holistic principles emphasize taking a view of the whole person – body, mind and spirit, however these are conceived – in the wider environment of family, neighbourhood, community, culture and society and, ultimately, through global connections, the Earth. In other words, true holistic practice is ecological in its nature and practice.

We need to go a little further into this notion of holism, because many doctors would claim to practise with regard to the whole person, and yet many complementary therapies lie outside conventional medicine. So there are different meanings of holism, depending on whether you are practising within the medical model or beyond it. Pietroni (1991: 25) expands this:

> Of course, 'whole-person' medicine is a concept that all doctors are, or should be, familiar with. But the 'whole' we choose to recognize is too often determined by the prevalent biomedical model, which embraces both reductionism and mind-body dualism. Holistic medicine is indeed about whole-person medicine but its strength and vitality lie in the fact that its definition of what constitutes a 'whole' person is drawn from a number of different disciplines and not solely the biological sciences. It is unfortunate that the term holistic medicine has become

almost synonymous with alternative medicine and it is important to distinguish between these two epithets.

We need to examine another linked idea. This is 'connectedness'. Holistic practice entails making connections. Pietroni links this rather neatly with theories about how the different components of the ecological system relate to each other. He points out that the theoretical assumptions that drive the conventional medical model are similar to those inherent in traditional natural science, that is, they are positivist and essentialist.

Before we move on to summarize the other perspectives, a practice example will enable us to appreciate the differences between biomedical and holistic approaches.

Practice example

Biomedical and holistic approaches

Johann has been to the doctor and almost simultaneously approached his complementary therapy centre for help with being unable to sleep and feeling depressed. The doctor listens briefly to Johann and decides the cause of his problem is his stress and depression. He prescribes antidepressants and sleeping pills for Johann. The complementary practitioner adopts a holistic view and asks Johann to describe to him:

- the circumstances in which he becomes stressed
- how this affects him
- how it affects his partner
- how it affects other family members
- how it affects his work
- how he feels he can tackle his stress and prevent himself becoming depressed.

The practitioner is not seeking a simple connection between cause and effect. He recognizes the complexity of the relationship and interaction between Johann's experiences and perceptions and his circumstances. He and Johann then discuss what support he needs in order to manage his stress and cope with his tendency to become depressed.

We can see the influence of holistic ideas in the WHO *Constitution* of 1948, which defines health as 'a state of complete physical, social and mental well-being and not merely the absence of disease and infirmity' (Nutbeam, 1998: 12).

Social Perspectives

Social perspectives on health promotion are based on the view that wider environmental factors play an important part in a person's health. Health is defined from the viewpoint of a positive state of wellbeing rather than the absence of a sign or symptom of disease. Social perspectives on health emphasize the interaction between a person's health and the wider social environment and relate closely to the educational and empowerment approaches identified by Tones and Tilford (2001).

Community Action Perspectives

The community action model (Kemm and Close, 1995: 30) is based on the notion that people take social action by campaigning for environmental improvements that will promote their health.

The empowerment model (Kemm and Close, 1995, p. 29) tends to be detached from the political and social realities of society and focuses on empowering individuals by providing them with relevant knowledge, skills and resources, so that they can choose how to improve their own health.

Integrated Perspectives

The integrated model of health promotion draws on medical, clinical and social perspectives on health, from an empowerment point of view, and enables people to direct their own health and wellbeing. Integrated health is a notion that, rather than focusing on the treatment of illness, emphasizes the development of optimum wellbeing. Ali's (2001: 2) book advancing integrated health practice states:

> Integrated health is the gathering together of all the factors that contribute to your continued well-being and balancing them to enable you to attain your full potential all the time. This takes the form of preventive measures to ensure your maximum freedom from disease and adverse conditions; the most advantageous curative procedures in the event of your falling ill, using the best of all the traditional and conventional techniques, and optimizing your condition to take advantage of your full potential.

Peters (2008: 20) notes that in the integrated approach, diagnosis and treatment are carried out on the basis of both conventional and complementary approaches. This reduces the risks associated with the use of one approach alone, which may lead to a harmful and potentially treatable condition being missed. Peters (2008: 21) maintains that an integrated approach to managing one's own healthcare entails thinking and working on three levels:

> maintaining self-regulation and building up resilience; using self-help and conventional medicine when necessary and using complementary approaches appropriately.

Self-help and self-care are linked ideas with a long historical tradition in many countries, often associated with notions of mutual aid and individual, family, group and community empowerment (Adams, 1990: 11). The traditional concepts of self-help and self-care are associated with preindustrial societies where, for the bulk of the population, health and social care services provided by the state are rudimentary or entirely absent and 'the role of professionals is largely limited to exhorting people to take responsibility for solving their own problems, with a little material and spiritual support for those whose efforts prove they deserve it' (Adams, 2008: 7). Nowadays, some industrialized societies have moved beyond this individualized model of health and welfare to a collective model whereby the state provides free healthcare services at the point of need, that is, as and when people need them. In a sense, traditional approaches to health such as reiki, which in Western countries have become known as 'complementary' and 'alternative', actually bring the history of self-care full circle, as Quest (2003: 17) argues in her book *Self-healing with Reiki*. According to Pike and Forster (1995: 39), the integrated model of healthcare and health promotion:

- does not exclude other models, but recognizes their complexity and locates them in the context of tackling people's lifestyles
- is rooted in sociological and psychological understandings
- is based on both treatment and broadly educational strategies
- combines treatment and education-based approaches
- targets individual, group and community domains (Adams, 2008)
- engages a range of organizations in the public, independent and private sectors. It does not rule out the previous models such as empowering people, but recognizes their complexity and locates them in the broader context of attempts to change people's lifestyles.

Chapter Summary

This chapter has reviewed biomedical, holistic, social, community action and integrated models of health promotion, highlighting the character of each and comparing the strengths and limitations of different models. Holistic, social and integrated models show the greatest congruence (harmony) with complementary and alternative approaches.

REVIEW QUESTIONS

1   What is the basic argument of Pietroni's *The Greening of Medicine*?
2   What five main perspectives on, or models of, health promotion are discussed in this chapter?
3   What are the main features of an integrated model of health promotion?

CHAPTER LINKS

For further discussion of the historical and ideas contexts of different medical systems in different parts of the world, see Chapter 13.

FURTHER RESOURCES

DH (Department of Health) (2004) *Choosing Health: Making Healthy Choices Easier*, White Paper, Cm 6374, London, TSO. Key government policy publication on health promotion.

Kemm, J. and Close, A. (1995) *Health Promotion: Theory and Practice*, Basingstoke, Macmillan – now Palgrave Macmillan. Useful text on approaches to health promotion.

Pike, S. and Forster, D. (eds) (1997) *Health Promotion for All*, Edinburgh, Churchill Livingstone. Good introduction to the subject of health promotion.

Web Links

www.dfes.gove.uk/qualityprotects (look under Work Programme, then Health Issues)

www.ncb.org.uk/healthycare

5 Policy and Legal Basis for Complementary Therapies and Alternative Medicine

ROBERT ADAMS

Learning outcomes

By the end of this chapter, you should be able to:

■ distinguish between conventional, traditional, complementary and alternative approaches

■ understand the policy basis for the legal regulation of practice

■ appreciate the factors contributing to practice regulation

Conventional, Traditional, Complementary and Alternative Approaches

Dominant conceptualizations of health services place complementary and alternative approaches to therapies, systems of medicine and particular remedies only in relation to conventional views of illness and treatment. This underrepresents the massive contribution of traditional medicine (TM) throughout many developing countries, where conventional health services are either nonexistent or exist only in a rudimentary form. It also reflects the somewhat marginal location of traditional sources of health and wellbeing in relation to the seats of power in health services, dominated as they are by the professions of conventional medicine.

The field of complementary and alternative approaches is led in different ways in different countries, which I term 'traditional' and 'modern'. These are not satisfactory labels, but they serve to highlight the contrasts between countries where beliefs rule over legal enactments and policies and those where the reverse is the case (Table 5.1). For example, as Table 5.1 indicates, Western developed countries rely on professional education and training courses, with their knowledge rooted in the libraries of research institutes, universities and colleges, to pass on the expertise of conventional health practitioners. In contrast, for thousands of years, the accepted manner of new practitioners acquiring expertise in TM has been from practitioner to practitioner. Many such practitioners are in a line of family practice that can extend back many generations.

Table 5.1 Traditional and conventional approaches to policy

	Traditional (TM)	**Conventional**
Policy	Led by practice wisdom	Led by policy
Education and training	Expertise validated by tradition; handed down from practitioner to practitioner	Expertise validated by qualification; course based
Knowledge and expertise	In head and hands of practitioner	Library based, in books
Regulation	Reputation based	Registration based (legal)

Activity

Put yourself in the position first of a conventional medical practitioner in a Western, industrialized and 'developed' country and then as a traditional medical practitioner in a nonindustrialized and 'developing' country. Spend a few minutes jotting down any differences you feel may exist in these two practice situations as far as the following two aspects are concerned:

- where the expertise of you as the practitioner is considered to lie, that is, whether it lies with you or somewhere else
- how your practice is regulated, in terms of how the society you live in maintains the standard of what you do and your standing as a practitioner.

Eastern and Western Philosophies and Health

Complementary approaches to treating illness and bringing about wellbeing have become increasingly popular in Western countries since the nineteenth century. An estimated 80% of people in the world (mainly in the developing countries) are dependent on complementary therapies or alternative medicines for their primary healthcare (WHO, 2002). Some commentators such as Stone and Matthews (1996: xvii) regard this as evidence of the growing credibility of these approaches and that they are 'now being taken seriously by orthodox health professionals'. Other more critical commentators, such as the journalist Shapiro (2008), view it as a sign of a massive confidence trick being played on the uninformed general public. Stone and Matthews, barrister and lawyer/complementary health practitioner respectively, see the nature of complementary approaches, rather than any inherent defect in them, as contributing to the controversies about them. In their view:

> the highly individualized, intuitive, and whole-person approach central to holistic complementary therapies is not amenable to the degree of certainty, objective assessment, and quantifica-

tion required for the efficient operation of existing legal mechanisms. (Stone and Matthews, 1996: xvii)

They argue that this situation will be greatly helped by a strengthened commitment to practitioners' ethics and ethics-led regulation in training and practice.

Contrasting Cultures of Treatment

The culture of complementary and alternative approaches differs from conventional medicine. The conventional medical practitioner maintains social distance from the patients and works in a hospital, where there is a quite distinctive hierarchical organizational model of practice. Complementary and alternative medicine can be a democratizing force that does not recognize professional or social barriers between the practitioner and the patient. Avicenna (Ibn Sina, 980–1037), the multitalented founder of Islamic medicine, taught his students to physically embrace their patients. Modern hand healers place their hands near or on the patient's body, so that the healing can pass through them. Some healers use the palm of the hand, others only use the finger tips.

The lack of social distance between practitioner and patient does not imply a trivializing of the treatment. To use the example of healing again, while the healer will sometimes encourage the patient to talk, as part of the healing, it is also the case that the practitioner may prefer to work in silence, so as to focus on the practice. For example, in the case of healing:

> the ideal is silence and for the healer to be an objective observer of what is happening, that is, the sensations that are being felt and where they are felt. If one can achieve this and become an interested observer one can often learn, not only about the patient, but also to interpret what is happening. Sometimes both the hands will be completely still, other times one hand is still while the other moves, or both may move. They may move with a gentle motion towards and away from the patient, or with an up and down movement. Whatever it is, there is normally a rhythm and it is rarely a jerky movement. (Baerlein, 1978: 89)

Practitioners: Training and Registration

In the UK, the seven professional groups of physiotherapists, occupational therapists, chiropodists, orthoptists, radiographers, medical laboratory scientific officers and dieticians were all regulated by the Professions Supplementary to Medicine Act 1960. The Osteopaths Act 1993 and the Chiropractors Act 1994 were modelled on the Medical Act 1983 and did not alter the fact that registration was still only required for professionals who worked within the NHS (Stone and Matthews, 1996: 58). As late as the mid-1990s, while members of these professions employed in the NHS had to be on a register held by their respective professional board, those in the private sector did not have to maintain their registration and non-qualified practitioners could also set themselves up (Stone and Matthews, 1996: 55–6). This culture of self-regulation already extended into, and had been strengthened in, the complementary medicine sector, by the Medical Act 1983 (Stone and Matthews,

1996: 46). However, at the same time, this Act formed part of two trends since the last quarter of the twentieth century (Stone and Matthews, 1996: 47):

1. towards registered GPs (entitled to call themselves 'doctors') learning complementary therapies
2. towards more registered GPs employing complementary therapists in their practices.

In the UK, while chiropractors and osteopaths must be registered with their respective regulatory body – the General Chiropractic Council or the General Osteopathic Council (GOsC), and there are moves towards statutory regulation of acupuncture and herbal medicine, a vast number of complementary and alternative approaches remain unregulated by existing legislation, and many have their own arrangements for self-regulation. For example, aromatherapy is governed by the Aromatherapy Organisations Council, representing the majority of practising aromatherapists. To summarize this complex picture, the field of complementary and alternative practice falls into three categories: unregulated, self-regulated and statutorily regulated (Table 5.2), to which we return in more detail below.

Table 5.2 Regulation, self-regulation and non-regulation of complementary practice

Unregulated	Self-regulated	Statutorily regulated
Practitioners can set up in practice without undertaking UK-wide agreed professional training and are not subject to legal regulation or professional registration, for example some alternative therapies	Practitioners register voluntarily with a self-regulated body, for example reflexology (see Ch. 27)	Practitioners cannot use the name of the practice or practise without statutory registration, for example osteopathy (see Ch. 26), chiropractic (see Ch. 25)

There are tensions between some areas of complementary practice and healthcare professionals. Pharmacists and doctors, for example, are likely to state that essential oils, apart from established medicinal preparations such as peppermint oil capsules, should only be taken orally under medical supervision. On the supply side, the Aromatherapy Trade Council (ATC), a self-regulating independent organization, represents about three-quarters of the suppliers of essential oils. The ATC regulates the marketing, labelling and packaging of single-drop dispensers on bottles of essential oils sold to the general public (Tisserand and Balacs, 1995).

In the nonindustrialized and developing countries, complementary therapies and alternative medicine have been well established for many centuries, yet in Western industrialized countries they remain controversial. In Australia, nearly half of more than 3,000 adults randomly surveyed had used at least one form of complementary or alternative approach in a non-prescribed way (MacLennan et al., 1996). Twenty years earlier, an Australian government report noted that the increasingly important contribution of complementary and alternative services corresponded with public doubts about conventional medicine (Webb et al., 1977).

In Quebec, many practitioners are self-registered and belong to a trade union, the Fédération des Professionnels, which acupuncturists joined in 1988, homeopaths in 1989, naturopaths in 1995 and osteopaths in 1996 (Crellin and Ania, 2002: 99). In one sense, of course, this only intensifies debates about standards, since the motivation towards building a large union with a strong, diverse membership is in tension with the need for strict professional regulation in each aspect of practice.

In the USA, the White House Commission on Complementary and Alternative Medicine Policy (WHCCAMP), set up in 2000 with a brief to ensure that social policy maximized the benefits of complementary and alternative medicine (CAM), examined four particular aspects:

1. research of CAM products
2. education and training of CAM practitioners
3. provision of information about CAM to healthcare professionals
4. guidance regarding accessing CAM services.

The WHCCAMP reported in 2002. Prominent among its views is the recommendation that more research is needed to establish which CAM treatments are safe and effective. This and its other 28 recommendations were heavily criticized by the National Council Against Health Fraud in its position statement published in 2002 and its analysis of the final WHCCAMP report.

In many countries, controversy has been associated with the use of certain substances in both conventional medicine and complementary preparations. For example, in August 2002, Health Canada published a warning of the major risks of liver dysfunction associated with using homeopathic and herbal products containing the ingredient kava. In 2003, after more than 80 people reported symptoms after taking a travel sickness pill manufactured by Pan Pharmaceuticals, Therapeutic Goods Administration, the medicines regulatory body in Australia, recalled more than 200 of Pan's products and suspended the company's licence for six months. The number of recalled products rose to more than 1,500, exported to about 40 countries, including the USA and the UK.

The situation of complementary approaches varies in different European countries, Scandinavian countries being more permissive than those nearer the Mediterranean. In 1997, the Committee on the Environment, Public Health and Consumer Protection, a committee of the European Parliament, initiated a study of complementary and alternative medicine that reported in 1998. Its main purposes were to:

■ evaluate the safety and effectiveness of CAM
■ review the different national approaches to the legal regulation of CAM practitioners
■ encourage research into the role and character of CAM
■ propose a directive to cover food supplements, often on the borderline between dietary and medicinal products.

The term 'alternative' in one sense applies to treatments and approaches that are not generally accepted by health professionals. As late as the 1990s, the British Medical Association and the General Medical Council (GMC) excluded them from the NHS (Maher, 1992: 122). Before 1987, the field of complementary practice was not formally represented in professional healthcare debates about the regulation of practice. In 1987, the British Complementary Medicine Association (www.bcma. co.uk) was established to regulate Chinese herbal medicine. In 1993, the Prince of Wales set up the Foundation for Integrated Medicine, now known as the Prince's Foundation for Integrated Health (www.fih.org.uk), as a means of advancing the cause of integrated approaches to health and wellbeing. A report by the Centre for Complementary Health Studies at Exeter University (Mills, 1997) provided a snapshot of the field of complementary and alternative approaches in the UK, which was updated three years later (Mills and Budd, 2000). In 2000, three concerns – the risk to people through poor practice, voluntary regulation and a credible although incomplete evidence base – led the House of Lords Select Committee on Science and Technology (2000) to produce a report on complementary and alternative medicine, which recommended statutory regulation of acupuncture and herbal medicine under the Health Act 1999. In 2004, the European Union (EU) published a European Directive on the licensing of herbal medicines.

A steering group was set up in 2006 by the Department of Health to develop guidelines for regulating acupuncture, traditional Chinese medicine and other herbal medicine, Ayurveda, Unani-tibb (a traditional medicine system originating in India, the Middle East and Greece), kampo (Japanese traditional medicine) and Tibetan medicine in the UK. It reported in 2008 (Pittilo, 2008).

There are three main regulatory bodies in the UK field of complementary and alternative approaches:

1. The General Regulatory Council for Complementary Therapies (GRCCT): This was launched in June 2008, with the aim of validating the status of registered practitioners, through a register which was operational from October 2007, each profession having its own Voluntary Self Regulatory group, sending a member to the Federal Regulatory Council of the GRCCT.
2. British Complementary Therapies Council for Voluntary Self Regulation: This was established in October 2008 to cater for therapies not included in the CNHC initiative.
3. Complementary and Natural Healthcare Council (CNHC): This was launched in summer 2008 and is modelled on the GMC and other similar professional bodies. It is separate from the professional bodies representing the therapies that it regulates, in the sense that the practitioners act in an advisory capacity and the CNHC is composed of lay members. It was set up following an independent process led by Dame Joan Higgins, and the Prince's Foundation for Integrated Health will regulate the fields of complementary therapies and alternative medicine. It follows the best practice model set out by the Department of Health in the White Paper *Trust, Assurance and Safety*, concerning the regulation of statutory health professions (DH, 2007). The functions of the

CNHC – which comprises eight lay people plus chair, advised by complementary practitioners, and funded from registration fees from practitioners – include registering practitioners and dealing with complaints, with suspension from the register as the ultimate sanction (dealt with by a second board).

There is a gap at present in the professional regulation of practitioners in the field. Anybody can advertise their services as a practitioner in many complementary therapies. A minority of approaches, such as osteopathy and chiropractic, are already subject to statutory regulation, which means that the terms 'osteopath' and 'chiropractor' are legally protected and cannot be used by non-qualified and registered practitioners. Quite apart from the preservation of professional standards, this has the advantage of keeping a tally of the number of active practitioners. Most of the osteopaths on the GOsC's Statutory Register practise in the UK. In some ways there is a fundamental gulf between complementary and conventional approaches to medicine, yet in other ways the boundary between them is becoming quite blurred. Most of the practice of complementary therapies lies outside government policy, the NHS and associated legal regulations. There are tensions for complementary medical practitioners between distancing themselves so far from conventional medicine that they carry no authority with the health authorities at one extreme, and at the other extreme joining the health service, becoming professions allied or supplementary to medicine and losing their right to diagnose.

In the 1980s, there was unease and even antagonism among many other European countries towards the UK, where unregulated and unlicensed practitioners could practise nonconventional medicine. This tension was made more pronounced by the Council Directive (89/49/EEC), which provided mutual recognition in different European countries of diplomas or equivalent qualifications awarded following at least three years' training in what was called a 'regulated profession'. This did not apply at the time to nonconventional practitioners in the UK, who therefore remained unregulated. The General System Directive (CD/92/51), which introduced mutual recognition of professional courses of less than three years, had more direct implications for nonconventional practitioners (Bannerman et al., 1983: 10). Instead of facing up to this diversity and confusion, the European Commission and the European Parliament distanced themselves from the situation and, as late as 1990, clearly stated that their responsibilities did not extend to healthcare delivery, including nonconventional therapies (Bannerman et al., 1983: 11).

Meanwhile, the field of nonconventional therapies continued to expand vigorously. Research indicates that by the late 1980s in France, for example, about 50,000 non-allopathic practitioners were offering complementary and alternative treatments (Maddalena, 1999). The Treaty of the European Union (the Maastricht Treaty), which brought the single European market into being, became operative on 1 January 1993. This allows employed and self-employed people to move freely throughout the EU and live where they choose. Two European Directives guarantee a single European market for homeopathic human and veterinary products.

In the twenty-first century, the European Parliament remains hesitant about advancing complementary and alternative medicine across the EU, reflecting the reality that, while the marketing of pharmaceutical products is subject to EU legislation, individual member countries remain responsible for the delivery of their own healthcare services (Gordon, 2005).

Factors Contributing towards Regulation

Superficially, it is easy to argue that the pressure towards better regulation of complementary approaches is to bring about better care for people. The reality is more complex, not least because the tight regulation of medicine and nursing has not eliminated poor practice and misconduct (Stone and Lee-Treweek, 2005: 68–9).

Activity

Consider for a few minutes whether you feel that therapies that lie closer to, or are further apart from, conventional medicine are more likely to be regulated by the state. Why do you think this might come about?

Stone and Matthews (1996: 89) argue that the closer therapies are to claiming to treat a wide range of health problems and disorders, that is, complete systems of medicine, the more of a threat they represent to conventional medicine. In this situation, they are more likely to need the protection of statutory recognition or regulation. Stone and Matthews (1996: 89–95) identify a number of factors that make approaches more likely to benefit from statutory regulation. We can use this as the basis for distinguishing between those circumstances that are more and less likely to benefit from the regulation of practitioners (Table 5.3).

Table 5.3 Factors related to regulation of practitioners

Factor	Less likely to benefit	More likely to benefit
1 Scope	Not complete system of treatment	Complete system of treatment
2 Mode of delivery	Does not resemble conventional medicine	Resembles conventional medicine
3 Overlap with conventional practice	No	Yes
4 Centrality to conventional treatment	Low potential for harm to patient	High potential for harm to patient
5 Research evidence	No	Yes
6 Knowledge base	No	Yes
7 Rigorous evidence-based training	No	Yes

Factor	Less likely to benefit	More likely to benefit
8 Measurable treatment	No	Yes
9 How long practising	No	Yes
10 Already a form of registration	No	Yes
11 Credible and high profile	No	Yes

The list below expands on the 11 main factors identified in Table 5.3:

1. The extent to which they are complete systems of medicine
2. The extent to which their mode of delivery resembles that of conventional medicine
3. Whether or not they overlap with, or have a distinct and separate identity from, conventional medicine
4. Their potential for harm, either directly or through preventing the patient from seeking more appropriate conventional treatment
5. The extent to which their practice is based on factual, especially scientifically researched knowledge
6. The extent to which they are based on a credible knowledge base
7. The extent to which practice must be preceded by the achievement of a rigorous standard through training
8. The extent to which they are based on a specific remedy or intervention that can be measured
9. How long specific practitioners have been practising
10. The extent to which they are subject to a form of professional regulation and/ or registration
11. The extent to which they establish and sustain credibility, whether through scientific validation, high-profile patronage or other factors.

It is important to recognize that the situation of complementary practitioners in relation to conventional medicine is complicated by the fact that in some ways the closer the area of practice to the territory of conventional practice, the more of a threat it presents to the status of the conventional practitioner. Stone and Matthews (1996: 94) argue that it is not the incompatibility of the approach with conventional medicine that is a barrier to regulation so much as its lay practice. It is less likely that medical practitioners will show an interest in areas such as aromatherapy than areas such as homeopathy and acupuncture, where there is more congruence with areas of conventional medical practice. These arouse more pressure from doctors for regulation when they are practised by lay practitioners. Another related point of interest, highlighted by Stone and Matthews (1996: 94), is that approaches such as acupuncture, which can be allied with medical applications, are prone to being adopted by medical practitioners, 'isolated from their alien philosophical underpinnings' and, in the case of acupuncture, 'stripped of its underlying traditional philosophy and used mainly for pain relief' (Stone and Matthews, 1996: 94).

Chapter Summary

This chapter has examined issues associated with the legal and regulatory basis for practice. Three particular barriers continue to prevent complementary and alternative approaches gaining ground:

- The lack of generic regulation of the many different categories of complementary and alternative approaches.
- Incorporation by orthodox medical practice, whereby orthodox medical practitioners simply take on selected complementary and alternative approaches and incorporate them into their own practice.
- Referral by orthodox medical practice, whereby orthodox medical practitioners recognize complementary and alternative approaches and refer selected patients to them. Ironically, this may reduce the strength of one of the main reasons why people turn to complementary and alternative approaches – because traditionally they are not part of the orthodox systems of medicine and healthcare.

Having drawn attention to the difficulties, this chapter has indicated that, in the UK, some areas of practice have made significant progress towards state regulation.

REVIEW QUESTIONS

1   What was the main purpose of the Professions Supplementary to Medicine Act 1960?

2   The Medical Act 1983 strengthened the self-regulation of complementary medicine. What is self-regulation?

3   What is the GOsC?

CHAPTER LINKS

For further discussion of different categories of complementary practice, see Chapter 3, and for comparisons between different medical systems, see Chapter 13.

FURTHER RESOURCES

Dimond, B. (1998) *The Legal Aspects of Complementary Therapy Practice*, London, Churchill Livingstone. An authoritative and informative guide.

Lee-Treweek, G., Heller, T., MacQueen, H. et al. (eds) (2005) *Complementary and Alternative Medicine: Structures and Safeguards*, Abingdon, Routledge. Useful collection of chapters on different aspects, including regulation and professionalism.

Stone, J. and Matthews, J. (1996) *Complementary Medicine and the Law*, Oxford, Oxford University Press. Detailed discussion of aspects of regulation of complementary approaches.

Resource file

Key Healthcare Policies

The health and social care services provide the legal, policy and organizational framework against which complementary and alternative services develop. While some of these latter services are completely independent of the NHS and the local authority social care provision, others are provided contractually, while others again are employed directly by health providers.

Key Legislation

The Health and Social Care (Community Health and Standards) Act 2003 created a new type of body in the NHS, transforming the existing NHS trusts that provided hospital care, for example, into foundation trusts, which perform the same function but are independent, not-for-profit, public benefit organizations. By 2007, 45 out of 257 acute trusts, 11 out of 20 specialist trusts and 6 out of 74 mental health trusts had become foundation trusts – a total of 62 out of 247, or 25%. Two important government aims are, first, to increase local financial flexibility over how resources are allocated and second – a matter of great relevance for complementary practitioners who wish to become involved – to decrease accountability 'upwards' towards central government and increase accountability 'outwards and downwards', that is, to encourage the direct participation of local people, including members of the general public, in the local management and provision of health services.

The National Health Service Act 2006, the National Health Service (Wales) Act 2006 and National Health Service (Consequential Provisions) Act 2006 bring together (the term often used is 'consolidate') previous legislation and provide the basis for organizing and delivering the NHS in England and Wales. Previous legislation now consolidated includes:

- National Health Service and Community Care Act 1990
- Health Authorities Act 1995
- Primary Care Act 1997

- Health Act 1999
- Health and Social Care Act 2001
- National Health Service Reform and Health Care Professions Act 2002
- Health and Social Care (Community Health and Standards) Act 2003
- Health Act 2006.

Health services are commissioned by primary care trusts (PCTs). The commissioning process entails procurement, which means a contract is set up and a pricing arrangement agreed. PCTs are free-standing statutory bodies in the NHS, which control local health services. Strategic health authorities (SHAs) monitor performance and standards of services.

Some areas of practice in health and social care are governed by National Service Frameworks (NSFs). *The National Service Framework for Older People* (DH, 2001) regulates the services for older people by setting minimum standards for the quality of their delivery. Any complementary services must be provided so that they match this NSF. Similar standards regulate services for children, young people and maternity services (DfES/DH, 2004).

Public Participation in Healthcare Performance

There are policy moves towards strengthening Section 11 of the Health and Social Care Act 2001, thereby increasing opportunities for people to be informed about the performance of their health services and contribute to decisions about policies and staff pay (DCLG, 2006: 16). Since 2001, there has been a rapid shift from the creation and implementation of patient and public involvement structures to local involvement networks (LINks).

Many of the above areas of debate and change are reflected in the White Paper: *Our Health, Our Care, Our Say* (DH, 2006). (White Papers outline government intentions.) This 2006 White Paper sets out a strategy for delivering:

■ greater emphasis on prevention and less on illness
■ shifting spending from large hospitals to smaller community hospitals and other units such as more walk-in centres, closer to local communities
■ improved NHS and local authorities working together to provide better joined-up and integrated health and social care services
■ democratized services with improved service user, carer and patient choice and say.

Among the detailed changes are the following:

■ new NHS 'Life Check' assessing lifestyle risks, actions to take and referrals where necessary
■ guarantee of registration at local GP practice
■ supporting self-care with increased investment in the expert patient programme
■ an information prescription that enables people to take better long-term care of themselves
■ a personal health and social care plan contributing to a person's integrated health and social care record
■ improved support, including respite arrangements, for carers
■ extended direct payments and piloting Individual Budgets for health as well as social care.

The White Paper is an attempt to promote partnerships between NHS bodies and local government departments such as those responsible for different aspects of services to improve the health and wellbeing of citizens, to achieve what the government calls 'joined-up' thinking and practice.

References

DCLG (Department for Communities and Local Government) (2006) *Strong and Prosperous Communities: The Local Government White Paper,* Vol. II, Cm 6939-II, London, TSO.

DfES/DH (Department for Education and Skills/Department of Health) (2004) *National Service Framework for Children, Young People and Maternity Services,* London, TSO.

DH (Department of Health) (2001) *The National Service Framework for Older People,* London, TSO.

DH (Department of Health) (2006) *Our Health, Our Care, Our Say: A New Direction for Community Services,* White Paper, Cm 6737, London, TSO

Further Resources

DH (Department of Health) (2004) *Standards for Better Healthcare,* London, TSO.

DH/Scottish Office/Welsh Office (Department of Health/ The Scottish Office/The Welsh Office) (1996) *Choice and Opportunity: Primary Care: The Future,* London, TSO.

Health and Social Care Act 2001.

Health and Social Care (Community Health and Standards) Act 2003.

NHS Executive (1999) *Primary Care Trusts: Establishing Better Services,* London, NHS Executive.

Patient and Public Involvement Team (2006) *A Stronger Local Voice: A Framework for Creating a Stronger Local Voice in the Development of Health and Social Care Services,* London, DH.

Promoting Health and Wellbeing

Understanding Health

There is no agreement among researchers, commentators and experts in the subject about what health and health promotion are (for further discussion, see Chapter 4). Associated with this is the reality that different ideas exist about the definition of health. From within the biomedical model, the World Health Organization's *Constitution* (WHO, 1948) defines health as 'a state of complete physical, social and mental well-being and not merely the absence of disease and infirmity' (Nutbeam, 1998: 12). The WHO *Ottawa Charter for Health Promotion* (WHO, 1986) defines health promotion as 'the process of enabling people to increase control over, and to improve their health' (Nutbeam, 1998: 12). The Ottawa Charter specifies three strategies for health promotion:

1. *Advocacy* for health: combined action by individuals and groups 'to gain political commitment, policy support, social acceptance and systems support' for particular initiatives (Nutbeam, 1998: 5).
2. *Enabling* everyone to achieve their full health potential.
3. *Mediating* between different societal interests with the aim of improving health (Nutbeam, 1998: 13).

The *Jakarta Declaration on Leading Health Promotion into the 21st Century* (WHO, 1997) confirmed the above and identified the following five combined strategies as most effective to:

- Promote *social responsibility for health*
- increase *investments for health development*
- expand *partnerships for health promotion*
- increase *community capacity* and *empower the individual*
- secure an *infrastructure for health promotion.* (Nutbeam, 1998: 13)

Health Development for People

Improving the health of citizens requires three things. The health services:

- should not just provide acute services such as hospitals to carry out medical treatments on people who are already ill.
- should promote citizens' health and wellbeing, so as to prevent them becoming ill in the first place.

- should encourage citizens' active participation and empowerment, by
  - giving them information about the issues
  - encouraging them to develop opinions
  - offering opportunities to tell decision makers what they think
  - providing feedback with how their opinions have shaped services
  - ensuring ways are found of taking account of the views of citizens from a diversity of ages, abilities, cultures and backgrounds.

References

Nutbeam, D. (1998) *Health Promotion Glossary*, Geneva, WHO.

WHO (World Health Organization) (1948) *Constitution*, Geneva, WHO.

WHO (World Health Organization) (1986) *Ottawa Charter for Health Promotion*, Geneva, WHO.

WHO (World Health Organization) (1997) *Jakarta Declaration on Leading Health Promotion into the 21st Century*, Geneva, WHO.

Further Resource

Pike, S. and Forster, D. (1997) *Health Promotion for All*, Edinburgh, Churchill Livingstone, pp. 125–40. A useful chapter covering practice issues regarding children and young people.

Managing your Own Practice

Part III
Managing your Own Practice

Introduction

Part III introduces and responds to the requirement that practitioners should have a knowledge and understanding not only of their own particular specialist area of practice, but of the practicalities of managing their practice. This is a crucial aspect of work that practitioners neglect at their peril. Complementary practitioners may work in a wide variety of practices, including completely independent work; working in partnership with health and social care services and with clients, patients and other people who use the services; and being contracted or employed by a health provider on a case-by-case, part-time or full-time basis.

Chapter 6 deals with some of the issues that arise in practice where the individual practitioner works with other professionals, for example on an interdisciplinary or multiprofessional basis. Chapter 7 tackles aspects of running a complementary practice, as a business, whether alone or working with other people. Chapter 8 examines the important hygiene, health and safety aspects that must be considered by all practitioners wherever they are working.

Working in Teams and with Different Professions

ROBERT ADAMS

Learning outcomes

By the end of this chapter, you should be able to:

■ define what is meant by teamwork

■ clarify different 'working together' arrangements involving different professions

■ distinguish different forms of disciplinary teams

■ assess the relative merits of different forms of teamwork

■ appreciate what makes for good team working

■ explore implications for practice

The title of this chapter covers two main areas: teamwork and joint work between different professional groups and organizations. These raise a range of possible topics, since complementary and alternative practice takes place in a variety of disciplinary and professional settings, and practitioners relate to other professionals in different ways. It is important to examine these different forms, since this enables us to appreciate the ways in which relationships between different areas of practice can be complex and demanding.

Where is Teamwork Relevant?

Teamwork is highly relevant both in complementary and conventional healthcare and medicine.

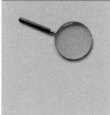

Practice example

Cass works as a healer in a multidisciplinary palliative care team (delivering end-of-life care to patients). The team comprises doctors, nurses, healthcare assistants and other healthcare professionals, who work closely with counsellors and social workers as well as different complementary practitioners. They aim not to 'cure' the patient, but to provide total care for and with patients and their families.

Complementary practitioners are likely to work in many different organizational settings and may also work with several different professionals in other organizations. In some of these relationships, the collaborations may be informal, yet in others a high degree of integration may exist. Sullivan and Skelcher (2002: 42–3) have studied these different forms of collaboration and identify loose networks of informal collaboration at one extreme, and, at the other, the merger of all professional activities into a single organization.

It is important to appreciate that complementary and alternative practitioners may seek employment in a health spa or complementary therapy clinic, they may go into partnership with other independent practitioners to run a complementary health centre, or they may practise singly and be available to work with different healthcare organizations. In any of these situations, practitioners are likely to come into contact with other professionals and to encounter teams and team working. It is necessary to be clear about the different models and methods of teamwork and to be confident about collaborative work with different practitioners and organizations.

Payne's excellent book about teamwork notes that primary care is an important location for multiprofessional teamwork (Payne, 2000: 180). Complementary practitioners often contribute to primary healthcare in the local health centre or GP surgery, the first point of call for many people.

What is a Team?

Activity

Reflect for a few minutes on what the word 'team' means to you, in the complementary practice setting. Try to jot down a concise definition of teamwork.

The word 'team' applies to work where there is a measure of shared agreement among staff about their values, aims, objectives and methods of achieving them. In the primary health centre, or the complementary health practice, the team, as Payne (2000: 181) notes, includes secretarial and administrative staff as well as professionals. The person who answers the telephone, or is behind the desk when the new client or patient arrives, is as important, at that moment, in projecting the values and purposes of the team, as are the professionals.

In practice, the word 'team' tends to be overused in work with people. Many settings where different professionals and other staff share offices at the same address may be loosely referred to as teams, yet they are simply sharing premises without working together.

Different Arrangements for Working Together

The term 'working together' is a more modest description than 'teamwork' for much work done by different professional groups, in parallel, working side by side with each other. However modest this may sound, since the 1970s, health and social services organizations in the UK have struggled with mixed results to achieve improvements in the arrangements for working together, in all areas of practice. This is particularly important in areas such as palliative care, mental health, physical and learning disability and work with children – all areas where complementary and alternative practitioners can make a significant contribution. Working together takes place in a range of circumstances, on a continuum (Table 6.1).

Table 6.1 Continuum of working together with people

Approach	What it means in practice
Liaison	Keeping in communication
Coordination	Links are made between essentially different approaches
Collaboration	Approaches are shared to a significant extent
Integration	Individual differences in approach are completely merged in a shared approach

Different Forms of Team Working

Let us return to the notion of the team. We find that health and social services increasingly are organized in teams and the focus on meeting the needs of individuals with particular illnesses and conditions brings together a variety of different professionals in these teams. Several words are commonly used to describe these teams, notably 'multidisciplinary', 'unidisciplinary' and 'interdisciplinary'. There is not complete agreement between commentators on the distinctions between these, but the following provides a starting point for further discussion.

Multidisciplinary and Unidisciplinary Teams

Cottrell (1993) distinguishes between multidisciplinary teams, wherein several disciplines share at different times the professional and managerial responsibility for different aspects of a case, and unidisciplinary teams, where one professional exercises professional leadership and managerial responsibility. Cottrell expresses doubts about the claims of a child psychiatrist that the unidisciplinary team works well, suggesting that the comprehensive range of assessments and interventions could not be offered and, contrary to claims of the psychiatrists, merely hid rather than resolving conflicts between the disciplines.

Cottrell tends to support the view of Ovretveit (1986) that multidisciplinary teams have many advantages, including:

> better service provision, easier access to the service for referrers (who do not have to deal with lots of different professionals), more colleague and peer support for team members, better planning of new developments and better management of different workloads. (Cottrell, 1993: 733)

Multidisciplinary and Interdisciplinary Teams

Jessup (2007: 330–1) has produced the following helpful distinction between multidisciplinary and interdisciplinary teamwork:

> Multidisciplinary team approaches utilise the skills and experience of individuals from different disciplines, with each discipline approaching the patient from their own perspective. Most often, this approach involves separate individual consultations … It is common for multidisciplinary teams to meet regularly, in the absence of the patient, to discuss 'case conference' findings and future directions for the patient's care. Multidisciplinary teams provide more knowledge and experience than disciplines operating in isolation.

> Interdisciplinary team approaches, as the word itself suggests, integrate separate discipline approaches into a single consultation. That is, the patient history taking, assessment, diagnosis, intervention and short- and long-term management goals are conducted by the team, together with the patient, at the one time. The patient is intimately involved in any discussions regarding their condition or prognosis and the plans about their care. A common understanding and holistic view of all aspects of the patient's care ensues.

From the above extract, we can deduce that multidisciplinary approaches tend to exclude the patient from case conferences, which focus on different professionals reaching clarification of their views of the patient's situation; while interdisciplinary approaches tend to integrate the approaches and views of different disciplines and offer the potential of arriving at a more holistic understanding of the patient's situation and needs.

Relative Merits of Different Forms of Teamwork

The multidisciplinary team has the advantage that it does not necessarily mean that differences of power and dominance between team members will adversely affect the consultation and decision-making processes. The interdisciplinary team meeting, however, may be dominated by the powerful personalities and/or senior staff and other junior practitioners may withdraw and not assert their view. On the other hand, the multidisciplinary team may not reach a concerted view, while from the viewpoint of the patient, the interdisciplinary approach is likely to lead to a more coherent outcome and therefore a more satisfactory one from the patient's point of view. A further advantage of the interdisciplinary team is that staff roles may become more flexible, as different practitioners become engaged in different aspects and some may volunteer to take on aspects of the practice in which they would not otherwise have been involved.

What Makes for Good Teamwork

According to Ovretveit (1997: 42), good teamwork depends in the first place on two things:

- *A well-designed base for the team to work:* this includes clarity about where the team members work from, points of contact, where records are stored, where clinics are situated.
- *A well-thought-out policy framework:* this needs to specify how the team is organized, how the work will be shared, what priorities will be and how much autonomy and flexibility each person has.

Part III

Activity

In the light of these two foundations for good teamwork, spend 10 minutes or so jotting down up to a dozen bullet points, which you consider to be the most important things you would consider in a checklist of things that would need to be clarified in setting out a policy and practice statement for good team working.

These are some of the main aspects of the framework for policy and practice that Ovretveit (1997: 43–5) suggests will need to be clarified in any teamwork setting:

- What needs are catered for
- What the responsibilities and role of the team leader are
- Who the team members are
- What the team purpose and work areas are
- What the catchment and boundaries are
- How clients/patients are referred to, or have access to, the team
- What team processes exist for decision making
- What coordination exists between the team and other (for example health and social care) services
- What supervision arrangements are made
- What case records and work records (for example staff meetings) are kept
- Team reviews
- Team targets and targets set at six-monthly intervals.

Clearly, the above list will need to be worked through differently, in order to meet the varying needs of different groups of practitioners and patients or clients.

Chapter Summary

This chapter has examined some of the main features of the great variety of ways in which professionals work together. Joint working takes place in a range of settings and between different groups of people, depending on the situation and the particular purpose. It is clear that there are many different ways in which professionals can collaborate. Also, it is apparent that effective team working depends on clarity about a great number of aspects, strategically and tactically, in policy and practice.

REVIEW QUESTIONS

1 What does the word 'teamwork' mean in complementary practice?

2 What is the main difference between coordination and collaboration?

3 In what main way does multidisciplinary work differ from interdisciplinary work?

CHAPTER LINKS

For discussion of the importance of good communication, see Chapter 10, and for discussion of the process of working, see Chapter 11.

FURTHER RESOURCES

Payne, M. (2000) *Teamwork in Multiprofessional Care*, Basingstoke, Palgrave – now Palgrave Macmillan. Excellent review of the literature, policy and practice issues concerning all major aspects of teamwork and multiprofessional work.

Sullivan, H. and Skelcher, C. (2002) *Working across Boundaries: Collaboration in Public Services*, Basingstoke, Palgrave Macmillan. Bird's eye view of the entire range of collaborative arrangements. Useful for sparking off ideas on aspects not covered in Payne.

Running a Complementary Practice as a Small Business

ROBERT ADAMS

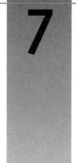

Learning outcomes

By the end of this chapter, you should have a grasp of how to:

■ prepare to run an independent complementary practice

■ market the practice

■ run the practice as a business

■ manage and administer the practice

■ deliver quality in the practice

Preparing to Run an Independent Complementary Practice

There are many decisions to make before setting out to do anything in practice. The preparation stage is probably the most time-consuming stage of all. Most initiatives take a relatively large amount of upfront investment and thereafter there is a tendency for strategic issues to be replaced by tactical ones. It would be misleading to say the workload is less once we move from planning to implementation, because work has a habit of filling all available spaces.

Making the Right Decision before the Start

It is important to make the right decision at the outset. There are different options for complementary practitioners:

1. to work as a member of a multiprofessional team
2. to practise independently as a sole practitioner
3. to join an existing complementary practice

4. to go into business by taking over, or founding, an independent complementary practice.

The first three options do not entail the work and the risk that the fourth involves. On the other hand, there may be advantages in setting up an independent practice, associated with the higher profile of the practice and the increasing opportunities for activities such as training, conferences and working with various media – writing, broadcasting and so on. Joining a multiprofessional team will not be without its challenges (see Chapter 6). A sole practitioner may find it as hard as any lone professional, not least because working alone requires the ability to self-motivate and be self-critical, as well as energy, commitment and self-discipline. Some sole practitioners work as a locum by supplying their labour as short-term relief in an established practice. Joining an existing complementary practice offers many benefits, not the least of which is that many of the day-to-day problems are taken care of. The growth of the spa industry, in the UK and other countries, gives a contemporary twist to the fashion for 'taking the waters' at spa towns, represented in England by Bath, Harrogate and Buxton, from Roman times to the present day (Cohen and Bodeker, 2008). There may be a room to be rented for a number of hours, sessions or days per week. There may be a shared receptionist who takes care of telephone and other personal calls, which the practitioner can catch up with between appointments. There may be a group of practitioners who can offer support and a measure of co-supervision and consultation. Much of this chapter is written on the assumption that the practitioner is pursuing the fourth, most challenging but potentially rewarding option.

Being Aware of One's Own Strengths and Weaknesses

It can happen that friends and relatives will have their say when one is making ground-breaking decisions about what to do. However, the practitioner is best placed to make the final decision and it is important to keep advisers and experts in their place. There are judgements to be made about one's strengths and weaknesses, but only one person is really closely involved in this particular initiative and that is the practitioner. This applies more clearly to professional judgements, of course, while some decisions will involve money and other similar resources such as the use of premises. These demonstrably are matters that involve other people, unless we are lucky enough to be sitting on an adequate pot of money over which we have sole control.

The assessment of our own strengths and weaknesses is important, because unless we know ourselves, there is little point in trying to help other people. So the judgements made about the business will spill over into professional decisions and vice versa. The personality of the person running a business is important, in the sense that the successful business relies on at least one person to take charge of the situation, solve problems rather than back away from them, be well organized and an efficient administrator, identify what needs doing at any one time and work at it until it is done. Running a business as the sole trader has certain unavoidable stresses associated with it and it is better to accept this at the preparatory stage and back off them, than to enter the business and find out too late that the stress is not for you.

Seeking Professional Advice and Support

This preparatory stage is the time to seek information, advice and support from other professionals, in the form of telephone calls, emails, internet searches for documents and, most of all, face-to-face frank discussions with people best placed to give independent advice. Much of this advice will not be related to one's area of professional practice. Unless you have run a business before, it will be about small business practice. There are government bodies that provide such information and the list of websites at the end of this chapter gives access to some of these, which will lead to others. There are also people with the expertise to give general advice, such as business advisers and officials in local banks. However, many of these people have a vested interest and their objective may be to attract business rather than to advise impartially and this needs to be borne in mind when approaching them.

On the professional side, there are many people involved in independent practice, either as individuals or in a complementary practice centre, and it is useful to approach them for advice. There is also a large group of professions grouped around the health services under a heading such as professions allied to medicine and among them there are many independent practitioners. The organization Occupational Therapists in Independent Practice has prepared a code of practice that provides a useful framework for independent practitioners in occupational therapy, which has more general relevance to other independent practitioners. This highlights the important aspects of independent practice that need to be considered. These come under the following three major headings: the practitioner, the business and the practice. I draw on these later in this chapter, where appropriate.

Marketing the Practice

Marketing may involve publicising the practice, but it does not stop there. Marketing is about identifying the market, analysing and specifying a target, devising ways of hitting that target and sustaining contact with the targeted market. Marketing is a focused, but wide-ranging activity, with its own specialized body of knowledge and expertise. It is easy to seize on a part of it and imagine that we have covered the entire field. Let us return to the five aspects we identified and attend briefly to each, recognizing that in this limited space we cannot do more than summarize.

Identifying the Market

Consider for a few minutes and jot down brief notes on the different sources you would draw on when marketing your practice.

There are many different sources of information that can be sought for the purposes of market research:

- the views of other practitioners in the locality
- the views of current patients or clients – these can be included in the information gathered when the history is first taken from the patient, or canvassed in a simple questionnaire to be completed anonymously and left in a box after they have had their consultation or treatment
- the views of potential patients or clients.

It is important not to collect information for its own sake. The priority is to gather information that will help to give a view of the market.

Analysing and Targeting the Market

It is important to reach a view about:

- what people want from complementary practitioners
- what people think about this practitioner and the practice
- what the competition is.

It will be necessary to devise a strategy to respond to the needs identified in the market.

Devising Ways of Hitting that Target

This is the point where the practitioner needs to decide how to respond to the market. Hopefully, a demand will be identified, but the question will be how best to tailor the service offered to meet that demand. It may be that people ask for flexible hours (in terms of early mornings and evenings), seven days as opposed to five, and a mobile service and this is more important than having a smart clinic. On the other hand, people may prefer to drive to a clinic and not have the mobile service delivered to their door.

Sustaining Contact with the Targeted Market

It is important to maintain the service and in order to do this, it will be necessary to keep checking that the expectations of patients and clients are still being met and are unchanged.

Running the Practice as a Business

In the first place, it is necessary to decide how to practise. There are three main options:

1. as a sole trader
2. as a partnership
3. as a limited company.

Let us review these briefly in turn:

- *Sole trader:* Most independent practitioners are sole traders. This is the most straightforward method of running the finances of the practice. An accountant will probably be needed, who will submit the self-assessed statement annually to HM Revenue & Customs (HMRC). It is sufficient to keep a straightforward account of income, expenditure and relevant expenses incurred in connection with the practice, with all receipts. The weakness of this method of trading is that should a patient or client wish to claim, or debts be incurred, then claims can be made against the personal assets of the practitioner.
- *Partnership:* Some independent practitioners who work well together may decide to operate their business as a group practice. In such circumstances, a partnership may seem attractive. This has the advantages that some of the basic costs of the business – premises, accountant – can be shared. The disadvantages, however, are that one partner's actions may affect others adversely. If one partner incurs debts in the practice partnership and does not pay them, the other partners are likely to be liable.
- *Limited company:* The size and/or complexity of the practice may be great enough to justify the decision to set up a limited company. It may be desirable to do this in any case, where there is a risk that claims may arise against the practitioner, for financial or professional reasons. The limited company gives some financial protection against such claims. The disadvantages are that running a company requires directors to be appointed, a company secretary and board meetings to be held and decisions recorded. At intervals, new information will arrive by post giving information about changes to employment law, national insurance and other items that may affect any employees of the business. Action must be taken to implement any such legal provisions. Also an accountant must be appointed to file annual accounts with Companies House.

Business Skills and Practice

The independence of the practitioner depends on sound business activities. The College of Occupational Therapists' (COT, 2005a) code of business practice states that it is important to give the business a distinctive identity and to run it professionally and fairly. This entails:

- Determining how the business is organized to deliver the service: whether through a limited company, partnership or by an individual practitioner as a sole trader
- Setting goals for the business and deciding on its scope and how the service is delivered
- Keeping financial records according to legal and HMRC requirements
- Maintaining a fair and clear structure of fees.

Rewards

The balance sheet of costs and benefits is not all on the debit side. There can be good financial rewards from complementary practice. However, when setting out, it is advisable to be realistic about the returns. Typically, the newly qualified practitioner in sole practice will be relying on the income from consultations. A typical working week may begin early and finish late, but realistically consultations will not begin before 10am and may finish at 6pm, with a break of one hour to have lunch and deal with administrative and other matters. Even though consultations may only be 40 minutes, it will be advisable to allow one hour, by the time people have taken off their coats at the start and said goodbye at the end and been shown out. The maximum number of patients or clients, on this basis, will be about 35 in a week. Let us put some notional prices on this estimate, purely as illustrations, to show how we calculate yearly income. If you charge £20–30 per person, this will produce gross income of £700–1,050 in a week. However, there will be occasions when you cannot see patients – perhaps two days per four weeks or half a day per week, when you have to attend practice meetings, in service courses or engage in other professional business. There will also be gaps between appointments. This inevitably will reduce gross income to £600–900 per week. It could even reduce it further, if you have to travel a distance to your consulting and treatment base. Allowing for public holidays, professional annual conferences and personal holidays of a total of four weeks per year produces a total of 48 earning weeks per year. This gives a total gross income of £28,800–42,000. This calculation allows for consultations of 40 minutes, but clearly these could be shorter. However, a proportionately lower fee would probably be charged, so the total might not be much different. Also, a significant proportion of unnotified cancellations needs to be taken into account, as any doctor's receptionist, dental surgery or music teacher who relies on giving private lessons will tell you. Obviously, this figure would rise and fall depending on the initial consultation fee you charged.

The gross income will be taxable, after deductions directly related to professional costs, which are likely to include membership of the professional body, equipment used solely in connection with the profession and so on. Practising from home can save an annual rental fee of several thousand pounds, if a room has to be booked at a neighbouring medical or complementary medical centre. Some practitioners make additional profits from the sale of products for home treatments. This applies, for example, to herbalists, naturopaths and homeopathic practitioners.

Managing and Administering the Practice

In the light of your own experience and what you would expect to be the case, think about and jot down a list of every kind of legal obligation you think a complementary business might have to satisfy.

The College of Occupational Therapists' (COT, 2005a) code of business practice draws attention to the legal obligations that the business must satisfy:

- Health and safety
- Taxation – HMRC
- National insurance
- Data protection
- Public and professional liability insurance
- Employer's liability insurance
- Customs and Excise
- Employment
- Complaints procedures
- National Occupational Standards, for example Care Standards
- Supply of goods and services
- Criminal Records Bureau (CRB)
- Equality and anti-discrimination
- Human rights.

Membership of a professional body is likely to entail the practitioner taking out professional indemnity insurance, which is essential as protection against any patient or client who makes a claim resulting from any faulty treatment provided. Employer's liability insurance is required by the business, which should provide cover for any liabilities with regard to employees. Until 1 October 2008, the insurance certificates had to be retained by employers for 40 years (Employers' Liability (Compulsory Insurance) Act 1969; Employers' Liability (Compulsory Insurance) Regulations 1998), and even though this has been abolished, employers are still advised to retain them for many years, as protection against claims made by employees, many years later.

Dispensing insurance is required for any herbal or unpackaged remedies the practitioner may supply. Liability for any defects in any packaged and sealed products should be covered by the manufacturer's or supplier's product liability, unless there is a question of professional negligence, in which case professional indemnity insurance should cover the circumstances.

Other forms of insurance are numerous, such as buildings, permanent healthcare, vehicle, legal and buildings insurances. It is advisable to take professional advice before embarking on insurance policies, as these can be expensive and, regardless of cost, may not meet the circumstances against which insurance is required.

Part III

Delivering Quality in the Practice

It is vital that while practitioners are devoting time to setting up an independent practice and running it as a business, they do not neglect their own professional practice. It is extremely important to ask oneself why people go to a complementary practitioner in an independent practice. Patients and clients do not just want to have their symptoms relieved, but often expect to have a positive experience in a setting where they feel unhurried and particular attention is being paid by the practitioner to them. The setting for this should be designed, furnished and structured so as to emphasize the potential for improving health and wellbeing.

It is necessary to bear in mind these points when setting up an independent practice. They should figure in the decisions taken about the location of the practice, its outlook, privacy, design and interior decoration and the detail of the layout of the waiting room, proximity to telephones ringing and so on.

The College of Occupational Therapists' (2005a) code of business practice draws attention to the need to ensure that you (and other practitioners in the practice, if it is multiple or shared) are qualified and competent to deliver the service. In areas of complementary practice where it is appropriate, it is important that the practitioner maintains registration and is subject to regulation alongside other similar practitioners in other sectors. It is also important that you and other practitioners follow the appropriate professional codes of practice, where these exist.

The independent practitioner needs to ensure that the independent practice mirrors the ethical and quality standards found in any other sector. There are many areas of practice which, while not legally necessary, are consistent with ethical practice accepted on a widespread basis. The following areas are noted in the College of Occupational Therapists' (2005a) code of business practice. The practitioner needs to:

- engage in continuing professional development to keep up with contemporary developments
- work with other professionals across professional boundaries when necessary
- maintain clear records to the relevant professional standards
- operate a complaints procedure
- deal with enquiries from clients and patients promptly, do the required work within reasonable time limits and provide relevant papers and reports where required.

Last, but not least, whether you practise from a room in your own home, occupy a room run by an independent practice, run your own independent practice or are working in a health service facility, it must be remembered that patients and clients judge the quality of your practice by the professional presentation of yourself and your premises. This brings us to health and safety, because a clean practice run by a presentable practitioner is more likely to be a hygienic and safe practice.

Health and safety are dealt with in Chapter 8, but are worth emphasizing in this connection. It is important to be aware that people using the premises appreciate when the proprietor takes more than a 'minimalist' approach to meeting legal requirements, including health and safety. A minimal approach often leads to increased accidents and illness and in the long run the business does not benefit. A smart, well-organized, clean premises, well above the minimum standards in terms of hygiene and health and safety, enhances the reputation of the practitioners using the premises.

Chapter Summary

This chapter has considered the main types of business arrangement most appropriate for complementary practice. It has examined the main issues that arise in running such a business, and explored some of the implications for the practitioner.

REVIEW QUESTIONS

1 One option for running the practice as a business is as a limited company. What are the other two options?

2 What is dispensing insurance?

3 What are the main distinguishing features of employer's liability insurance and professional indemnity insurance?

CHAPTER LINKS

For further discussion of legal aspects of health, safety and hygiene, see Chapter 8.

FURTHER RESOURCES

Aldred, E.M. (2007) *A Guide to Starting your own Complementary Therapy Practice*, Edinburgh, Churchill Livingstone/Elsevier Books. Good practical guide to setting up and running your practice as a business.

Burkholder, P. (2007) *Start your Own Day Spa and More: Destination Spa, Medical Spa, Yoga Center, Spiritual Spa*, Irvine, CA, Entrepreneur Press. Provides guidance on many practical aspects of developing and sustaining an independent practice, including researching the market, funding, the business plan, management, using the internet, marketing, and creating the atmosphere.

COT (College of Occupational Therapists) (2005) *Occupational Therapists in Independent Practice (OTIP): Code of Business Practice*, London, College of Occupational Therapists. Contains a great many practical hints, particularly on the professional aspects of practising independently.

Web Links

www.businesslink.gov.uk
www.dti.gov.uk
www.princes-trust.org.uk
www.business.gov
www.sba.gov

8 Hygiene, Health and Safety

ROBERT ADAMS

Learning outcomes

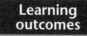

By the end of this chapter, you should:

■ appreciate the contribution of hygiene to safety and wellbeing

■ know the requirements of health and safety legislation

■ understand how risk management and risk assessment operate

It is important to recognize that health and safety are not a minimalist art, that is, where the practitioner does just enough to satisfy the minimal legal requirements. It is important, whether as employer or practitioner renting a room for a few hours a week in another premises, or practising in a room at home, to take seriously the responsibility to maintain a healthy and safe environment. In the wider sense, employers have responsibility for managing occupational health issues in the workplace and this means taking reasonable measures to promote the health and wellbeing of employees and prevent illnesses and injuries.

Hygiene, Safety and Wellbeing

Each complementary therapy presents its own specific requirements in terms of health and safety and there are some issues that apply generally across the field. We should bear in mind that complementary practice may take place in conventional healthcare settings and that in that case, the regulations applying in health services will also apply to complementary practitioners. Complementary practitioners are subject to the law, which requires that doctors must prescribe all medicines administered to patients and only a registered nurse (a nurse on the register of the United Kingdom Central Council for Nursing, Midwifery and Health Visiting) can administer medicines and supervise them (UKCC, 2002).

It is as important in complementary practice as in conventional healthcare to safeguard against hazards and risks in the treatment environment. A **hazard** is the manner in which a situation or an object may cause harm. A **risk** is the calculated chance that harm will occur.

One of the greatest hazards is in the risk of infection to patients and clients. This can occur in any public setting frequented by numbers of people. It is particularly a characteristic of hospitals, clinics, health centres and complementary health centres, where people – practitioners, patients, clients, relatives and friends – gather together in settings focusing on the treatment of ill and vulnerable people.

Practice example

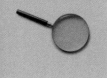

Sharon runs a small complementary practice. She wants to ensure that all possible hazards and risks to hygiene and health and safety are minimized. She holds regular meetings with all staff to ensure that nobody thinks health, safety and hygiene are mainly or solely the responsibility of professionals, but are shared by everybody using the premises.

Responsibility for health and safety in the workplace is shared by all staff, including administrative and clerical staff as well as practitioners. It is important for any person who notices a hazard to health and safety to bring it to the attention of a staff member who can tackle it.

Activity

What is infection? Consider for a few minutes what the word 'infection' means to you.

Infection is the process of invasion of the body by organisms that produce disease – whether bacteria or viruses. While all surfaces, and the air around us, are full of these organisms all the time, some of them are more dangerous than others and a small number – made notorious by mass media coverage of **MRSA** (methicillin resistant *Staphylococcus aureus*) – are quick to invade the body and are potentially lethal. The most vulnerable parts of a person's body to such infections are the urinary tract, the skin – particularly any open wounds – and the respiratory tract. Precautions in the complementary health clinic or centre need to take particular account of these.

A complementary practitioner working in a health service setting such as a health centre run by a primary care trust will need to understand what is meant by the following important terms:

■ **Cleaning** is the process of physically removing contaminants, which does not necessarily entail eliminating them.
■ **Disinfection** is the process of reducing contaminants, but will not eliminate microbial infection.
■ **Sterilization** is the process of eliminating viable microorganisms from an object.

■ **Clinical waste** is waste that has been in contact with bodily fluids such as blood. This must be incinerated.

Beyond this, infection prevention and control depend on everybody who uses the complementary health clinic or centre taking active responsibility for sustaining a safe, healthy environment. A GP notes that:

> All healthcare personnel, patients, family members and both formal and informal carers must be encouraged to practise effective hand washing. The single most important thing we can do to prevent infection and the spreading of illness to others is to clean our hands. Thorough hand antisepsis removes or destroys the transient microorganisms that can cause disease. Hands may be washed under running water using soap for 10–30 seconds or decontaminated with a water-less, alcohol-based gel or hand rub for 15–30 seconds, which is only recommended for hands that are not visibly soiled. (Stuart-Cole, 2007: 219)

Disposable gloves and aprons may be used, but are only useful alongside, not instead of, other measures such as hand washing. Practitioners and other staff should cover cuts and grazes with dressings, wear protective aprons and gloves and dispose of these after treating each patient or client. Items that come into contact with the patient should be cleaned thoroughly after each use. Crockery and cutlery should be washed thoroughly. It is important to be aware that protective clothes do not ensure complete protection to the wearer, as there is always the likelihood, for example, of tiny punctures in gloves, undetectable by the human eye, through which infection can enter. The clothes worn by practitioners when entering and leaving the clinic are also a particular site of potential infection. Ties are not usually worn by males when treating patients, and it is desirable for short sleeves to be worn so that hand washing can extend up the forearm.

Infection control policies will be in place in any health service setting where complementary practitioners are working and it is necessary to be aware of these. These will include regulations governing the cleaning, disinfection and decontamination of equipment, the handling of food and the disposal of waste.

Food hygiene is particularly important in complementary practice. Microorganisms do not respect human divisions between conventional and complementary settings. The preparation of food and drink on the premises, whether for staff or patients and clients, needs to be undertaken with a continuous awareness of the risks of food poisoning that may result from any lapses in hygiene.

Health and Safety Legislation and Regulations

Employers – for example those running a complementary healthcare centre – have responsibility for the health and safety of their employees and any other people, including clients, patients and suppliers. Legislation, Statutory Instruments (secondary regulations by government departments and agencies following on from legislation) and regulations govern these aspects. The main legislation is the Health and Safety at Work etc Act 1974 and Table 8.1 gives brief details of this and other major relevant regulations. The Health and Safety Executive (www.hse.gov. uk) and Environment Agency (www.environment-agency.gov.uk) are the main government bodies responsible for health and safety.

Table 8.1 Health and safety and related legislation and regulations

Employers' Liability (Compulsory Insurance) Act 1969	Deals with liability of employers for injury to persons or damage to property on the premises
The Health and Safety at Work etc Act 1974	Comprehensive legislation requiring employers to safeguard the health, safety and welfare of their employees
Management of Health and Safety at Work Regulations 1999/1992	Covers risk assessment and health and safety procedures for employers and self-employed people
Display Screen Equipment Regulations 1992	Deals with hazards in connection with use of display screens
Manual Handling Operations Regulations 1992	Covers the health and safety aspects of lifting and handling
Provision and Use of Work Equipment Regulations 1992	Governs the use of equipment so as to protect users from hazards
Control of Substances Hazardous to Health Regulations 1994	Deals with employers' duties to control and put in place proper systems for the use of hazardous substances and protection of employees
Reporting of Injuries, Diseases and Dangerous Occurrences Regulations 1995	Self-employed practitioners and employers are responsible for reporting and recording incidents and accidents

Risk Assessment and Management

Employers have a duty to protect their employees from hazards at work and to ensure their health and safety. This duty extends to clients and patients visiting the premises, people who accompany them and members of the general public. Employers are also responsible for providing clean toilets and washing facilities, meeting fire safety standards, making sure employees use IT equipment safely and reporting dangerous incidents and accidents at work. As part of these responsibilities, they must carry out risk assessments, put up necessary notices and ensure a basic level of comfort at work.

Risk Assessment

We live in an era when risks are perceived as dangerous not only to the individual service user or carer, but to the agency and the professional, in that people, their carers and surviving relatives may be inclined to sue the providing agency for any claimed shortcomings in services. There is an inbuilt tendency for organizations to develop defensive procedures designed to protect themselves against litigation, rather than to develop policies and practices that maximize the potential and actual benefit to clients or patients.

The procedure for assessing risks focuses on the steps to be taken, rather than critically appraising the options for risk taking. These steps are:

1. Identifying hazards
2. Deciding who could be harmed
3. Deciding how they could be harmed
4. Assessing risks
5. Taking appropriate steps to deal with risks
6. Recording findings of the risk assessment
7. Monitoring the risks and assessing them regularly
8. Taking appropriate action.

Risk Management

Risk management covers the actions entailed in dealing with risks. It is important to carry out a risk and hazard assessment in order to minimize any risks to people using the premises. Table 8.2 gives an example of a risk management chart displayed in a prominent position in a small kitchen and eating area at a family centre, where meals are being served to children, parents, staff and visitors.

Table 8.2 Hazard and risk action sheet

Identified hazard	Risk	Precautionary action required
Environment	High	Report/do not report any incident
Hygiene in family centre	Medium	Wash hands
Personal hygiene	High	Prepare food in designated areas Sterilize all utensils between use Wash hands
First aid	Medium	Check first aid boxes daily Ensure first aid trained staff on duty daily Ensure all staff know location of nearest pharmacy, doctors, health centre and hospital Ensure all staff know numbers of emergency medical services
Fire	Medium	Carry out fire drills weekly Alert all staff to location of extinguishers and fire blankets Ensure all staff know numbers of emergency services

Identified hazard	Risk	Precautionary action required
Electricity	Low	Building rewired this year Ensure all staff know procedures and first aid for electric shocks Ensure contact details of electricity suppliers and electricians displayed prominently in centre

Safety: Moving and Handling

One particular aspect of safety entails how patients and clients are moved and handled. This particularly applies in complementary approaches that involve 'hands-on' manipulation of the person's body, for example through massage, osteopathy and chiropractic. Employers have responsibilities for assessing risks in relation to moving and handling and to minimize those risks. This involves providing the means to make lifting manageable and providing sufficient training to enable lifting and handling to be carried out. At the same time, practitioners have a responsibility to take part in any training that is offered.

Chapter Summary

This chapter has dealt with those aspects of hygiene, health and safety that have a direct bearing on complementary practice. Practitioners have to be as vigilant as all other workers in the health and social care services, to ensure that the highest standards of hygiene and health and safety are maintained.

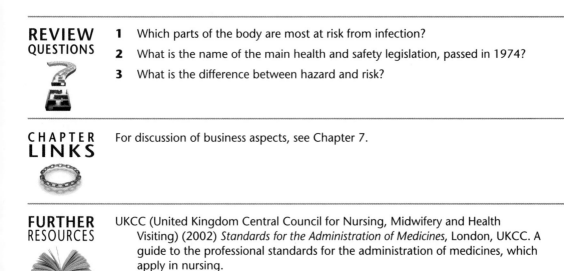

REVIEW QUESTIONS

1   Which parts of the body are most at risk from infection?

2   What is the name of the main health and safety legislation, passed in 1974?

3   What is the difference between hazard and risk?

CHAPTER LINKS

For discussion of business aspects, see Chapter 7.

FURTHER RESOURCES

UKCC (United Kingdom Central Council for Nursing, Midwifery and Health Visiting) (2002) *Standards for the Administration of Medicines*, London, UKCC. A guide to the professional standards for the administration of medicines, which apply in nursing.

Web link

www.hse.gov.uk and www.environment-agency.gov.uk – Government agencies responsible for health and safety and the working environment.

Part III

Resource file

Legislation Directly Affecting Complementary Practice

Freedom of Information and Data Protection Acts

More than 100,000 public bodies are covered under the Freedom of Information Act 2000, including government departments and local authorities, voluntary and private organizations.

People have the right to ask for information about themselves and their treatment. A person's right to this information continues to be governed by the Data Protection Act 1998. This can only be refused on certain, strictly governed grounds, such as if it is 'vexatious' or likely to cause serious physical or mental harm to the person asking.

A request is submitted in writing and the public authority normally has 20 working days to respond.

The Data Protection Act 1998 introduces strict guidelines on how data (information) on people is stored. This is particularly important for health and social care practitioners in agencies where there are many items of personal information about people who use services and carers, some of which refer to intimate aspects of people's health and lives. Under the Act, there are eight principles governing the proper handling of data. Data must be:

- lawfully and fairly processed
- processed for limited reasons
- relevant and adequate but not excessive for its purpose
- accurate
- kept only as long as is necessary
- processed so as not to undermine the person's rights
- secure
- only transferred to another country with adequate protection.

NB: There are tensions for complementary practitioners between satisfying the legal requirement for disclosure and meeting their professional responsibilities to protect the confidentiality of matters to do with the treatment of carers and service users, including patients. This is particularly the case when practitioners share information in the course of their daily work.

Note: This is adapted from a similar resource file in Adams, A. (2007) *Foundations of Health and Social Care*, Basingstoke, Palgrave Macmillan.

Further Resource

Wadham, J. (2001) *Blackstone's Guide to the Freedom of Information Act 2000*, Oxford, Blackstone Press.

Consent to Treatment

The client or patient should always be asked before assessment, treatment or any touching of the body to give informed consent. This consent should be in the form of signing and dating a written consent form, unless the person is physically unable to give this consent. Informed consent is consent that is given after the full implications of the assessment or treatment have been thoroughly explained to, and understood by, the client or patient.

A person has the freedom of choice over whether to accept or refuse treatment. In the absence of other evidence, judges tend to grant that a competent person has freedom of choice. It cannot be assumed that a person can only refuse when they have no mental health problems. In the case of *Ms B* v. *An NHS Hospital Trust* (2002), Ms B was completely paralysed and asked the High Court to rule that continuing her ventilation against her wishes was unlawful. The judge granted this declaration on the grounds that Ms B was competent to make all the decisions relevant to her circumstances (Brayne and Carr, 2008: 138–9).

The Mental Capacity Act 2005 (summarized from Brayne and Carr, 2008: 144–5) gives a comprehensive framework for assessing whether the person is competent to make decisions. It provides legal stages for taking action where the person does not have the capacity to make decisions. The following principles govern the decision as to whether the person has this capacity and the subsequent process (Brayne and Carr, 2008: 144):

1. A person must be assumed to have capacity unless it is established that he lacks capacity.
2. A person is not to be treated as unable to make a decision unless all practicable steps to help him to do so have been taken without success.
3. A person is not to be treated as unable to make a decision merely because he makes an unwise decision.
4. An act done, or decision made, under this Act for or on behalf of a person who lacks capacity must be done, or made, in his best interests.
5. Before the act is done, or the decision is made, regard must be had to whether the purpose for which it is needed can be as effectively achieved in a way that is less restrictive of the person's rights and freedom of action.

Reference

Brayne, H. and Carr, H. (2008) *Law for Social Workers*, 10th edn, Oxford, Oxford University Press.

Dealing with a Complaint

The regulatory frameworks covering complementary health and alternative medical services in the UK cover health, social work and social care services. The legal and administrative arrangements for these services are slightly different in the different countries of the UK – England, Northern Ireland, Scotland and Wales. The Care Quality Commission (CQC) is the regulator of the quality of health and social care services in England and Wales, created under the Health and Social Care Act 2008. In April 2009, the CQC replaced the now defunct Healthcare Commission, Mental Health Commission and Commission for Social Care Inspection.

The National Health Services (Complaints) Regulations 2009 deal with complaints by patients or clients. A complaint is an extremely important factor contributing to the quality of future services. Potentially, complaints can improve services in key aspects which hitherto have functioned less than adequately.

Most assessment and treatment of people are satisfactory to all parties – patients, clients and their carers and relatives. There are occasions, however, when the treatment does not go according to the wishes and expectations of those involved. Practitioners need to know what procedures people should follow if and when they wish to make a complaint.

People who receive assessments or treatments from complementary practitioners have the right to complain, either to the practitioner or the complementary service, or to the health service provider where the complementary practitioner works.

It is important that practitioners issue patients and clients with full information about their assessment and treatment and what these entail, so that they can give informed consent before the start (see above). Part of this information should include written and accessible information about how to complain – bearing in mind that it should be available in different languages and formats for people whose first language is not English and those who have sight or hearing impairments. If the practitioner works in an NHS setting, that setting is required to have a complaints procedure. In a complementary practice, there should also be a written and publicly displayed complaints procedure and patients or clients should be made aware of this.

People who wish to make a complaint may be inhibited about doing this, perhaps because they do not wish to offend the practitioner, or because they do not want to be excluded from the possibility of receiving further services.

The sequence of complaints should be made clear to patients and clients. At first, the patient or client may make the complaint to the practitioner delivering the service. In most cases, it is to be hoped that the complaint will be resolved at this point, so that the person making the complaint does not feel it necessary to pursue the complaint any further.

Subsequently, the patient or client has the right to complain to the body commissioning the service, if it is based in an NHS setting. This could be the primary care trust or other organization. This organization will normally have a complaints manager. The complaint may be made verbally or in writing. The complaint normally should be made within 12 months of the date of the event complained about, or as soon as it becomes apparent to the patient or client. The time limit can be extended where the patient or client had good cause not to complain within this period.

The complaint may be investigated and resolved at this point to the satisfaction of the patient or client. If it is not resolved, the patient or client has the right to refer the complaint to the parliamentary and health service ombudsman. This person is completely independent of the NHS and the government. The telephone number of this person is 0345 015 4033.

Help to patients and clients wishing to make complaints is available from the Patient Advice and Liaison Services (PALS) and the Independent Complaints Advocacy Service. PALS cannot progress the complaint for the person wishing to complain. NHS Direct and the Citizens Advice Bureau can also give advice on making a complaint.

Working with Patients and Clients

Part IV
Working with Patients and Clients

Introduction

Part IV looks at the basics of actually working with patients and clients. Chapter 9 explores the ethical issues and skills base of working with patients and clients. Chapter 10 discusses two aspects of communication: written forms of communication and 'live' communication. Written records are an essential feature of complementary practice and it is vital to understand how the different legal and related regulatory procedures affect these. 'Live' communication, in terms of interaction, is important, as it is necessary to be able to talk and interact with patients, clients and colleagues skilfully and effectively. Chapter 11 examines the idea of 'process' and sees how this is applied in stages of work, from the first meeting, including history taking, through to evaluation. Chapter 12 deals with the question of evidence-based practice, discussing different approaches to validating this and examining the main arguments about the credibility of practice. It also explores what becoming 'research aware' and 'research-minded' entails, from the viewpoint of the practitioner.

Ethical and Value Bases for Practice

ROBERT ADAMS

Learning
outcomes

By the end of this chapter, you should be able to:

- understand what is meant by values and ethics
- appreciate the nature of the general statement of values for healthcare
- grasp the relevance of some related examples of codes of practice
- discuss the content of an ethical code for complementary and alternative practice

Values and Ethics for Complementary Practice

Values are beliefs, standards and ideals about what is considered desirable or worthwhile. The values that concern us here are those ideas that form the foundations for a standard of practice. They are not necessarily ideas that translate straight into techniques for practice, that is, ideas about what to do and what works. They are more abstract and removed from practice. They are ideas linked with other fairly abstract notions of, for example, justice, right and wrong. They tackle questions of what it is right and just to do. As such, values are matters of opinion rather than fact.

Given that values are matters of opinion – often strongly held – it follows that there will be disagreements over these, between people who practise and between complementary practitioners and other professionals, including those with whom they have other serious disagreements. Just as some areas of complementary and alternative practice are disputed by some sectors of conventional health and medicine, so we would expect that the value base for practice is also the subject of dispute. Having acknowledged this, there are some values that underlie all professional practice. Values underlie the codes of ethics that many professions set out for their practitioners to follow. A **code of ethics** is the set of rules and standards of conduct that professionals should follow. These ethical codes tend to embody principles, which are applied directly in practice.

Codes of Practice in Traditional Medicine: a Long History

Most of the people in the world only know traditional medicine (TM). These people, and the health remedies and systems on which they rely, remain largely excluded from the realm of conventional medicine. Yet traditional practices predate conventional modern health services and, in keeping with this, the written history of statements about ethical practice dates back at least to the ninth century and Arab traditional medicine. A book on medical ethics was written by Ali al-Rahawi (854–931) entitled *Adabal-Tabib*, which translates as *Ethics of the Physician*. In summary, this took the view that the responsibilities of the physician are extremely grave, as the person who safeguards the body and soul, or spirit, of the person. This notion of the physician as responsible not just for alleviating symptoms but having a holistic responsibility for the person is common in TM.

Different ethical standards apply across a variety of professional areas and they also apply in different ways in different geographical locations. The huge diversity of complementary and alternative approaches makes it difficult to generate one statement of ethical standards. However, it is important that clients and patients can have confidence that they will receive a common standard of treatment across the entire range of practice and that this will be compatible with other branches of the health and social care services.

Examples of Relevant Codes of Ethics for Practice

In society as a whole, there are codes of ethics governing personal as well as professional conduct. Many religious, social and community organizations have statements that set out rules and procedures governing the expected behaviour of their members. So just as a code of ethics is a set of rules for expected personal conduct, a professional code of ethics also governs professional practice. It consists of a set of principles that links morality with publicly recognized standards of acceptable professional conduct. Ethical standards are at the core of professional practice and are linked with a professional's personal as well as professional values. Ethical standards, therefore, reflect the basic values of the particular profession. We need to arrive at a general statement of values for complementary therapies and alternative medicine, which can be linked with their ethical principles and standards for practice. We can see from this statement that ethical practice refers to standards of practice that reflect professional values and codes of conduct.

In order to be more specific about ethical principles and standards, we need a general mission statement for complementary approaches, with which we can link a statement of core values. A commonly agreed statement of the values of all healthcare professionals, as upheld by their regulatory bodies, has been published (Chief Executives' Group, 2007), on the basis that, regardless of the nature of their practice, they should be able to explain to others the ways in which they share the duty to protect and promote the interests and needs of patients and clients. These values are:

- Openness with patients and clients and respecting their dignity
- Respecting the right of patients and clients to be involved in decisions about treatment
- Honesty and trustworthiness
- Providing good standards of practice
- Acting quickly to safeguard against harm
- Cooperating with colleagues within the profession and with other professionals.

This list of value statements has a lot in common with the some of the statements of codes and principles of practice to which we now turn. Drawing on the mission statements and codes of ethical practice of different professional groups in health-care, social care and social work would probably produce a list of ethical standards and principles that would meet the requirements of the field of complementary therapies and alternative medicine. Alternatively, this chapter puts several codes of practice alongside each other (Table 9.1), such as the code published in 2007 by the Nursing and Midwifery Council (NMC) and implemented in 2008, the code of ethics and professional standards of the College of Occupational Therapists (COT, 2005b) and the code of practice of the General Osteopathic Council (GOsC, 2005).

The primary purpose of complementary therapies and alternative medicine is to enhance people's health and wellbeing and quality of life. The three core areas of nursing and midwifery, as reflected in the code of practice, can be summarized as:

- The priority concern with caring for people
- Promoting the health of individual patients, clients, their families and the community
- Demonstrating integrity of practice consistent with professional standards.

The code of ethics of occupational therapists can be summarized around four core areas:

- Respecting and responding to the needs of clients
- Providing adequately recorded services to clients
- Maintaining the basis for professional standards of integrity
- Sustaining and developing professional practice.

The code of practice for osteopaths emphasizes four core areas:

- The priority of caring for patients with integrity, honesty and respect
- Ensuring that the rights of patients are preserved at all times
- Justifying public trust and confidence in professional practice
- Respecting, maintaining and safeguarding information about patients.

Table 9.1 Comparing conventional and complementary codes of practice

Nursing and midwifery	Occupational therapy	Osteopathy
Making caring a priority, treating people as individuals, respecting dignity	**Client autonomy and welfare**	**Making care of patients a priority**
Treating as individuals	Respecting client autonomy	Acting honestly, being trustworthy
Respecting confidentiality	Meeting duty of care	Acting politely and considerately
Collaborating with patients	Maintaining confidentiality	Respecting dignity and privacy
Ensuring consent	Protecting client	Providing appropriate care and treatment
Maintaining professional boundaries		Not abusing one's professional position
	Services to clients	**Respecting rights of people to be involved fully in decisions about their care**
Working with others, protecting and promoting health of people, families, carers, wider community	Dealing with referrals	Guaranteeing patients' rights, e.g. to stop treatment or examination at any time, or bring a chaperone
Sharing information	Providing adequate services	Obtaining consent before examining or proceeding
Team working	Keeping proper records	Listening to, and respecting, patients' views
Delegating	**Personal/professional integrity**	Giving patients full information and ensuring they understand
Managing risk	Maintaining integrity	
Basing care on best evidence	Sustaining professional manner	**Justifying public trust and confidence**
Updating skills	Ensuring fitness to practise	Working within limits of your competence
Keeping clear, accurate records	Balancing personal profit and professional service	Not allowing your personal views and values to prejudice care of patients
	Advertising professionally	Developing your knowledge and skills
Being open, honest, acting with integrity, upholding the profession	Giving information and representing people	Responding promptly to complaints and criticisms
Acting with integrity	**Professional competence and standards**	Acting quickly to protect patients from your other colleague being not fit to practise
Tackling problems	Maintaining professional competence	Respecting other professionals' skills and collaborating with them
Acting impartially	Dealing with delegation	Dealing promptly with superseding health professionals
Upholding the profession	Committing to lifelong learning	
	Providing for student education	**Respecting, maintaining and protecting patient information**
	Sustaining research and service development	Taking full, accurate case histories
		Keeping full, accurate records
		Keeping patient information confidential
		Keeping patient records secure

Source: COT, 2005; GOsC, 2005; NMC, 2007. Reproduced with permission

A Code of Ethical Complementary and Alternative Practice

The four main areas identified for osteopaths provide a good basis for a general code of ethical practice for the entire field of complementary therapies and alternative medicine.

Part IV

Activity

Use what you have read above to help you to generate your own list of no more than six general headings, as the basis for a professional code of practice for complementary and alternative practitioners.

The discussion of ethical aspects below draws on the diversity of this field and also incorporates relevant aspects of the statements from healthcare and other related professions. It needs refining in any particular area, of course, although key themes and ideas to be shared are highlighted below in italic.

Complementary approaches are rooted in many different philosophies and knowledge bases, so they are well placed to *value the diversity* and *enhance the health, wellbeing and quality of life of patients, clients, their families and the community*. In this spirit, complementary and alternative practice should be *inclusive* and *nondiscriminatory*.

Practising with Integrity and Respect for People

The fundamental principle is that all *work with* and *care for patients and clients, their families, carers and the community* should be the priority for practitioners. Also, *respecting the unique worth of each person* is a basic human value, which the professional takes to a further level – ensuring that whatever issues and problems the client or patient discloses, the practitioner gives them due worth. This respect is a goal that may be in tension with meeting the requirements of human rights, anti-discrimination and equality-based legislation, since one person's interests, for example in a family, may conflict with those of another.

Integrity refers to practising in a trustworthy way. It is vital that clients and patients can give the same trust to practitioners as to conventional medical practitioners. The practitioner should act with *honesty* and *trustworthiness* at all times. Part of the respect for the client or patient should consist of *politeness* towards, and *consideration* for, their views and feelings.

The provision of appropriate care and treatment takes the form of ensuring that patients and clients are treated with *dignity* and that their *privacy* is protected. Aspects of examination and treatment can be invasive and it is easy to forget that some people will be extremely sensitive to examinations of their bodies. Together, these aspects amount to the practitioner *not taking advantage of their professional position* and *not exploiting the relative lack of power of the client or patient* and the degree of trust they invest in the practitioner.

Upholding the Rights of Patients and Clients

The principle of preserving the rights of patients and clients is rooted in the United Nations' Universal Declaration of Human Rights (UN, 1948), similar European conventions (European Convention on the Protection of Human Rights and Fundamental Freedoms 1950) and the Human Rights Act 1998 in the UK. These generate the linked principle that at all times *patients and clients should participate fully in decisions* about the work done with them. It should never be imposed on them without their *informed consent*. The notion of informed consent is crucial in the human rights field. **Informed consent** means that the practitioner has to explain the consequences of a particular decision, treatment or intervention, so that the person understands the nature of the consequences – possible, probable or certain – of anything that is or is not done.

It follows from this that *patients and clients should have the right to interrupt or permanently stop any examination, treatment or other work* with them at any time.

Practitioners should ensure that patients and clients have the right to bring a chaperone with them to any appointment. Practitioners may find it preferable to initiate this by suggesting it to them.

Practitioners should listen carefully to the views of patients and clients at all times. They may disagree with patients or clients, but they should always respect their views, making sure they have access to the fullest information and understand as much as possible of what is happening. There should be strict adherence to the principle that *practitioners should not allow personal views to prejudice the services they provide to patients and clients*.

Justifying the Trust of Patients, Clients, Families, Carers and the Community in Practitioners' Expertise

Practitioners should act in ways that build up the confidence and trust of patients and clients in their practice, as well as other people – the family, carers and the wider community. This requires the practitioner to clarify the interface between what they feel confident in practising and what they do not feel confident to practise. This is about the practitioner remaining self-aware and self-critical throughout practice. There is no shame in the practitioner admitting to patients or clients that there are limitations to personal expertise. This is no different to the general medical practitioner referring the patient to a consultant in a particular medical specialism. The most important aspect of this is for the practitioner to develop a clear notion of the boundary between the territory of personal expertise and areas beyond that. It is necessary for the practitioner to convey to patients and clients the area of *fitness to practise*. This notion of fitness to practise extends further. Each practitioner will be aware of their own fitness to practise and the limits of this expertise.

Practitioners should welcome the potential contribution that working with other professionals, in both complementary and conventional practice, offers to patients and clients, their families, carers and the wider community. They should *collaborate with other professionals and respect other professionals' expertise*, that is, their understanding, knowledge and skills.

Expertise is something that develops throughout one's career. The practitioner demonstrates expertise in every thought and action. Expertise is the term used to refer to this. The expression **showing expertise** refers to applying appropriate knowledge, understanding and skills in practice and taking responsibility for continuing professional development. Thoughts that feed into actions are the professional expression of the practitioner's capacity to engage in continual critical reflection on practice. Practice is the outward expression of this process of inner reflection. **Practice** reflects the integrative process of gathering knowledge and understanding and incorporating this into actions, upon which the practitioner continually reflects. It is part of the professionalism of the practitioner to regard professional development – the continued development of knowledge and skills – as a continuing responsibility and not as something that stops at the point of qualification.

Practitioners should *recognize and deal promptly with any complaints or criticisms* from patients, clients, families, carers or members of the wider community. Sometimes it will be necessary to deal with such matters that affect the practitioner's own practice and on occasions it may be necessary to respond to circumstances where a colleague or other professional is not fit to practise. The practitioner should deal with such circumstances promptly and professionally.

The situation of many areas of complementary approaches to practice is vulnerable, because they are not subject to statutory (legal) regulation. Practitioners not subject to legal regulation still have an equivalent responsibility to maintain their professional and personal development. All practitioners face the twin challenges of initial qualification followed by continuing professional development. Many complementary practitioners work in organizational and physical isolation from each other.

Respecting, Maintaining and Safeguarding Information about Patients

Practitioners are responsible for carrying out *adequate assessments* of patients' and clients' circumstances and needs. This entails taking *comprehensive case histories* and paying attention to gathering and checking details to ensure that these are full and accurate. This responsibility for accuracy and completeness extends to the absolute necessity of maintaining *full and accurate records*.

The fact that practitioners are expected to keep personal details of patients and clients makes essential the *security of personal records*. There is an absolute expectation that procedures will comply with data protection legislation and procedures (see Chapter 10). It is important that practitioners safeguard the confidentiality of clients and patients. *Confidentiality* is a principle closely related to respecting and treating each person so as to meet their unique expectations and needs. However, this is in tension with the principle of *professionals sharing information* between them and this tension needs to be managed in any complementary practice, in much the same way that it needs managing more generally in healthcare. Apart from exceptional circumstances, information should only be shared with the consent of the patient or client.

Chapter Summary

This chapter has explored the meanings of the key concepts of values and ethics and discussed how they relate to practice. In the process, it has outlined a number of key ethical principles that form the basis for ethical practice. A general ethical code that applies across the entire field of complementary therapies and alternative medicine has been devised, drawing on a number of statements of ethical standards in key areas of conventional and complementary practice.

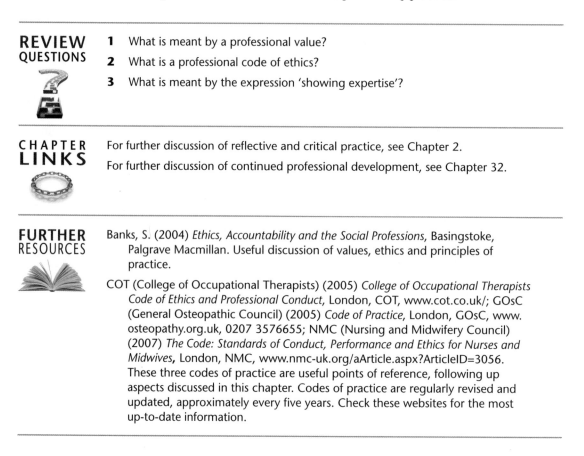

REVIEW QUESTIONS

1   What is meant by a professional value?

2   What is a professional code of ethics?

3   What is meant by the expression 'showing expertise'?

CHAPTER LINKS

For further discussion of reflective and critical practice, see Chapter 2.

For further discussion of continued professional development, see Chapter 32.

FURTHER RESOURCES

Banks, S. (2004) *Ethics, Accountability and the Social Professions*, Basingstoke, Palgrave Macmillan. Useful discussion of values, ethics and principles of practice.

COT (College of Occupational Therapists) (2005) *College of Occupational Therapists Code of Ethics and Professional Conduct*, London, COT, www.cot.co.uk/; GOsC (General Osteopathic Council) (2005) *Code of Practice*, London, GOsC, www.osteopathy.org.uk, 0207 3576655; NMC (Nursing and Midwifery Council) (2007) *The Code: Standards of Conduct, Performance and Ethics for Nurses and Midwives*, London, NMC, www.nmc-uk.org/aArticle.aspx?ArticleID=3056. These three codes of practice are useful points of reference, following up aspects discussed in this chapter. Codes of practice are regularly revised and updated, approximately every five years. Check these websites for the most up-to-date information.

Communicating with People and Record Keeping

ROBERT ADAMS

By the end of this chapter, you should be able to:

- define different forms of written and interpersonal communication
- understand the protocols governing recording as a means of communication
- draw on research that confirms the importance of talk to communication
- specify other ingredients of good communication

What is Communication?

Communication is the term used to refer to written and spoken messages between people. In this chapter, I deal mainly with interpersonal interactions between people involving communication, so there is just a brief section on written forms of communication.

Written Communication

Written communications are important, of course, and include not only letters but the records kept by practitioners as well. Through records, agencies and professionals can monitor people's health and note patterns – particularly unusual patterns – of ill health or conditions, thereby enabling action to be taken, often preventively. In a group practice, records also allow different practitioners to work together and enable assessments, planning, intervention and evaluation of practice to be carried out.

In legal terms, the record kept of a client or patient is governed by a legislative framework that covers the responsibilities of individual practitioners, organizations, groups and agencies. The laws governing record keeping include:

- Common Law Duty of Confidence (where an individual has not given consent for the purpose of use of the information provided by that individual)
- European Convention for Protection of Human Rights and Fundamental Freedoms 1950
- Data Protection Act 1998
- Crime and Disorder Act 1998
- Human Rights Act 1998
- Caldicott Standards
- Various laws in healthcare throughout the four countries of the UK.

The Caldicott Standards are the outcome of a review set up in response to concerns about the risks to patient confidentiality of information in the NHS in England and Wales (Caldicott, 1997), and were adopted across the health and social services. Caldicott set out transparent principles and procedures governing good practice (including safe storage and transfer of confidential information) and the appointment of a senior person in each health and social services organization – known as the Caldicott guardian – to protect the confidentiality of patient information.

Recording in Practice

Practitioners and agencies have a duty in common law to protect the confidentiality of personal information that is held about an individual. Records are legal documents that can be used in legal proceedings and read by patients and clients. It is important, therefore, to ensure that the information kept about people helps them rather than potentially harming them. The information needs to be:

- factually accurate and not based on rumour or false information
- used responsibly in order not to violate people's confidentiality.

The Data Protection Act 1998 governs the sharing of information between professionals and between agencies. Basically, professionals need to ensure that the information gathered and stored about patients and clients is sufficient for its purpose and not excessive beyond this, and is not kept beyond the time when it is useful in the interests of patients and clients.

We have discussed what makes for good recording of our communications. Now we need to be able to identify what makes for good communication, in the sense of good interaction with people. So we shift our focus, from keeping records to the interactions with the people with whom we work – whether colleagues, patients, clients, carers, relatives or others. As well as records, our interactions with people lie at the heart of our practice.

Activity

1. Spend a few minutes trying to think of somebody you know who you regard as a good communicator.
2. Consider what it is about this person that enables you to reach this judgement.

3. Jot down brief notes on the ingredients of this person's good communications. For example, is it to do with things they say, do, or is it to do with their skills?

Face-to-face Communication

'Face-to-face communication' refers to the attitudes, intentions, emotions and meanings exchanged when people interact, using words, gestures, body language (the way we sit, our facial expressions and gestures) and the settings in which communication takes place. Work with people entails us learning how to communicate effectively and this necessarily is complicated by the many factors feeding into the situation:

- our previous experiences
- the other person's previous experiences
- how sensitive and aware we are to the mood of the other person
- what our own mood is
- our knowledge of human interaction
- our level of communication skills.

What Makes Good Communication?

Roter and Hall (2006: 4), two researchers who have examined how communication between doctors and patients can be improved, argue that two main ingredients contribute to the quality of this communication:

1. the talk that takes place between them
2. the expert knowledge of the professional.

Clearly, expert knowledge plays a crucial part in this and other parts of this book deal with this. This chapter examines talk, and the surrounding conditions in which it takes place. This leads us to go beyond and behind talk, as it were, because the setting in which talk happens and the unspoken ways in which people communicate alongside or instead of talk are also extremely important.

We can learn a good deal from the accumulated wisdom of researchers and professionals about how to communicate well with people. We can also learn from the mistakes of others. No healthcare profession has been criticized as severely as doctors and the point has often been made that people in power may use the relatively scarce and poorly understood commodity of their professional knowledge to reinforce their power, rather than to empower other people and ensure that they understand their situation and make informed decisions. Before seeing what we can learn from research into doctors' communication with their patients, I want to emphasize the importance of language as a tool in the exercise of power.

Language and Communication

Language is not only a neutral vehicle used to convey meanings, but can also be a tool wielded in the interests of acquiring and maintaining power. It can be used to exclude and oppress people, or to prevent them gaining access to information.

People communicate using language and through other means such as body language, to which the label 'nonverbal communication' is usually applied. Language is far more than simply the means by which people pass messages between each other. It can be used in a simple way, but it can be used, for example, to reinforce other means of control and oppression. In short, language can be abused, that is, used as a means of abusing people. Language can be used in the power battles between people. The expression 'information is power' arises from observing how people retain and measure out communications in situations where they want to exercise power. It is a short distance from this to the statement that 'language is power'.

Doctors Talking with Patients

Doctors and other health professionals can wield language as a means of maintaining their professional power. At its crudest, medical terminology may be used by professionals as a means of baffling laypeople and thereby excluding them from interactions. Patients may be told, in effect: 'This is for your own good. If I tried to explain how it works, you wouldn't understand. So take it and don't ask questions.'

The way is open for complementary and alternative practitioners to make their mark by maintaining high-quality, open communication with their clients/patients. Let us see what we can learn from research into how doctors communicate with their patients.

Talk is important

We tend to take the talk between health professionals and patients for granted as quite routine. 'Good morning, how are you feeling?' 'Well enough, thank you.' What is important is what remains unsaid, the hesitations, the eye contact or lack of it. The skill of the practitioner lies in creating space for the patient to say what lies behind this routine exchange. 'Well enough' may actually be spoken in a doubtful tone. If the practitioner asks a carefully phrased follow-up question, the patient may reveal a further layer of doubts, worries or problems. Have a look at the following:

'Good morning, how are you feeling?'

'Well enough, thank you.'

'Do sit down. Are you feeling better than last time?'

This is an invitation to the patient but it is focused. It offers the patient an opportunity to give further information, but asks the question in such a way that the onus is on the patient to self-evaluate. The focus is on whether this practitioner–patient relationship is productive and therefore leading to the patient feeling better.

This keeps the interchange professional. It is not an open invitation to general conversation. It says to the patient that the practitioner is interested, but within the defined boundaries of their previous appointments.

The patient or client is the expert

There is another vital ingredient in good communications and this is to appreciate that what the patient or client says is the first point of reference for the practitioner in working out how to help. There is a phrase in social care that refers to the client as an 'expert through experience'. This is the person's unique position in the practitioner–patient/client relationship. It is necessary for the practitioner to rely on professional expertise and bring this to bear on the situation, but not so as to ignore or contradict the experience of the client/patient. This does not mean that the practitioner has to follow the person's perception even when it appears patently mistaken, but it has to be taken properly into account when assessing, planning and implementing the plan.

Making the link between the person's presenting situation or problem and their general condition

There is a need for the practitioner to develop a holistic view of a person's situation. The way this is done varies according to the nature of the approach. In acupuncture, for example, the first proper encounter between the practitioner and the patient takes the form of a quite lengthy history taking, where the practitioner goes through a much wider set of enquiries than might be suggested by a simple query from a patient, such as 'Can you take away the pain in my shoulder?'

This question may lead any practitioner to enquire as to what has contributed to this pain. Has the person fallen on the shoulder recently? Does the person have to carry the daily shopping a long distance in a heavy bag? One writer I knew developed a shoulder strain through sitting awkwardly at a desk for many hours a day. In a quite different set of circumstances, a headache may have many physical causes, some of which are minor but others may be serious, especially if the headache is major or prolonged and linked with other symptoms such as dizziness, nausea or sight disturbances. On the other hand, a person who, literally, complains to the practitioner about a headache on the lines of 'My life is a headache' is indicating that there may be other personal, family or social factors that amount to a headache. The headache may be a metaphor for other kinds of problems. (A metaphor is a figure of speech – a way of describing something that takes a quality from a quite different field and applies it to the situation. For example, 'my brother is a donkey' is not literally true, but invites the listener to take one or two (assumed) qualities from the donkey and apply them to my brother. In this case, it is slightly vague, but possibly I mean the donkey is stupid and/or stubborn and so is my brother.)

Writing from within the medical situation, Roter and Hall (2006: 12) discuss the need to establish the connection between the person's presenting illness and their mental state.

*Ensuring the means of communication adequately conveys the emotions
of the patient or client*

It is important to recognize that as part of the holistic approach to working with a person, the practitioner takes all aspects of the person's perceptions, experiences and situation into account. As part of all this, it is necessary to grasp not only what the person is thinking, but what they are feeling as well.

Roter and Hall (2006: 15) note that some medical practitioners may have a rather neutral and distant style of communication, but recognize that, in spite of this, the patient's emotions may still get through to them. In this connection, the practitioner needs to be aware that while words are the most accurate way of conveying what we are thinking, we often communicate our feelings through nonverbal means. Thus, our feelings may be conveyed by our physical expression, our sighs as we speak, the pitch and tone of our voice, the way we hesitate or our voice cracks when talk about sensitive matters. Our physical appearance gives information about how we are feeling, through our gait (the way we walk briskly or shuffle, stride straight up or stoop), our sitting position, either tense and defensive with arms folded and head down, or with legs spread out and arms down at our sides in an open and relaxed manner. Our eyes and facial expressions convey a good deal. Do we smile and look straight at the person we are addressing? Do we engage their eyes throughout? At crucial points in the encounter, do we look away, out of the window, up at the ceiling, or down at the floor? Is our voice strong and confident, hesitant or thoughtful and measured? These are all questions not just for the patient or client but for the practitioner. It takes more than one person to communicate and the interaction between the practitioner and the person shapes the encounter. If the practitioner begins the session with every indication of being tired, stressed and too busy, this affects the patient or client, may inhibit responses and severely restrict the value of the session to both parties.

The Ingredients of Good Communication

The social setting makes a crucial contribution to the quality of communication. Situations can be structured so as to make the patient or client feel disempowered, or to encourage the person to relax and talk about personal aspects. Within the setting, good communication is more than a matter of technique. It depends on two components:

1. The practitioner's skills in engaging with patients/clients. By engagement we mean how effectively the practitioner makes a professional relationship with the person.
2. The quality of the interaction between practitioner and other people.

'Interaction' refers to all the physical and verbal signals that people exchange, which either sustain and reinforce or undermine and ultimately break their relationship. Ingredients in this process include speech, tone of voice, choice of formal or colloquial language, body language, gestures, facial expression, and how the practitioner dresses and behaves.

'Body language' is the term used by professionals who work with people. Argyle (1988) has studied interaction and observes how body language can include how people make eye contact, which in turn is affected by factors such as social class and culture. In some groups, it is accepted that avoiding eye contact when replying indicates a less than honest reply. In other groups, a person may find direct eye contact intimidating and may prefer to interact without making eye contact, especially with a stranger who is a professional. In some cultures, it is forbidden for some people to make eye contact with strangers.

Talk in History Taking

One thing that research tells us is the crucial importance of storytelling in conventional and complementary or alternative practice. It is important for complementary practitioners to appreciate that one sign of successful graduation to the position of a legitimate professional in the eyes of the patient or client is the trust they put in the ability of the practitioner to know their ills and how to tackle them and improve health and wellbeing. It may be an unrealistic expectation, but it is often there. Roter and Hall (2006: 6–7) put it thus: 'People expect the doctor to know them in a fundamental and intimate way, and doctors need to know their patients in order to truly care and cure.'

In order to match this high expectation, communication needs to support two complementary activities:

1. The desire of the patient to tell the story of the illness or condition
2. The need of the practitioner to gather sufficient information to enable a full and accurate assessment and plan to be made.

Interviewing

The professional social work literature provides much knowledge and understanding that contributes to good communication. Thompson (2003: 120), for example, describes an interview as any formal or semi-formal discussion between a practitioner and a person using services. He identifies four main stages in the interview: planning, engaging, responding and ending.

Planning involves establishing the setting, ensuring that the patient/client is feeling relaxed, and creating a non-stigmatizing atmosphere that encourages the person to be open. *Engaging* entails listening and responding appropriately. The practitioner must be *responding* appropriately all the time. The skills of sensitivity, warmth, empathy (showing an understanding as a professional, rather than expressing sympathy as a friend) and active listening (checking out the meaning of what is said and seeking clarification where appropriate rather than just listening) are required, as well as a nonjudgemental attitude (not expressing views that imply approval or disapproval, but accepting and trying to understand what is being said). The professional is also expected to take responsibility for stating the purpose of the session, keeping it on track and *ending* it at the right point.

Chapter Summary

This chapter has been concerned with communication, which is at the heart of complementary practice with clients or patients. Good communication is an essential component of good practice and is as important as the expert knowledge of the practitioner. Communication is multifaceted and it is important to develop skills in communicating that take account of what research evidence tells us about the most effective ways to communicate.

REVIEW QUESTIONS

1   What is the main responsibility of the Caldicott guardian?

2   What is the main purpose of the Data Protection Act and what date was it passed?

3   According to Thompson, what are the four main stages of the interview and what does each consist of?

CHAPTER LINKS

For further discussion of the process of working with people, see Chapter 11.

FURTHER RESOURCES

Davies, H. and Fallowfield, L. (1991) *Counselling and Communication in Healthcare*, Chichester, J. Wiley & Son. Practical advice on the use of communication skills in work with people.

Roter, D.L. and Hall, J.A. (2006) *Doctors Talking with Patients/Patients Talking with Doctors*, 2nd edn, London, Praeger. Thoughtful and thought-provoking text, with many messages about communicating in practice, based on research into the interaction between doctors and patients.

Thompson, N. (2003) *Communication and Language: A Handbook of Theory and Practice*, Basingstoke, Palgrave Macmillan. Useful handbook for practice.

Process of Working with Clients and Patients

ROBERT ADAMS

Learning outcomes

By the end of this chapter, you should be able to:

■ grasp how critically reflective practice connects with the process of working with people

■ understand different approaches to the process of working with people

■ appreciate the main stages of the work

■ discuss the key aspects of each stage

It is not accidental that this chapter is placed midway in the book, in the part that deals with the ideas that contribute to our understanding of how we work with people. We start by making some links between what goes on as we develop the habit of critically reflective practice and the process of our work with patients and clients.

Critically Reflective Practice Connects with the Process of Working with People

It is important to grasp the fact that as we develop as a critically reflective practitioner, we shall develop certain skills. We saw in Chapter 2 that reflective practice embodies three main aspects of being critical: self-awareness, which is more of a quality, and critical analysis and evaluation, which are activities or actions. Let us examine these in turn, using an example from practice as the starting point.

Reena has seen her patient Min for several weeks. She feels the need to reflect on the point reached before booking further appointments with Min. She casts around for a framework of ideas and procedures to help her to carry out this process systematically and rigorously. She reads about the related notions of self-awareness, critical analysis and evaluation and how they relate to each other and contribute to critically reflective practice.

Let us examine these notions, to help us understand how they may help her:

- **Self-awareness** is the knowledge and understanding we have of our own values, beliefs and actions. It goes without saying that the critically reflective practitioner is self-aware. Self-awareness is not just an essential component of being critically reflective, it is crucial to interaction with other people. So, it is a foundation of complementary practice with patients and clients.
- **Critical analysis** refers to the set of describing and analytic skills upon which we draw when we engage in the process of reflecting on practice in the light of our existing knowledge and understanding and posing questions about how well we have done and whether we could do differently and better next time.
- **Evaluation of practice** is the term used to refer to how we judge our practice and the practice of others. Self-evaluation is closely related to self-awareness and self-criticality, since evaluation is an activity drawing on critical skills.

These three components feed into the development of critically reflective practice and should be taken as continually present in the following discussion. It is crucial for this not to be read simply as a technical description of the sequence that practitioners go through in their practice. Practice is not just about the application of techniques, or following prescriptions or procedures. Practice engages our values, knowledge, understanding and creativity, and is crucial to complementary practice. Complementary practitioners rely on this creativity in order to understand their patients and clients and endeavour to meet their needs. Let us now go briefly through the sequence of stages this entails. We use the word 'process' to refer to this, so first we need to understand what is meant by this.

Understanding Different Approaches to the Process

'Process' refers to the different stages of work with people. Process is a term with different meanings, which provide a variety of viewpoints of the sequence of practitioners' work with people. Process means different things in different settings. We often use the word in everyday speech. Table 11.1 lists some of these meanings.

Table 11.1 Different meanings of process

Type of meaning	Key aspects
Time passing	Over a period of time
Sequence of events	In a work process
Change	Changes that alter the state or situation of the person
Education	Awareness raising or knowledge development
Investigation	A question is posed and research is carried out to try to tackle and, if possible, answer it
Problem solving	A problem is identified and tackled
Therapy or remedial treatment	Use of treatment or therapeutic technique
Integrative	Bringing together different kinds of understanding and skills in practice

What the Process of Working with Patients and Clients Entails

In the conventional medicine setting, practitioners are exploring the illness or condition of the patient to try to find out what is wrong, intervene and, hopefully, rectify it. In the complementary therapy and alternative medicine setting, a variety of possible processes may be envisaged. The focus, as with conventional medicine, may be on diagnosing an illness or condition and effecting a cure. Or it may be on improving health and wellbeing in a person who is not suffering from a particular illness or condition. Again (as in the case of the Alexander technique), the process may be mainly educational. A clue to the focus and the way those taking part in administering and receiving the treatment lies in the differing use of the terms to refer to the person receiving it, and the model used and the nature of the key process regarded as taking place, as Table 11.2 shows.

Table 11.2 Models of complementary approaches

Model	Key process	Person receiving
Pathological	Treating illness	Patient
Quality of life	Enhancing wellbeing	Client

The major approaches to traditional medicine, traditional Chinese medicine (TCM) and Ayurvedic or traditional Indian medicine (TIM), have two aspects:

1. they can be used as whole systems approaches
2. their components can be used as single aspects of complementary and alternative medicine, such as massage, special diets and herbal remedies.

In their holistic aims, both TCM and TIM have the purpose of balancing mind, body and spirit. As we shall see in Chapter 13, this notion of restoring harmony

Part IV

and balance is shared by more than one traditional perspective on health and wellbeing and its restoration. For example, both TCM and TIM are based on similar beliefs about how the different elements of the body ideally exist in harmony. The role of the practitioner is to identify how they may be out of balance and restore them to harmony. Figure 11.1 shows how this is visualized in TIM.

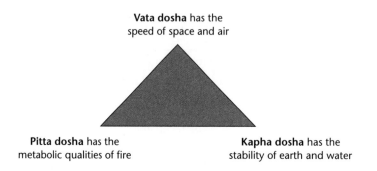

Vata dosha has the
speed of space and air

Pitta dosha has the
metabolic qualities of fire

Kapha dosha has the
stability of earth and water

Figure 11.1 Balance between the doshas in traditional Indian medicine

An excess of one of the doshas is called a 'vriddhi' and a deficit is a 'kshaya'. Both are signs of illness or another condition. The process of the practice is devoted to the physician restoring any imbalance that occurs between the doshas (see Chapter 13).

Main Stages of Practice

This sounds very different to conventional medical practice, but in fact underlying this practice is a model commonly used in healthcare. In this, conventional and complementary/alternative practitioners begin by taking a history to try to assess the situation of the patient or client. They reach a view – a diagnosis – and arrive at a treatment plan to tackle the situation. They intervene and in future modify the plan where necessary. Afterwards, they carry out an evaluation in which they review progress.

Activity

Reflect for a few minutes on this summary and try to clarify, in one or two headline words for each, the main stages of the process of the work.

Conventional practitioners can describe this general process thus: assessing, planning, implementing and evaluating. Now we shall go into a little more detail to clarify what each stage entails.

Gathering Information/Taking a History

The process of working with patients/clients is conventionally rooted in a successful first meeting and history taking. This contributes to assessment/diagnosis.

Planning

In complementary practice, planning tends to be carried out with the patient or client. Together they negotiate on the basis of judgements, wishes and expectations, that is, what each would like to happen and what each expects to happen.

Implementation

This involves the carrying out of the programme of treatment that has been negotiated and agreed.

Review/Evaluation

It is not always the case, but often circumstances make a review necessary after a period of time has elapsed. Six weeks or several months may pass and the practitioner has built into the process a review session. It is appropriate to do this when several treatments have been carried out, to enable the practitioner and the client/patient to give their views about any outcomes, desirable or otherwise.

In the light of the initial review, the practitioner and client/patient may decide that more work is needed. They may return to the assessment and add further needs, which generate fresh tasks to be carried out. Here are three additional headings suggested by this:

- More refining of assessment
- More intervention
- Further review after a further three months.

In theory, this could go on indefinitely, as new needs constantly may be identified during the further work. The important findings from this are, first, that the list of stages may be much longer and more detailed than we anticipated, and second, a significant chunk of the sequence is circular rather than linear, that is, we can envisage that it may loop back after the review stage to reassessment and through further work.

Evaluation takes place at the conclusion of the treatment. I know of one case where after the initial intensive, weekly acupuncture treatment, the frequency of treatment for an older person with arthritic hands dropped to once a fortnight and then to once a month. After a year, the practitioner talked with the patient, who wanted to continue. Years later, the patient attends every six months, for a 'maintenance' treatment, which she still finds very rewarding. (This is quite common in acupuncture and other complementary therapies.)

Reminder: client/patient involvement

It is vital to keep the client/patient centrally involved in the process of the work. There is agency-wide commitment in the health services to patient involvement, and in adult social care, a similar commitment exists to maintain participation by service users and carers in steering the direction of their own services. People are encouraged to opt for controlling their personalized budgets, which means they direct the resources to the needs they identify.

The next chapter illustrates the importance to the practitioner of the evidence base from research and argues that the practitioner needs to develop confidence and expertise in the journey towards becoming more research aware and research-minded.

Chapter Summary

In this chapter, we have seen that the process linking the stages of assessment, planning, implementation and review/evaluation is complex, because of the complexity of the job of working with people. The detail of working in each particular area will become apparent when working through these stages as a specialist student or practitioner.

REVIEW QUESTIONS

1   What different meanings can you think of for the word 'process'?

2   What are the four main stages of the nursing process, applied here in complementary practice?

3   What are the key processes in the following two processes of complementary practice: pathological and quality of life?

CHAPTER LINKS

For more discussion of the idea of critically reflective practice, see Chapter 2.

For more discussion of continuing practice development, see Chapter 32.

FURTHER RESOURCES

Christensen, P.J. and Kenney, J.W. (eds) (1995) *Nursing Process: Applications of Conceptual Methods*, St Louis, MI, Mosby. Useful discussion illustrating the process of nursing in practice, with some lessons for other healthcare professions.

Kenworthy, N., Snowley, G. and Gilling, C. (eds) (1999) *Common Foundation Studies in Nursing*, Edinburgh, Churchill Livingstone. Helpful summary of ideas and practices concerning the nursing process.

Yura, H. and Walsh, M.B. (1988) *The Nursing Process: Assessing, Planning, Implementing, Evaluating*, Norwalk, CT, Appleton & Lange. Chapter 4 covers a classic, extensive, detailed list of examples of the nursing process in practice.

Researching Practice

ROBERT ADAMS

By the end of this chapter, you should be able to:

■ understand what is meant by research

■ appreciate debates about 'what works' in complementary and alternative approaches

■ discuss the relative merits of the major research strategies and methods

■ explore what is entailed in practitioners becoming research aware and research-minded

What is Meant by Research

Research is the term used to refer to systematic attempts to focus on particular aspects of a subject and, rather than relying on opinions, establish patterns, processes, outcomes or effectiveness.

Research is increasingly referred to as the only legitimate basis for what is called **evidence-based practice** (EBP) in the health and social professions. However, this raises three questions that are constantly debated. What sort of research is considered legitimate? Is some research more legitimate than others? How do we judge the boundary between legitimate research and the rest? Although important, these are questions that would sidetrack us from our main interest in this chapter, which is to deal with two aspects of researching practice:

1. the general matter of the evidence base for practice, in the research carried out over the years by professional researchers
2. the practicalities of practitioners and students, perhaps as part of a course, carrying out their own small-scale research projects into practice.

This chapter aims to enable you to develop your views about these two topics and to answer the questions that precede them. Let us begin with two contrasting examples of the use of the word 'effectiveness'.

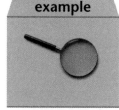

Practice example

Fay was in her thirties, confined to her bed, in the terminal stage of cancer. Her consultant, doctor and nursing staff all supported her receiving complementary therapy as part of her palliative care. She was very thankful, as she said the treatment relaxed her, contributed to her pain relief and enabled her to enjoy visits by relatives and friends.

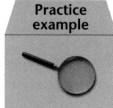

Practice example

Edvard had suffered from lower back pain for years and neither surgical interventions nor pain control using drugs gave him relief. He tried various alternative medical approaches and found them helpful in alleviating the pain.

Research into Approaches and Treatments

The example of Fay illustrates how complementary therapies – which may be ineffective in improving treatment outcomes in terms of the illness or condition – may nevertheless improve the patient's quality of life. The example of Edvard, more conventionally, illustrates how alternative medicine may be claimed to be an effective treatment in alleviating an illness or condition – in this case used as a substitute for conventional medicine – in areas such as specific problems of pain relief.

Traditional experimental research into complementary therapies and alternative medicine commonly attempts to test the efficacy and safety of particular approaches or treatments. This may take the form of objective measures of, say, levels of blood pressure before and after treatment. Alternatively, it may rely on people's experiences – how they report what they feel. Thus, research may investigate people's perceptions of whether particular treatments make them feel better. In the case of patients suffering from arthritis or cancer who have massage, they may feel comforted, rather than there being a claim to cure the condition. The effectiveness of a treatment may lie in the extent to which it improves the patient's comfort in the here and now, rather than in improving the eventual outcome of the disease. In judging the validity of a particular treatment, it is necessary to be clear about the grounds on which this is judged.

Debates about 'What Works'

Many sources of advice and information about complementary approaches exist. There is a gap, however, between the generally assertive and confident nature of the public literature and the scientific and research base. Some writing attempts to steer between these two extremes. Bratman (2007), for example, in association with the Complementary Medical Association, has written an encyclopedic and seemingly authoritative study on the effectiveness of different approaches. However, the weakness of this is that it summarizes the research findings in each area, but does not give any sources. This means that it is impossible to trace back his conclusions to their evidence base. A much more clearly evidenced book (Spencer and Jacobs, 1999) goes through a succession of major conditions and illnesses and gives a well-researched, evidence-based commentary on each, detailing their nature and sources. Spencer and Jacobs do not simply list possible types of complementary treatment, but evaluate the validity of each in the light of current research.

We need to bear in mind that debates about which particular treatments are more effective take place in the wider context of differences between researcher, commentators and professionals about:

- the origins and nature of illnesses and conditions
- conceptions of health and wellbeing
- notions of what health and wellbeing mean in the wider setting of the family and the community.

Different Research Methods

It is important to become familiar with the meanings of terms commonly used in research and these are listed in Table 12.1.

Table 12.1 Terms connected with research

Clinical trial	Detailed study of a small group of patients undergoing a particular intervention
Double-blind trial	Study in which neither the professional nor the person treated know which treatment is given to which person
Observational study	Study of the effects of a particular treatment, without a control group
Placebo-controlled trial	A study where one group of people are given the treatment and the other group are given a **placebo** (a dummy treatment that looks just like the real one)
Randomized controlled trial (RCT)	A study where people receiving treatments are allocated by chance (randomly) to one of at least two treatment groups
Reliability	Reliable methods of research are those which repeatedly produce similar, in theory identical, results
Single case study	A study of the treatment given to one person
Case series	A number of case studies of people subjected to a single treatment
Validity	A study which, when we check it out, perhaps by other means, seems, according to our common sense, to achieve what we aimed to do when we started

There is a hierarchy of research methods, in that some are more highly regarded by researchers and medical professionals than others. The most highly regarded is the double-blind, placebo-controlled study, but it is more suited to testing clearly measurable effects of one particular application under laboratory-controlled conditions. It is probably less suited to testing those complementary approaches that are more holistic or 'energy based', but it can be modified to fit those areas of complementary practice that lie closer to conventional medical intervention.

Typically, research in a novel area of practice is likely to begin with the practitioner or researcher having a hunch or question based on personal observation of practice. This may lead to a case study being carried out, perhaps followed by a case series. At the next stage, small-scale exploratory research may follow, as the prelude to setting up a formal, large-scale RCT trial.

Since the mid-twentieth century, a considerable volume of RCT trials have been carried out into a variety of complementary approaches. Bratman's summary of the evidence for the use of complementary approaches is based on more than 10,000 double-blind, placebo-controlled studies, which represents a considerable body of research. Double-blind studies are suitable for eliminating factors that tend to confuse the results of particular treatments. Bratman's (2007: xii–xv) discussion of these factors is summarized in Table 12.2.

Table 12.2 Factors confusing the results of research

Observer bias	Distortions in the judgements by observers, including medical practitioners, when they know which is the real treatment and which is the placebo
Rosenthal effect	Researchers influencing the opinions of research subjects about their treatments by communicating their expectations to them, through suggestion or even, when briefing them with identical words, through subtle changes in tone of voice
Reinterpretation effect	Patients tending to emphasize improvements and play down problems because they think that is what their doctors want to hear
Placebo effect	A widely known effect, where patients given a 'dummy' treatment report feeling improvements
Memory distortion	Practitioners and patients selectively recalling the successes and conveniently forgetting the occasions when they are less successful
Cognitive dissonance	Practitioners whose living depends on an activity, or who state out loud that their treatment works, will avoid cognitive dissonance (the discomfort of being aware of two simultaneous and different views) by ensuring that other evidence in their world supports the view on which their world depends
Illusion of agency	A practitioner may tend to seek evidence of having brought about the improvement, even though in reality the condition or disease has run its course and the body has naturally recovered
Regression towards the mean	Because people's test scores tend to vary and those with abnormal scores tend to be selected for research, over a period they will tend towards the mean (normal score for most people) and so this effect may be attributed to the treatment

Study effect	In industry, this was called the Hawthorne effect, after a famous study in the USA. It happens when patients being studied take greater care because they feel more important through being part of a research study
Dropping out	The converse of the study effect, patients with bad effects may tend to drop out of the research

There is still less evidence to support the use of particular complementary approaches than to support specific conventional medical treatments. Bratman (2007: viii) argues that despite this, there are three reasons why complementary approaches should still be considered:

1. complementary approaches may offer benefits not available through any conventional treatment
2. complementary approaches may offer benefits with less side effects than conventional treatments
3. many people feel better taking a 'natural' remedy, for example herbal or complementary therapy, than a drug.

Some herbal treatments and supplements can interact harmfully with specific drugs. This is sometimes used as an argument against using herbs or supplements, whereas it is the combination of different treatments that is harmful, rather than one or the other on its own.

Let us build briefly on the example of Edvard, cited above. There is evidence to support the use of complementary therapies in integrated care. The following examples of effectiveness in specific areas may be used to advance evidence-based practice:

- Use of massage with cancer patients: Smith et al. (2003) found a significantly lower rate of psychological and neurological complications for people receiving massage therapy during chemotherapy.
- Use of aromatherapy in pain and mood relief: Kowalski (2002) found slight decreases in pulse and blood pressure scores, pain, mood and anxiety relief, as well as improved wellbeing when lavender therapy used.

Becoming Research Aware and Research-minded

Practitioners in the health and social services are being encouraged by government and their professional bodies to become more research aware and research-minded, as part of the agenda of building a culture of EBP. Towards this end, it is important for complementary practitioners to be committed to building the evidence base for future effective practice. Without the continual efforts of practitioners to provide evidence of 'what works' in their practice, there will be no basis on which other people can take encouragement for the further support of complementary approaches.

The goal of encouraging practitioners to become involved in research is easier to state than to carry out. Research can seem daunting, especially to the beginning practitioner. Yet it is desirable to build a research dimension into practice, so that it becomes part of the continuous process of professional development and is associated with lifelong learning.

In order to be an active researcher, it is necessary to be familiar with the principles and practice of research. Interestingly, we often talk about *doing* research but *being* a researcher. The practice of researching as a practitioner brings these two aspects together – it is about being as well as doing.

Research carried out by practitioners must conform to ethical standards. Most health settings require new research projects to go through the process of applying for and being granted ethical approval. One of the main purposes of ethical approval is to ensure that the research satisfies legal requirements regarding the safeguarding of data, the protection of the rights of the subjects of research and specifying what will be done with the data collected.

Practicalities

Students need to be familiar with what research entails and it is good to go through the process of doing a small piece of research while on a course. This breaks us in to the practicalities of researching. It is good to understand in advance the principles on which research is based and the process of research. Let us follow through these two aspects:

Principles of research:

- Ethical – respecting all participants
- Confidential – respecting people's personal information
- Equal – treating all people equally, without discriminating.

Process of research:

- Design
- Planning
- Gathering information
- Analysing
- Writing up
- Sharing with other people.

Being an active researcher involves qualities and areas of expertise that we introduced in Chapter 2, among which are the following:

- Being critical
- Being sensitive
- Being reflexive
- Being open-minded.

Chapter Summary

This chapter has tackled the arguments associated with adopting an evidence-based approach in complementary practice. It has also examined briefly what is involved in practitioners becoming research active. It should be borne in mind that EBP is a goal that is likely to involve a longer term process, rather than being achieved in the short term.

REVIEW
QUESTIONS

1   What do the initials EBP stand for?

2   What is a double-blind trial?

3   What is an RCT?

CHAPTER
LINKS

For further discussion of the qualities and areas of expertise associated with an evidence-based approach to practice, see Chapter 2.

For further discussion of reading and critically reviewing research publications, see the resource file below.

FURTHER
RESOURCES

Bratman, S. (2007) *Complementary and Alternative Health: The Scientific Verdict on What Really Works*, London, Collins. Useful discussion of the technical aspects of research in the field of complementary practice that are relevant to adopting an evidence-based approach.

Lewith, G., Jonas, W.B. and Walach, H. (2002) *Clinical Research in Complementary Therapies: Principles, Problems and Solutions*, Philadelphia, WB Saunders. Deals with the important questions concerning the place of research in complementary practice.

Spencer, J.W. and Jacobs, J.J. (1999) *Complementary Alternative Medicine: An Evidence-based Approach*, St Louis, MI, Mosby. Contains a useful, brief discussion of many relevant issues to consider when adopting an evidence-based approach.

Part IV

Resource file

Developing Expertise in Criticality and Research

A critically reflective practitioner in a particular complementary approach needs to be confident in dealing with published material on topics relevant to practice. This is a necessary part of ensuring that one's practice is evidence based. Here we examine aspects of the necessary skills to bring this about.

Reading Critically

Critical reading is the term used to describe what we do when we reach an independent view of a piece of written work and evaluate its strengths and weaknesses. It is an important skill for a complementary practitioner to acquire. The reason is that you need to feel confident that you can appraise (evaluate) the worth of an article about complementary therapy or alternative medicine.

The first stages in developing your critical reading skills are as follows:

- Select a short article or chapter about complementary therapy. Do not be intimidated by it. Tell yourself that even if you do not know as much as its author, you, as the reader, are in a position to reach a judgement about how well it is written.
- Decide that you will read it through and reach a judgement about two aspects:
  - How well it is written, that is, how clearly written you think it is.
  - How good the content is, that is, how far the content matches up to the aims of the piece of written work.
- In order to reach a critical judgement, you will need to read slowly through the piece of written work, as follows:
  - Read the entire article through first.
  - Now read the article through again, taking in the arguments. Keep a notepad by you and try to summarize in a single sentence the main point of each paragraph, or series of two or three paragraphs. Try to make sure that by the

end of it you have no more than one side of A4 filled with notes.
- Keep details of the page number by each of the particularly important or interesting points. Make sure you can find each of these again. Highlight a particular keyword to help you, or make a note of it in your notepad.
- Now skim through the article, checking quickly and ask yourself two questions: is there anything the writer has written that you strongly agree with? Is there anything that you strongly disagree with? Jot down on a separate piece of paper these two questions and underneath briefly try to summarize your reasons, referring to the content of the article. Highlight and quote from the article at least one thing the author says to back up each of your points of agreement and disagreement.

Forming Habits to Help you Read Critically

1. *Develop a questioning attitude:* Take the idea you have read about and sit for a few minutes thinking about it. Do you agree with it? Does it agree with your own experience? Has it particular strengths or weaknesses? Jot down notes on this, under your notes on the ideas from the book.

2. *Put the idea in the wider context:* Spend time thinking about the wider context. Does the idea link with other ideas of other people you have read or heard about? Jot their names down.

3. *Doodle on a sheet of paper:* Put the original idea in the centre and put a circle round it. Jot down related ideas on the sheet, putting closely related ideas nearer and more important ones in larger letters. Make links between the ideas using lines. You can use different colours for ideas that correspond and differ.

4. *Go networking for ideas:* Have a look in the library for the names of people who have written about these other ideas. Or go to the internet and type

the ideas in. For example, if you are studying user participation, you can access the SCIE website (www.scie.org.uk/) and type in user participation (see resource file at end of Chapter 2).

5. *Make links with other ideas:* Use the above procedures so that you follow the original idea along threads of reference until you decide you have enough.

6. *Review your work:* Spend a few minutes looking back over the notes you've made and jot down any thoughts that occur to you. Try to relax and let thoughts bubble to the surface. Jot down 'off the wall' ideas as well as the more 'rational' thoughts. This will help you when you come to discuss, present or write about the topic later.

7. *Sign off your work:* Put the date either at the top or the bottom of your notes.

Using Critical Judgements

There are two important components of using your own critical judgements: evaluating a report of a piece of research and writing your own review. Let us consider these in turn.

Evaluating a Report of a Piece of Research

In order to make a judgement about the quality of research evidence for practice, you need to be able to carry out a review of the research. Most commonly, the research will be written up in the form of a report or article in a journal. So your review will be what we call a 'literature review'. Sometimes a review of the literature will take the form of a long piece of written work examining critically all the references the person can find on a particular topic. In this case, your literature review will be of just one article or report summarizing the research. In order to evaluate the research, you need to follow a systematic procedure, which we now outline.

Your purpose

You are carrying out a literature review of one or more pieces of research. Let us assume there is only one. You are assessing a piece of research from the point of view of its integrity, rigour and usefulness.

What makes a good literature review? It should:

■ give a clear picture of what the research is all about
■ explain the main features of the research
■ analyse the ideas presented in the research report
■ examine the strengths and weaknesses of the research.

Where do we start?

First, identify the kind of research it is. Karen Hucker's (2001: 6–7) clearly written book on research in work with people distinguishes six of the main ones (I have put an example of each in brackets):

■ *basic* (researching a topic 'for its own sake'. This could involve writing a history of a voluntary agency, with a view to answering certain key questions such as why it developed in a particular way)
■ *applied* (hoping to apply the results to improve practice)
■ *strategic* (exploring a new area of policy)
■ *scholarly* (examining the effectiveness of a new drug or therapy)
■ *creative* (testing the contribution of interior design to recovery rates from illnesses and operations)
■ *longitudinal* (following the development of a generation or 'cohort' of babies born on a particular day, or twins born in particular circumstances).

Ingredients of good research

Not all research is equally rigorous or helpful. Good research usually includes the following ingredients:

■ *Introduction/summary/synopsis/abstract:* words referring to the brief statement of what the research is about.
■ *Aims/questions/hypotheses:* what the researchers are trying to find out.
■ *Methodology:* the theories, perspectives or ideas which underlie the methods.
■ *Methods:* the techniques used to collect the information, such as interviews or questionnaires.
■ *Results:* the description of what information was actually collected.

- *Analysis/discussion:* discussion and interpretation or explanation of results.
- *Conclusions:* a final statement of what has, or hasn't, been achieved.
- *Recommendations:* suggested practice implications of the research.

Aims and objectives of the research

- Have you checked out the aims and objectives of the research?
- Have you clarified the actual focus of the research, as opposed to its stated focus in the aims and objectives near the start?
- Do these differ in any ways?
- Did the researchers admit that in some way the research fell short of achieving its aims and objectives?

Methods and methodology of the research

- Summarize the methods used.
- Were the methods wholly quantitative (which can be expressed in numbers), wholly qualitative (which can be expressed in any categories and terms the researcher chooses, to help understanding) or a mixture of both?
- Discuss in your review the relative merits of these, in relation to the research you are reviewing. Find out whether the research contains elements of both.
- Are the chosen methods appropriate to the aim of the research?
- Have the researchers shown convincing evidence to you that they understand method and methodology issues?
- Have the researchers taken into account the views of patients and/or people who use services and their carers?

Analysis of research issues

- What limitations were identified by the researchers?
- Did these undermine the usefulness of the research?
- What were the findings of the research?

Evaluation of the research

To test the evidence base for practice, ask the following questions:

- Is the study valid? Validity means that the research method produces information relevant to the subject being researched.
- Are the results reliable? Reliability means that if repeated in the same circumstances, the research would produce the same results.
- Will the results improve practice?
- Were the conclusions drawn appropriate to the research?
- How significant and useful were the conclusions?

Remember, if you are a student presenting your review of the research report or article, you may need to show:

- An understanding of the research process.
- An appreciation of how the research tackled ethical issues, such as researched people being exploited, taken for granted or not having the aims of the research explained to them properly and an opportunity to give, or withhold, informed consent. Informed consent is agreement in the light of the person having sufficient information to be able to understand the full implications of consenting or not consenting.
- You have examined issues of diversity and anti-discriminatory practice.
- You can state your conclusions clearly.
- You have used the right convention (for example Harvard; see resource file at end of Chapter 2) to present your bibliography correctly.

Writing a Critical Review

This may be of anything, but most commonly it will be of a book or article.

Essentials:

- You need peace and quiet and space and time around you to think properly.
- Switch off your mobile phone.

- Tell people to go away.
- You are thinking. Thinking is as much work as digging the garden or cleaning the bathroom. Without space and time, your mind is like a muscle that can't expand.
- Exercise your mind by thinking critically and it will grow stronger every time you use it. Again, think of your mind as a muscle. The more you exercise your mind, the more confident you will become.

Preparation:

- Read the item through and take notes of the major points.
- Make particular note of anything you strongly agree or disagree with.
- Spend time afterwards thinking about how the item relates to anything else you have come across or read.
- Write down a list of the strengths and a list of the weaknesses of the item.
- Spend time writing down points of interest that either agree or differ in the two items.
- If you have time, look up any other similar items and check whether they agree or disagree.

Writing:

- Put yourself in a creative mood.
- Become confident.
- You are about to give your opinion. Your opinion is as valuable as anybody's.

- Don't hold your views back. Don't be afraid to commit yourself.
- Spend a few minutes jotting down the main points you want to make, in note form, not in full sentences.
- Look at the points you've made and try numbering them in a logical sequence.
- Try different sequences. You may want to go through the strengths first and the weaknesses second. Or, it may work better with your strongest criticisms first.
- Write a simple sentence summarizing each point.
- Make each sentence the first sentence in a short paragraph. Write two or three more sentences explaining each key point.
- Try to round off at the end with a paragraph summing up whether, on balance, you like or dislike the item, whether its strengths impress you more than its weaknesses, and whether you think the author could have tackled it another way. Don't be afraid to suggest this.

Note: This resource file is adapted from similar resource files in Adams, A. (2007) *Foundations of Health and Social Care*, Basingstoke, Palgrave Macmillan.

Reference

Hucker, K. (2001) *Research Methods in Health, Care and Early Years*, London, Heinemann.

Philosophical and Scientific Basis for Practice

Part V
Philosophical and Scientific Basis for Practice

Introduction

This part of the book tackles the ideas and scientific knowledge that form the basis of practice in many of the established complementary approaches. This is not a comprehensive picture but does give an indicative picture of the science behind practice and offers information about resources to guide further learning on particular topics.

Many complementary approaches rely for their effective practice on the practitioner having a basic grasp of anatomy and physiology. However, different approaches regard the body in different ways, depending on their philosophical basis for practice. One way to approach the understanding of the human body is to present anatomy and physiology purely as scientific knowledge. However, the variety of perspectives on understanding the body, mind and spirit are associated with different understandings of how illnesses and conditions arise and may be tackled.

Chapter 13 provides an overview of the main currents of historical thought and development. Chapters 14, 15, 16 and 17 deal with different aspects of anatomy and physiology as they apply in many areas of complementary and alternative practice. These four chapters use brief practice examples from the author's own experiences to illustrate how knowledge of anatomy and physiology is applied to complementary practice, rather than taking a traditional biology textbook approach to the subject. It is worth noting that the main purpose of Chapter 14 is to provide a basis for the knowledge and understanding required for chapters that fall under the heading of manipulative and body-based approaches. Chapter 18 indicates how differential diagnosis – the process of identifying the most probable condition among the differing probabilities of the range of possible conditions – can be applied to patients and clients. It offers the opportunity for the practitioner to bring together knowledge and understanding in an integrative way when working with them.

Roots of Traditional, Complementary and Alternative Medicine

ROBERT ADAMS

Learning outcomes

By the end of this chapter, you should be able to:

■ outline the basis of traditional medicine (TM) in the ancient world

■ trace the spread of TM and other remedies

■ trace the main currents of ideas about TM through the major civilizations

■ grasp the key ideas and assumptions of TM and related remedies

■ appreciate Western sociological perspectives on traditional and professionalized approaches to health and wellbeing

■ provide a snapshot of worldwide use of TM and complementary approaches

Basis of Traditional Medicine in the Ancient World

For thousands of years, TM has made a vital contribution to the morale, health and wellbeing of people in many countries where access to conventional medicine and treatments is restricted or nonexistent. The spread of TM is extremely broad, far broader than that of conventional medicine. A global survey by the World Health Organization (WHO, 2001) identifies more than 190 countries where TM is practised. Some idea of the broad scope of herbal remedies within these countries can be gathered from the fact that the WHO has amassed an inventory of more than 20,000 different herbal remedies (Azaizeh et al., 2006: 230). However, it is only where the only option is TM, because no conventional medicine exists, that the nature and identity of TM remains clear and uncontested. In practice, in many countries, the boundary between conventional medicine and its alternatives inevitably tends to blur and there are two reasons for this:

1. in developing countries, herbal remedies have been the first and only source of treatment for illnesses for centuries
2. in developed countries, many modern conventional drugs have their origins in traditional herbal remedies.

In contrast with people's primary reliance on TM in many developing countries, in developed countries, complementary and alternative medicine (CAM) is seen as a supplement, enhancing the quality of life. In many parts of the world, where traditional practitioners carry out procedures on people suffering from life-threatening conditions, treatments can make the difference between life and death. Some forms of CAM, which have become integrated into conventional health services in developed countries, have their origins in ancient TM practice. Homeopathy is one of these areas of practice and its origins can be traced back to the work of Galen and Hippocrates in ancient Greece (Saad et al., 2005: 476).

Spread of Traditional Medicine and Other Remedies

Space does not permit a history of TM and CAM. Present-day practice takes place against the backcloth of thousands of years of TM, which has evolved in ancient civilizations in different parts of the world. Much of this history predates written records, so we have to rely on archaeological evidence. Herbal remedies have been found, for example, in the remains of human settlements dating back 60,000 years (Saad et al., 2005: 475).

More recently, we can be certain that two traditions of medicine were established in China and India, which predated Western medicine by more than a thousand years. The family tree of systems of herbal medicine (Figure 13.1) shows how these systems of traditional Chinese medicine (TCM) and traditional Indian medicine (TIM), themselves several millennia old, were influenced by other ideas, notably from ancient Greece. All these influences fed into developments in Tibet and Arab countries. This is not to say that traditional medicine did not exist in these parts of world before this. There is every likelihood that people sought traditional remedies in many different countries for the ills they suffered and knowledge grew over the centuries about which treatments were most effective. By the Middle Ages – about 1000 AC – traditional medicine was well established at the heart of the civilizations of China, India, Tibet and Arab countries.

Much of the extensive history of these different systems of medicine is hidden, because a great deal of traditional medicine is transmitted orally through the generations. The access of later practitioners to earlier traditional medical expertise also was restricted because of secrecy surrounding theories and prescriptions. The publication of manuscripts and books cataloguing herbal and other medical practices began to erode the jointly enmeshed traditions of secrecy and expertise, and the Unani medicine system from ancient Greece, which influenced TCM and TIM, was translated from Greek into Arabic and found its way into Arab traditional medicine. Later, treatises of Arab medicine were translated into Latin, which was the common language that enabled priests, lawyers, physicians and academics in many countries to communicate with each other. Renowned Arab scholars and practitioners, such as al-Tabari (838–870), al-Razi (846–930) and Ibn-Sina (980–1037), known in the West as Avicenna, were responsible for advancing Arab medicine and its associated sciences. In Arab countries, medicine made notable advances before the Middle Ages in Europe. The first pharmacies were established in Baghdad as early as the eighth century. In that period, al-Rahivi wrote about a peer review process in medicine – duplicate notes of the physician on the patient's treatment were passed to the local council of other physicians who scrutinized performance. If considered unsuitable, the patient was able to take out a law suit. Avicenna wrote classic texts on herbal and dietetic medicine, including *The Book of Healing*. His *Canon of Medicine* (published *c.* 1025) was translated into Latin and Hebrew, passing through many editions in the fifteenth and sixteenth centuries, thus making it available and influential in European medicine (Saad et al., 2005: 476).

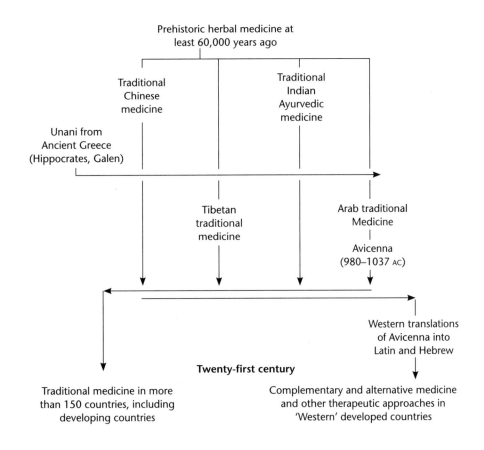

Figure 13.1 Family tree of traditional medicine
Source: Adapted from Saad et al., 2005

Part V

As traditional medical practice spread to Western countries, a separation took place between traditional herbal medicine and those medical practices that were taken up by the growing medical establishment of physicians in Europe and North America. The eighteenth-century Enlightenment – the spread of ideas about reasoned scientific research as the basis of knowledge – coincided with the spread of industrialization and modern wealth built on mass production and modern methods of communication. The Enlightenment refers to a philosophical and scientific movement that promoted reason and science as sources of knowledge, wisdom and understanding, rather than faith in religious and other beliefs. By and large, science and rationality have become associated with conventional medicine and complementary and alternative approaches have been detached from the mainstream health services of developed countries. Despite being widely studied and practised (Smith, 1997; Godagama, 2001; Lad, 2001, 2006; Pole, 2006), Ayurvedic medicine, for example, has never become established in the UK and USA, in the sense that its practitioners cannot achieve registration as legally regulated professionals. The acupuncture of TCM, however, has developed a Western form, with some non-Chinese practitioners being trained in its techniques. In Yorkshire, for example, in 2008, it is possible to receive acupuncture treatment from a Chinese practitioner, trained in Hong Kong and China, who is in private practice within a health centre. It is also possible to be referred by a consultant to an English-trained practitioner, who works as a qualified physiotherapist in the NHS and whose services, therefore, are free.

Main Ideas and Assumptions of Traditional Medicine

We cannot do justice in this limited space to the great complexity of different approaches. The following provides a brief summary of some of the different approaches referred to in Figure 13.1.

Ayurvedic Ideas and Medicine

Ayurveda is an ancient Sanskrit word, comprising *ayur* meaning 'life' and *veda* meaning 'knowledge'. Ayurvedic, or traditional Indian, medicine is an ancient system that now occupies a place in Western countries, such as the USA and the UK, as an 'alternative' medical practice rather than 'alternative and complementary' as TCM is. I suggest the following two reasons for this:

1. the subjection of TCM to a greater degree of scientific scrutiny, which has enabled some of its components such as acupuncture (particularly for pain relief) to become better accepted in Western health services
2. the readiness of practitioners to accept TCM as a system that more easily adapts to the wide span of people's illnesses, conditions and health and wellbeing issues.

The notion of holism is reflected in the Ayurvedic principle of interconnectedness. Associated with the idea of interconnectedness is the notion of the person's body and mind being in harmony with elements of the universe. The Ayurvedic practitioner combines the use of a variety of different herbal, animal and mineral prescriptions with the assumption that there are three body types or **doshas** (bearing some resemblance to the three body types in Western psychology – thin, muscular and fat, which correspond respectively to the personality types of ectomorph, mesomorph and endomorph). The three doshas are:

- Kapha – water and earth
- Vata – ether and air
- Pitta – fire and water.

The most important combinations of these produce the following body types:

- Mono types: in which kapha, vata or pitta dominate
- Dual types: in which vata-kapha, kapha-pitta or vata-pitta dominate
- Equal types: in which there are equal proportions of vata, pitta or kapha.

Ayurvedic practice works on the basis that diseases or other conditions of being unwell arise when the person is:

- out of harmony within themselves, that is, there is a lack of balance between the three doshas represented in their body types (Figure 13.2)
- out of harmony with the external environment, which is a reference to the connection between the person and the universe.

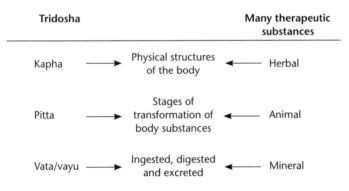

Figure 13.2 Ayurvedic assumptions and treatments

Comparing Traditional Chinese and Indian Medicine

Chapter 20 discusses the philosophical basis for TCM. I shall refer in passing to these ideas, with the aim of putting them alongside TIM, to highlight some points of comparison (Table 13.1).

Part V

Table 13.1 Some points of comparison between TCM and TIM

	Traditional Chinese medicine	Traditional Indian medicine
Aims	To promote health and quality of life	To promote health and quality of life
Focus	Holistic: focusing on the patient as a person rather than on the disease or condition	Holistic: focusing on the patient as a person rather than on the disease or condition
Philosophy	Five elements of the material world: water, fire, earth, metal, wood. Four bodily humours	Five elements in the universe. Three forces (doshas) governing all life: kapha, pitta, vata
Physician	Gives treatment to keep energies circulating and balancing yin and yang	Treats to maintain balance between the three doshas and therefore health

Source: Adapted from Patwardhan et al., 2005

Unani (Islamic or Arab) Medicine

Islamic or Arab medicine is also referred to as 'Unani', which is the Arab word meaning Greek. Unani was influenced by Greek, Roman, Indian, Persian and Chinese beliefs and expertise. By the Middle Ages, Arab societies had well-developed traditions of medicine, doctoring, hospitalizing people for operations, using nurses to care for them and pharmacists to administer treatments with herbal and other preparations. There was some evidence of what we would call modern evidence-based practice linked with experimental research. Clinical trials, experimental medicine and testing on humans and animals were not unknown.

The Unani system of medicine contributes to a globally recognized tradition of medicine extending back to the Greeks, Hippocrates and Galen, and through Persia, now known as Iran, where cranial surgery was carried out three centuries before 0 AC. The practice of Unani passed to many other countries and, by the eighth and ninth centuries, combined the influence of Greek, Chinese, Ayurvedic and Persian traditional systems of medicine (Chishti, 1991). By the eighth century, medical and pharmacological practices were distinguishable, an important contribution being the work of an Arab alchemist Abu Musa Jabir ben Hayyan, in Iraq, who wrote a book about poisons and their antidotes (Saad et al., 2006: 433).

The Unani system of medicine attends to the physical and mental health of the patient. One of the specialized areas of medicine is devoted to mental problems and some minerals such as gold are used in the treatment of conditions such as depression and anxiety (Bajaj and Vohora, 2000).

Unani and Ayurvedic Views of the Elements

The Unani and Ayurvedic systems both believe that the elements of the body are reflected in four liquids and associated humours and that the health of the body is sustained by the balance between the four humours, each associated with substances with particular characteristics. We can find the essence of the

Ayurveda system reflected in British medicine in the Elizabethan era of the sixteenth century, written about but by no means created by Robert Burton in 1621 (Burton, 1932), since both draw on the work of ancient theorists such as Galen. A good deal separates the Ayurvedic, Unani and Elizabethan views of people's personalities and their relationships both with their bodily characteristics and the wider environment, but, greatly simplifying, we can show some common assumptions they share in Table 13.2. It should be borne in mind that these are types, not individual people, and most people are assumed to display a mix of humours. In Ayurvedic, Unani and Elizabethan medicine, treatment commonly aims to restore the balance of the humours and thus achieve an adjustment of mood, health and wellbeing.

Table 13.2 The elements and humours of the body

Humour	Element	Nature	Body type	Mood
Blood	Air	Moist and hot	Fat/face flushed	Sanguine
Yellow bile	Fire	Dry and hot	Thin/colours up when angry	Choleric Quick tempered
Black bile	Earth	Dry and cold	Thin/pale Introspective	Melancholic 'Depressive'
Phlegm	Water	Moist and cold	Fat/pale	Phlegmatic 'Laid back'

Diagnosis is carried out principally by measuring the pulse (nabz) and physically examining the patient's urine and stools. Unani medicine is associated with preventing or treating ill health through restoring the balance between the humours discovered through this process of investigation. There are four main approaches to treatment: regimenal therapy (Ilajbil tadbeer) programmes such as massage, Turkish baths, douches and exercise; dietary therapy (Ilajbil ghiza); surgery (Ilajbil yad); and pharmacological therapy (Ilajbil dava), mainly using herbal prescriptions, with some use of substances, some more recently derived from minerals. These forms of therapy are administered with careful attention to the following:

- Maintaining fresh air
- Sustaining food and drink
- Balancing:
  - Periods of waking and sleeping
  - Retention and excretion
  - Mental activity and rest
  - Physical activity and rest.

Despite concerns about quality and reliability, the Unani medicine system is well established as a primary source by many people in developing countries. It is

Part V

still preferred by rich as well as poor people in India (Izhar, 1989). Modern issues about the safety of traditional Arab medicine are made more pronounced by fears about the effects of plants grown on soils contaminated by poisonous chemicals or microorganisms. This has led to the recommendation that minimum standards should be laid down for sourcing, harvesting, processing and clinically testing herbal products (Saad et al., 2006: 435), as well as subjecting them to appropriate licensing and regulation (Azaizeh et al., 2006: 234).

There is evidence that many herbs used as the source of traditional remedies have been disappearing. Only 23 of over 800 plant species used in traditional Arab medicine are still in use in pharmaceutical products (Azaizeh et al., 2006: 232). Additional factors weakening the base of traditional Arab medicine in the Middle East include climatic changes that threaten the destruction of some plant species and a loss of expertise among practitioners through the lessening of the traditions of skill transmission by pastoral and other practitioners to a new, younger and more urban generation of practitioners (Azaizeh et al., 2006: 234).

Western Sociological Perspectives on Traditional and Professionalized Approaches to Health and Wellbeing

We round off this chapter with a brief reference to how Western sociological perspectives contribute to our understanding of traditional and professionalized approaches to health and wellbeing. From what we have said above, there are obvious contrasts between Western and non-Western approaches to illness, health and wellbeing. Western and non-Western ideas of disease causation are compared by Ryan and Pritchard (2004: 19). In Western societies, disease models are based on naturalistic views of causation – infection, stress, organic deterioration and accidents. In non-Western societies, disease models based on supernatural views comprise three main groups of theories:

- theories of mystical causation through impersonal forces, for example mystical retribution, fate, ominous sensations
- theories of animistic causation through personalized forces, for example spirit aggression, soul loss
- theories of magical causation or the actions of evil forces, for example witchcraft or sorcery.

For thousands of years, TM and lay approaches to coping with birth and ageing existed side by side in communities. Cant and Sharma (1999) argue that most sociologists have unrealistically narrowed their attentions to cover Western countries, especially the USA and the UK. Over the past two centuries, healthcare in Western countries has become professionalized and largely medicalized. The healthcare system in the UK is built around the National Health Service, which was set up under the NHS Act 1948 as part of the welfare state.

Many of the health services in the UK have remained free to anybody in the population. Some aspects of health provision have remained privatized and because of the way privatized medicine is priced, its availability is rationed largely according to the means of purchasers. So better off people have unequal access to it.

There are different explanations of the reasons why complementary approaches have expanded and now assume an enhanced importance in Western countries. This can be seen in terms of different sociological perspectives, which are summarized in Table 13.3.

Table 13.3 Sociological perspectives on expansion of complementary and alternative medicine

Perspective	How it applies to complementary approaches
Modernist	Modernist perspectives emphasize rationality and scientific research into medicine aiming to find objectively proved cures for diseases, which means these perspectives are sceptical of alternatives to conventional medicine, such as TCM. The Weberian (based on the work of Max Weber, the sociologist) argument is that conventional medicine established its dominance through its success in pushing complementary and alternative approaches to the periphery
Functionalist	Functionalist perspectives adopt a defence of the high status of conventional professions of medicine, by arguing that surgeons, consultants and doctors deserve their privileged position because they are working for the good of society and not for any personal reward. Traditional (complementary and alternative) practitioners are suspect, to the extent that they do not accept the biomedical model of conventional medical practice
Marxist	Complementary and alternative medical approaches – including traditional medicine – have been replaced in industrialized – including Western – countries by conventional medicine, buttressed by the biomedical model of health. Conventional medicine reinforces the privilege and power of the ruling class by reproducing social inequalities in health, through people's unequal access to health, as demonstrated by persistent inequalities in illness and death rates
Feminist	Radical and socialist feminists combine in their analysis of the male-dominated conventional medical professions becoming dominant and replacing the power of both women and men as traditional healers
Late modernist and postmodernist	The growth of complementary approaches reflects the development of a plurality of different models of conventional and 'alternative' (including traditional medical systems such as TCM, Ayurveda or Unani) medicine. Consumers (patients and clients) can move between these and use more than one approach at a time on a 'mix and match' basis. In short, there is no single dominant approach, equally acceptable throughout all countries

We can see in Figure 13.3 how the different authors reflect these different perspectives.

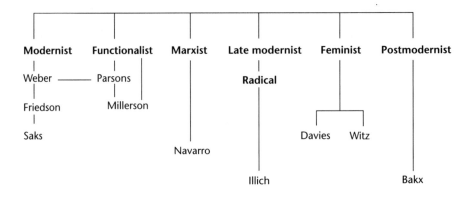

Figure 13.3 Complementary approaches: perspectives and authors

For the following summary, I have drawn extensively on the excellent and very simply explained review of different authors in Haralambos and Holborn (2008: 292–8).

Saks (1998) argues that the rise of the biomedical model is associated with, and partly contributed to, the development of modernity, that is, the growing reliance on rational, 'scientifically based' ideas and practice, which flowed in the wake of the Enlightenment. This led, from the nineteenth through into the mid-twentieth century, to the marginalization of complementary and alternative approaches not based on the biomedical approach. However, in the era of post-modernity, this process was challenged, partly because of accumulating evidence that the biomedical model had not brought about significant changes to the outcomes for people with chronic conditions such as Alzheimer's disease, or abolished all threats to the lives of people – epidemics such as HIV/AIDS and SARs. In addition, in the twenty-first century, of course, there is evidence that hospitals, as prominent symbols of healthcare under the biomedical model, have, to an extent, become 'toxic' as centres for spreading epidemics such as MRSA and *C. difficile*. They have thereby fulfilled the analysis of the radical critic Illich (1977) on the ways in which conventional professionals disempower and disable people, on the increasing dominance of technocratic elites such as biomedical professionals in conventional medicine (Illich, 1975a), and on the increasing medicalization of life's everyday problems and professional responses to them, linked with the growing incidence of medical, that is, drug-induced and hospital-based, sicknesses and fatal conditions (Illich, 1975b).

Bakx (1991) distinguishes between popular (informal caring), folk (alternative therapies) and biomedical approaches. Haralambos and Holborn note that Bakx argues that people's renewed interest in folk, that is, complementary and alternative, approaches reflects their ability, as consumers, to choose. In a postmodern world, people regard biomedical approaches as simply one option among many. Haralambos and Holborn also discuss the Weberian (see Table 13.3) argument, put forward by Saks (1998), that interest-based politics motivates biomedical professionals and complementary practitioners to protect their interests, leading to two contrasting trends: towards the distancing of approaches viewed as alternative, and towards incorporating certain practices, for example acupuncture by nurses and physiotherapists and homeopathy by registered practitioners who are also doctors, as complementary within the biomedical healthcare professions.

We can see how TM has been supplanted by orthodox medicine in many countries, notably Western countries. Ways of dealing with illnesses and conditions that formerly were based on the expertise of lay practitioners have been subjected to the processes of professionalization and medicalization. This applies to many of the stages of later life, such as ageing. It also applies to learning and physical impairments (disability) and many mental health problems. For example, the adoption of the medical model of depression means that the first line of explanation and treatment for the depression experienced by a lonely, housebound 'housewife' is medically based and drug based, rather than examining the social origins of depression and the implications of this for treatment (Brown and Harris, 1978).

From the twentieth century onwards, there have been accelerating trends in the globalization of illnesses and healthcare. Globalization refers to the tendency of things to spread throughout the world. In the health field, illnesses and conditions that affect people in developed countries – obesity, heart conditions and certain cancers associated with higher standards of living and food consumption – are spreading to some developing countries. Trends towards globalization highlight tensions between traditional, lay, 'complementary and alternative' approaches to health and medicalized, 'orthodox' approaches.

'Medicalization' refers to the process whereby areas of social life not otherwise associated with medicine are being taken over by health professionals. 'Professional' refers to several traits that, it is argued, distinguish professions from non-professions. Millerson (1964) equates medicine with the traditional profession of the law. Parsons (1959, 1965) regards medicine as contributing to a well-regulated society by delivering health services to people according to doctors' impartial, professional diagnosis of their needs. Friedson (1970) bases the analysis of the nature of professions on Weber's view, arguing that professions try to achieve professional dominance by social closure. This entails doctors, for example, restricting membership to the profession to people from a similar background, maintaining a high status and compelling other competing health carers into subordinate roles. Turner (1995) builds on this Weberian view, arguing that doctors use their professional aspirations as 'an occupational strategy to maintain certain monopolistic privileges and rewards' (quoted in Haralambos and Holborn, 2008: 294). Witz (1992) argues from a feminist viewpoint that many healthcare providers have had their position systematically damaged by the dominance of doctors, for example homeopaths were marginalized and nurses and midwives were subordinated (Haralambos and Holborn, 2008). Celia Davies (1981) writes of the ways in which nurses have been subordinated to physicians and surgeons as these male-dominated professions grew in power since the Industrial Revolution.

There have been some trends, however, towards doctors losing some of their professional power. Haug (1973) argues that this is because a better educated general population means that doctors are less able to dictate how people should

Part V

be treated, as seen in the growth of self-help and the growing significance of complementary therapies and alternative medicine in people's lives. McKinlay and Arches (1985) argue that some loss of status of doctors is happening, through the closer regulation of doctors' work by management, often referred to as 'managerialism'. Another attack on the dominance of doctoring is the growth of clinical nursing (Haralambos and Holborn, 2008). Some nurses working in GP surgeries are taking on more of the tasks traditionally carried out by doctors – taking blood pressure and moving towards 'nurse prescribing'. The power of the medical practitioner is symbolized by scribbling a seemingly indecipherable prescription for the patient to take to the pharmacist, akin to the spell cast by the witch doctor in a nonindustrial society. We round off this brief visit to the socio-logical literature by referring to the Marxist view. Haralambos and Holborn (2008) illustrate this with reference to Navarro (1978), who argues that higher status professions such as conventional medicine occupy more entrenched positions of power in a capitalist society.

A Snapshot of Worldwide Use

This brief overview cannot convey the richness and variety of the uses of trad-itional and complementary/alternative systems of medicine throughout the world. The WHO (2001) worldwide survey recorded significant usage in the 123 coun-tries surveyed, the survey of remaining countries being constrained not by lack of activity in those countries but by a lack of WHO resources (WHO, 2001: ix). According to this survey, Ayurvedic medicine is still widely practised in South Asia, especially India, Bangladesh, Nepal, Sri Lanka and Pakistan. Chinese medicine, especially acupuncture, is 'the most widely used traditional medicine' and 'is prac-tised in every region of the world' (WHO, 2001: 2). Unani medicine is practised not only throughout Arab and other Mediterranean countries, but also in South Asia. For example, in Pakistan, Unani is reported as widely used, with 70% of the popul-ation, especially in rural areas, using traditional and complementary/alternative medicine and approximately 52,600 registered Unani medical practitioners.

In the USA, more than 40% of the adult population had used at least one complementary/alternative therapy, an increase from 33.8% in 1990 (WHO, 2001: 65). This included treatment dispensed in 1993 by the following (WHO, 2001: 66):

1. 45,000 licensed chiropractors, seeing 10–15% of the US population
2. 32,000 doctors of osteopathy (60% of whom practised in primary care), responsible for delivering about 10% of the total healthcare services in the USA
3. 6,000 acupuncture practitioners, with 3,000 allopathic doctors taking courses in acupuncture
4. 10 Ayurvedic clinics in the USA.

Chapter Summary

Traditional systems of medicine have their origins in ancient civilizations and flourish in the modern world. In developing countries, they continue to provide the first line of primary health services, often in the absence of any alternative. In developed countries, the situation is reversed. Conventional medicine holds the foreground and traditional systems of medicine and many different therapies provide a vast array of complementary and alternative approaches.

REVIEW QUESTIONS

1   Where, traditionally, has Ayurvedic medicine been practised?

2   What was the philosophical movement known as the Enlightenment?

3   What is professionalization in the field of health?

CHAPTER LINKS

For a discussion of the importance of lineage, see Chapter 30.

FURTHER RESOURCES

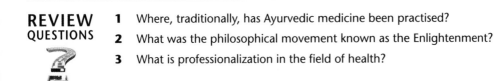

Chishti, H.G.M. (1991) *The Traditional Healer's Handbook: A Classic Guide to the Medicine of Avicenna*, Rochester, VT, Healing Arts Press. A relevant study of traditional medicine.

Haralambos, M. and Holborn, M. (2008) *Sociology: Themes and Perspectives*, 7th edn, London, Collins, especially Chapter 5. A useful commentary on sociological perspectives on the health services in Western societies, with a helpful survey of perspectives on complementary and alternative medicine.

Loeffler, A. (2007) *Allopathy Goes Native: Traditional Versus Modern Medicine in Iran* London, Tauris Academic Studies. Useful comparative study, showing how, in Iran, conventional Western medicine has adapted to the practice of traditional medicine.

Part V

14 Basic Functional Anatomy

JACQUELINE RICHARDS

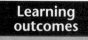
Anatomy is an enormous subject. In this chapter, the basic biomechanics of the body will be discussed. Should further anatomy information be required, please refer to the textbooks recommended at the end of the chapter.

Basic Anatomy

Body Planes

In order to describe the direction of movement, the body is divided into three planes (Figure 14.1). The body is positioned in the anatomical position, which means the body is facing forward, hands at the side with the palms facing forwards and feet pointing straight ahead (Figure 14.2). The sagittal plane is vertical and extends from front to back. The coronal plane or frontal plane is vertical and extends from side to side. The transverse plane is a horizontal plane and divides the body into upper and lower components.

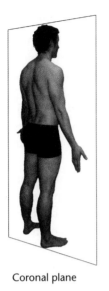
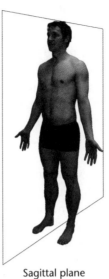
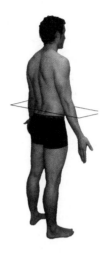

Coronal plane   Sagittal plane   Transverse plane

Figure 14.1 Body planes

Superior (towards the head)

Anterior (front)   Posterior (back)

Proximal (part of the body   Lateral (away from
closest to the midline)   the midline)

                                                   Medial (towards
                                                     the midline)

Distal (part of body
farther away from
the midline)

Inferior (towards the feet)

Figure 14.2 Anatomical language

General Rules of Body Movement

The definitions of body movement can be applied to most joints in the body, however, there are exceptions to the rule.

Flexion and extension occur in the sagittal plane. 'Flexion' is described as movement at a joint so that the anterior surfaces approximate. 'Extension' is described as movement at a joint so that the posterior surfaces approximate. The exception to this rule is the knee, whereby flexion of the knee is described by the posterior surfaces approximating and extension is described by the anterior surfaces approximating.

Adduction and abduction occur in the coronal plane. 'Adduction' is described as movement at a joint so that the distal segment moves towards the midline. 'Abduction' is described as movement at a joint so that the distal segment moves away from the midline. The term 'lateral flexion' is used when the segment is part of the midline of the body and moves from side to side.

Rotation occurs in the transverse plane. Rotation can be described as 'medial rotation', towards the midline of the body, or 'lateral rotation', away from the midline of the body.

Basic Biomechanics

The neuromusculoskeletal system can be likened to a machine. These components can combine to produce infinite movements and postures. The study of these movements is called 'biomechanics' or 'functional anatomy'.

In order to understand biomechanics, each section of the body needs to be discussed separately. The skeleton is divided into the axial and appendicular skeleton. The axial skeleton consists of the skull, spine and the sacrum. The appendicular (refers to an appendage, for example the upper and lower limbs, or anything attached to a major part of the body) skeleton consists of the upper and lower limbs.

The Axial Skeleton

The spine protects the spinal cord, aids movement and locomotion and supports the erect posture. It has four curves: two curves are concave anteriorly, called kyphoses, and two curves are concave posteriorly, called lordoses (Figure 14.3). The thoracic and sacral kyphoses develop intrauterine and are present at birth. The cervical and lumbar lordoses develop once an infant begins to lift its head and sit up. The spine is curved to provide strength and elasticity, to act as a shock absorber to dissipate vertical compressive forces, and to reduce the demand on the surrounding musculature.

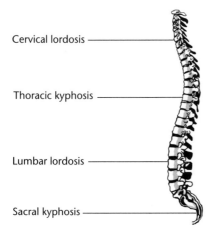

Cervical lordosis

Thoracic kyphosis

Lumbar lordosis

Sacral kyphosis

Figure 14.3 The curves of the spine

Typical vertebrae

A typical vertebra consists of a vertebral body and a vertebral arch. The vertebral body is anterior and functions as the weight-bearing component of the vertebra. The body increases in size from C1 to L5. An intervertebral disc separates each vertebral body, except at C0–C1 and C1–C2. The vertebral arch consists of two pedicles, which form the lateral aspect of the arch, and two fused laminae, which form the posterior aspect of the arch. When all the vertebrae are aligned, the vertebral canal is formed.

The vertebral arch has projections of bone that serve as attachment sites for ligaments and muscles as well as sites of articulation with adjacent vertebrae. These projections include the spinous process, which projects posteriorly, the transverse processes, which project laterally, and the superior and inferior articular processes, which project upwards and downwards from the vertebral arch respectively (Figure 14.4).

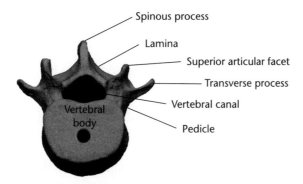

Spinous process

Lamina

Superior articular facet

Transverse process

Vertebral canal

Vertebral body

Pedicle

Figure 14.4 A typical vertebra

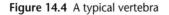
Part V

Functional spinal unit

A functional spinal unit consists of two adjacent vertebrae and all the components required for movement. These components are the intervertebral disc, which acts as a cushion between the vertebrae, the ligaments that stabilize the vertebrae, the muscles that surround the vertebrae, and the spinal nerves that exit between the vertebrae (Figure 14.5). In Figure 14.5, the ligaments and muscles have been removed to illustrate the interaction between two vertebrae and the intervertebral disc.

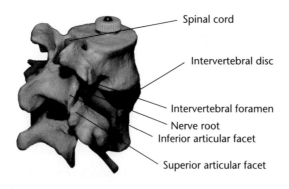

— Spinal cord

Intervertebral disc

Intervertebral foramen
Nerve root
Inferior articular facet

Superior articular facet

Figure 14.5 A functional spinal unit

Muscular control of range of motion

When a muscle is activated and required to lift a load, it shortens. Contraction that permits the muscle to shorten is termed 'concentric contraction'. Controlled lengthening of a muscle is termed 'eccentric contraction'. For example, lifting a coffee cup from the table requires the biceps brachii muscle to shorten to get the coffee cup from the table to your lips. However, when you want to put the coffee cup back on the table, the biceps brachii muscle is still active. The biceps brachii muscle will control the movement of replacing the cup, thus although it is still active, it is lengthening.

When each joint is moved through its range of motion, the following are required:

1. A muscle to initiate the movement.
2. A muscle to control the movement.
3. A limiting factor, which can be the bones in the joint itself, the ligaments and joint capsule that surround the joint or the elastic limitations of the muscles moving the joint.

The cervical spine

The cervical spine is a very mobile part of the body and has the greatest disc height to body ratio to increase the range of motion possible between the vertebrae. The cervical spine consists of seven vertebrae, five of which are typical cervical spine vertebrae and two of which are atypical vertebrae.

The five typical vertebrae are C3 to C7. They have the same structure as all other vertebrae, but with a few distinct features. Each transverse process has a transverse foramen, which contains the vertebral artery. The vertebral artery passes through the transverse foramen from C6 to C1. The cervical spinous processes are bifid to allow more surface area for muscle attachments.

The two atypical vertebrae are C1 (atlas) and C2 (axis) (Figure 14.6). The joint between the occiput of the skull and C1 is designed for a rocking motion of the head, for example jutting your chin forward and pulling your chin back. The joint between C1 and C2 is designed for maximum rotation around the dens of C2, and 50% of cervical spine rotation occurs at this joint. Table 14.1 outlines the ranges of motion of the cervical spine, where all normal ranges are measured using a digital inclinometer and taken from the neutral anatomical position.

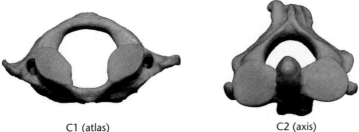

C1 (atlas)   C2 (axis)

Figure 14.6 C1 and C2 vertebrae

Table 14.1 Ranges of motion of the cervical spine and the muscles that initiate, control and limit the movement

Motion	Normal range	Muscles
Flexion	80–90°	■ Initiated by concentric contraction of neck flexors ■ Controlled by eccentric contraction of neck extensors ■ Limited by the elastic limits of the neck extensors as well as supraspinous, interspinous and ligamentum flavum ligaments
Extension	70°	■ Initiated by concentric contraction of neck extensors ■ Controlled by eccentric contraction of neck flexors ■ Limited by facets and anterior longitudinal ligament
Lateral flexion	20–45°	■ Initiated by sternocleidomastoid, scalenes, trapezius ■ Controlled by eccentric contraction of contralateral (opposite side) musculature ■ Limited by facets, uncinate processes and intertransverse ligaments
Rotation	70–90°	■ Initiated by rotatores, multifidus, sternocleidomastoid, scalenes, trapezius ■ Controlled by eccentric contraction of contralateral musculature ■ Limited by facets, uncinate processes and intertransverse ligaments

The thoracic spine

The thoracic spine is the least mobile part of the spine, partly due to the ribs stabilizing the thoracic spine and partly due to the shallow intervertebral discs. The thoracic spine consists of twelve vertebrae. Although each thoracic vertebra is built the same, there are differences in the articulation between the body of the vertebrae and the rib heads. There are twelve pairs of ribs. All ribs articulate with the vertebrae posteriorly. Ribs 1–7 articulate through costal cartilage with the sternum anteriorly, ribs 8–10 articulate with the margins of the cartilage above and ribs 11–12 are called 'floating ribs' as they do not articulate with anything anteriorly. The ribs protect the viscera or organs and aid breathing. Table 14.2 outlines the ranges of motion of the thoracic spine, where all normal ranges are measured using a digital inclinometer and taken from the neutral anatomical position.

Table 14.2 Ranges of motion of the thoracic spine and the muscles that initiate, control and limit the movement

Motion	Normal range	Muscles
Flexion	20–45°	■ Initiated by concentric contraction of rectus abdominis ■ Controlled/limited by eccentric contraction of erector spinae and elastic limits of muscle tissue
Extension	25–45°	■ Initiated by concentric contraction of erector spinae ■ Controlled by eccentric contraction of rectus abdominis ■ Limited by bony impact and muscles
Lateral flexion	20–40°	■ Initiated by concentric contraction of ipsilateral (same side) erector spinae and quadratus lumborum muscles ■ Controlled by eccentric contraction of contralateral (opposite side) erector spinae and quadratus lumborum muscles ■ Limited by facet, capsules and ligaments
Rotation	35–50°	■ Initiated by concentric contraction of ipsilateral erector spinae, multifidii and rotatores muscles ■ Controlled by concentric and eccentric contraction of abdominal oblique muscles ■ Limited by ligaments, facets and bilateral segmental and nonsegmental muscles

The lumbar spine

The lumbar spine is subject to greater loads than the rest of the spine, so it receives a lot of attention clinically and experimentally. It is largely responsible for trunk mobility and therefore experiences significant mechanical demands that require powerful muscle action. There are five lumbar vertebrae. They can be distinguished from other vertebrae by their large size. Table 14.3 outlines the ranges of motion of the lumbar spine, where all normal ranges are measured using a digital inclinometer and taken from the neutral anatomical position.

Table 14.3 Ranges of motion of the lumbar spine and the muscles that initiate, control and limit the movement

Motion	Normal range	Muscles
Flexion	40–60°	<ul><li>Initiated by concentric contraction of psoas and abdominal muscles</li><li>Controlled by eccentric contraction of erector spinae (sacrospinalis)</li><li>Limited by ligamentum flavum, posterior longitudinal ligament, supraspinous and interspinous ligaments</li></ul>
Extension	20–35°	<ul><li>Initiated by concentric contraction of sacrospinalis (gravity helps)</li><li>Controlled by eccentric contraction of abdominal muscles</li><li>Limited by anterior longitudinal ligament and spinous process and facet impaction</li></ul>
Lateral flexion	15–20°	<ul><li>Initiated and controlled by quadratus lumborum (erector spinae may have both concentric and eccentric roles)</li><li>Limited by facet impact, ligaments and fascia</li></ul>
Rotation	3–18°	<ul><li>Initiated by concentric contraction of abdominal obliques and assisted by contralateral (opposite side) mutifidii and rotators muscles</li><li>Controlled/limited by eccentric contraction of ipsilateral (same side) multifidii and rotators muscles</li></ul>

The sacrum and coccyx

The sacrum consists of five fused vertebrae. It is triangular in shape with the apex pointing inferiorly. It is curved and is concave anteriorly, creating a kyphosis. The coccyx consists of four fused vertebrae and it articulates with the apex of the sacrum.

The Appendicular Skeleton

The pelvis

The pelvis consists of three bones – two innominate bones and the sacrum. It is a three-joint complex comprising two sacroiliac joints and the pubic symphysis. The sacroiliac joint is most probably the least understood and most controversial joint of the body. It is not designed for a wide range of motion and its mobility is limited to approximately two degrees. The two surfaces of the joint are not smooth, but have a groove and a crest that lock together for stabilization of the joint. No muscle acts specifically to produce active movements at this joint. The sacroiliac joints are presumed to be stress-relieving joints in the pelvic girdle and aid locomotion.

Part V

The pubic symphysis is an extremely strong joint, which is well stabilized by its design as well as by ligaments surrounding the joint. The joint moves passively when the pelvis moves during locomotion.

The hip

The hip is one of the largest and most stable joints of the body. The accetabulum or the pelvic side of the joint is deep and lined with cartilage to act as a shock absorber, thus the joint is made stable at the expense of range of motion. The head of the femur fits into the accetabulum and is surrounded by strong ligaments and bursa (a fluid-filled cushion). There are many large muscle groups that move the hip (Table 14.4).

Table 14.4 Muscles acting on the hip joint to initiate movement

Actions	Muscles
Flexion	Iliopsoas (primary hip flexor), sartorius, rectus femoris, tensor fascia lata, gracilis and pectineus
Extension	Gluteus maximus (primary hip extensor), gluteus medius and hamstrings
Abduction	Tensor fascia lata, gluteus medius and minimus and piriformis
Adduction	Hip adductors, pectineus and gracilis
External rotation	Piriformis, gamelli, obturators and quadratus femoris
Internal rotation	Tensor fascia lata, gluteus medius and minimus and gracilis

The knee

The knee joint is well stabilized by ligaments and muscle. It is a flexible joint to assist locomotion and foot placement during walking.

The ankle and foot

The components of the foot and ankle work together to form an intricate functional unit. The unit is an important part of the kinematic chain that works together to provide propulsion during locomotion and balance. The foot and ankle play an important part in weight bearing. The bones of the foot and ankle lock together with the help of ligaments to produce a flexible, but stable surface for weight bearing.

The shoulder complex

The shoulder complex consists of three joints and one articulation, which function in unison to produce shoulder movement. There are three anatomical joints – the glenohumeral joint, the acromioclavicular joint and the sternoclavicular joint.

There is one physiologic articulation between the anterior surface of the scapula and the thoracic cage, the scapulothoracic articulation, which is an integral part of shoulder function. The anatomy of the shoulder allows for a large range of motion, at the expense of stability. The function of the shoulder is to work in unison with the elbow to allow accurate hand placement.

The shoulder is complex and relies on small muscle groups to produce the full range of motion. It is difficult to investigate exactly what would initiate, control and limit shoulder movement; however, there are four major shoulder muscles that are active in all ranges of movement. These muscles are the supraspinatus, infraspinatus, teres minor and subscapularis – collectively called the rotator cuff muscles (Table 14.5).

Table 14.5 Rotator cuff muscles of the shoulder and their actions

Rotator cuff muscle	Action
Supraspinatus	Initiates abduction and supports the shoulder joint
Infraspinatus	Lateral rotation of the arm at the shoulder joint and stabilization of the shoulder joint capsule
Teres minor	Lateral rotation of the humerus at the shoulder joint
Subscapularis	Medial rotation of the arm at the shoulder joint and assists in adduction. Stabilization of the shoulder joint

The elbow

The elbow consists of two joints. Flexion and extension occurs at the humeroulnar joint, and elbow rotation, otherwise known as supination and pronation, occurs at the humeroradial joint. The function of the elbow is to work in conjunction with the shoulder for accurate hand placement.

The wrist and hand

The wrist and hand consist of a series of complex, intricate and delicate joints. These joints act as a single unit to provide dexterity and precision.

Activity

The ranges of motion in Tables 14.1, 14.2 and 14.3 are given in degrees and are determined using digital inclinometers. This is not practicable in a practice setting as the equipment is costly and time-consuming to use. Reflect and make brief notes on other methods of measurement that can be used in a clinical setting to get an idea of range of motion.

Tables 14.6, 14.7 and 14.8 give clinical ways of testing movement.

Part V

Table 14.6 Cervical spine range of motion

Motion	Notes
Flexion	Extreme range of motion is normally found when the chin is able to reach the chest with the mouth closed; however, up to two fingers width between chin and chest is considered normal
Extension	Normally the plane of the forehead and the nose is nearly horizontal
Lateral flexion	NB: Ensure that the ear moves towards the shoulder and not the shoulder towards the ear. How far the ear is from the shoulder can be measured
Rotation	The chin does not quite reach the plane of the shoulder

Table 14.7 Thoracic spine range of motion

Motion	Notes
Flexion	Can use tape measure to measure difference between two points from standing to forward flexion: measure from C7 to T12 standing, then get the person to flex forwards and measure again. The measurement should increase by at least 2.7cm. Finger floor distance (FFD) can also be noted
Extension	Can use tape measure. Difference in measurement standing to extension: C7 to T12 = 2.5cm
Lateral flexion	Run hand down the side of the leg as far as possible without flexion or extension. Can measure FFD

Table 14.8 Lumbar spine range of motion

Motion	Notes
Flexion	NB: Some people can touch their toes even with no movement in the spine, for example gymnasts and ballet dancers where the movement comes from the hips and not the back. Should move from normal lordosis to at least straight or slightly flexed curve. Difference in measurement standing to flexion: T12 to S1 = 7–8cm
Lateral flexion	Run hand down side of leg as far as possible without flexion or extension. Can measure FFD

Chapter Summary

This chapter has explored the basic biomechanics of the body. It has referred to the body planes and body movement, the components of a functional spinal unit, the axial and appendicular skeleton, the basic biomechanics of each spinal section of the axial skeleton, movements in each spinal section of the axial skeleton and the functions of each joint of the appendicular skeleton.

REVIEW QUESTIONS

1 Can you name the following?
   – the planes of the body, with a brief description of each plane
   – the movements of the body, giving examples of each movement
   – the curves of the spine, specifying when each curve develops
   – the movement at each of the atypical cervical vertebrae.

2 What initiates, controls and limits movement in each area of the spine?

3 What is the function of the pelvis and how do the joints differ from normal synovial joints?

4 What musculature acts around the shoulder complex?

CHAPTER LINKS

For further discussion of problems of the musculoskeletal and integumentary systems, see Chapter 17.

FURTHER RESOURCES

Anatomy

Drake, R.L., Vogl, W. and Mitchell, A.W. (2005) *Gray's Anatomy for Students*, Toronto, Elsevier.

Palastanga, N., Soames, R.W. and Field, D. (2006) *Anatomy and Human Movement: Structure and Function*, Oxford, Butterworth Heinemann.

Sambrook, P., Schrieber, L., Taylor, T., Ellis, A. (2001) *The Musculoskeletal System*, London, Churchill Livingstone.

Biomechanics

Kapandji, I.A. (1974) *The Physiology of the Joints*, New York, Churchill Livingstone.

Levangie, P.K. and Norkin, C.C. (2001) *Joint Structure and Function: A Comprehensive Analysis*, 3rd edn, Philadelphia, PA, FA Davis.

Magee, D.J. (1997) *Orthopaedic Physical Assessment,* 3rd edn, Philadelphia, PA, WB Saunders.

Part V

15 Cardiovascular, Respiratory and Urinary Systems

JASON TSAI

Learning outcomes

By the end of this chapter, you should have a basic understanding of:

- the anatomy and physiology of cardiovascular systems
- cardiovascular system disorders
- the respiratory system and commonly seen disorders
- the anatomy and physiology of the kidney and its functions
- urinary system disorders

This chapter deals with some of the basic functions of the cardiovascular, respiratory and urinary systems. It uses practice examples to illustrate how these systems function. The purpose of these practice examples is to illustrate some of the major pathological aspects of these systems. Several of these highlight how the complementary practitioner should respond to conditions that require conventional medical intervention. It is important for the complementary practitioner to recognize and work confidently across this boundary between complementary and conventional practice.

Cardiovascular System

Anatomy and Physiology

The heart is like a pump that keeps the blood flow running smoothly and continuously in the blood vessels and bringing oxygen and nutrients to every cell.

There are four chambers in the heart – right atrium, right ventricle, left atrium and left ventricle (Figure 15.1). Apart from the four chambers, there are valves to keep the blood flowing in one direction when the heart contracts. Several blood vessels are connected to the heart so that the supply of oxygen and nutrients to the cells and disposal of waste through blood flow can be performed.

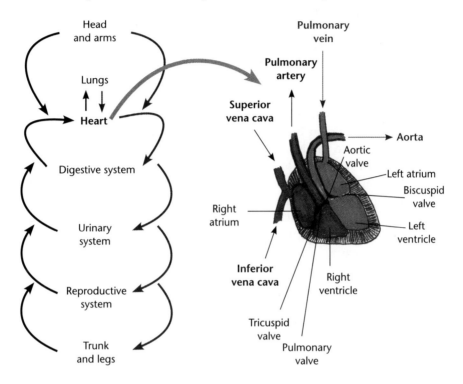

Figure 15.1 The heart and circulatory system

There are three different types of blood vessels – artery, vein and capillary. An **artery** is a blood vessel that carries blood away from the heart to the peripheral capillaries. A **capillary** is a small blood vessel, between an arteriole (small artery) and a **venule** (small vein), whose thin wall allows the diffusion of gases (mainly oxygen and carbon dioxide), nutrients and wastes between plasma and interstitial fluid. A **vein** is a blood vessel that carries blood from the capillary bed towards the heart. **Interstitial fluid** is the fluid in the tissues that fills the spaces between cells.

We now outline how the heart's circulatory system works. The aorta, the large elastic artery, carries oxygenated blood (blood full of oxygen) from the left ventricle through small arteries, arterioles and capillaries to the cells. Deoxygenated blood (blood lacking in oxygen) is then carried through capillaries, venules, small veins, the superior vena cava (SVC) and the inferior vena cava (IVC) and back to the right atrium of the heart. This pathway through which blood is carried from the heart to the body and back to the heart is called the 'systemic circuit'. When the right atrium contracts, blood in the right atrium is pumped into the right ventricle. When the right ventricle contracts, blood is pumped into the pulmonary (of, or relating to or affecting the lungs) artery. The tricuspid valve prevents blood from flowing back into the right atrium when the ventricle contracts. After contracting, the atrium or the ventricle needs to relax so that another contraction can take place. When the right atrium relaxes, blood flows in from the SVC and the IVC. When the right ventricle relaxes, blood will not flow back to the ventricle from the pulmonary artery because the pulmonary valve only allows blood to flow in one direction. So when the right ventricle relaxes, blood can only flow into the ventricle from the right atrium. The pulmonary artery carries deoxygenated blood from the heart to the lungs, and gas exchange takes place in the lungs (this will be discussed later in the respiratory system section). After gas exchange, blood becomes oxygenated through our breathing activity. Oxygenated blood is then carried away from the lungs to the left atrium of the heart by the pulmonary vein. The pathway through which the blood is carried from the heart to the lungs and back to the heart again is called the 'pulmonary circuit'. When the left atrium contracts, blood is pumped into the left ventricle, and then into the aorta when the left ventricle contracts. The mitral valve, also known as bicuspid valve, is in between the left atrium and the left ventricle and the aortic valve is in between the left ventricle and the aorta.

Cardiovascular System Disorders

We now move on to discuss a range of heart problems.

Arrhythmias

The heart beats regularly because there is a natural pacemaker in the heart to control the heartbeat. This natural pacemaker is a small area of tissue located in the right atrium called the sinoatrial node (SA node). The SA node sends electrical impulses that initially cause both right atrium and left atrium to contract, and then it activates the atrioventricular node (AV node), which is the only electric connection between the atria and the ventricles under normal conditions. The impulse will then spread through both left and right ventricles via the bundle of His and the Purkinje fibres to cause both ventricles to contract. And then the pulse can be felt.

When the SA node is not functioning properly, or another electric impulse is sent from somewhere other than the SA node, then the rhythm of the heartbeat will be affected and arrhythmia happens. Arrhythmia means an irregular rhythm of heartbeats, which can be tachycardia (faster than normal, more than 100 beats/min) or bradycardia (slower than normal, less than 60 beats/min). We might or might not be able to feel the arrhythmia. The most common symptom of arrhythmia is palpitations, which can be due to stress or heart problems. Some palpitations may be harmless, but many of them are indicative of adverse outcomes, or even sudden death. It is therefore important that we differentiate the underlying causes of arrhythmias, and, if in doubt, we should refer the patient to medical professionals. The simplest and most specific diagnosis to assess the heart rhythm is by an electrocardiogram (ECG).

Mr M, 58 years old, is the ex-CEO of a dot com company. He suffered a stroke three months ago due to a cerebral haemorrhage. Table 15.1 shows his typical daily food and drink consumption for the past 15 years.

Table 15.1 Eating patterns and cerebral haemorrhage

Time	Food/drink intake
06.45	2 rashers of bacon, 2 sausages, 1 tomato, 2 pieces of toast with butter, 1 poached egg, baked beans, 1 cup of English breakfast tea with white sugar and full fat milk
09.00	1 cup of coffee with brown sugar and full milk, 1 chocolate bar
11.00	1 cup of coffee with brown sugar and full milk, 1 small chocolate muffin
13.00	2 rounds of sandwiches with bacon and eggs, 1 cup of black coffee
15.00	1 cup of tea with white sugar and milk
18.00	Roast beef /lamb/pork, mashed potato (or 6 roast potatoes), carrots and broccoli
21.00	A bowl of cornflakes with full milk

Explore the possible factors that resulted in the cerebral haemorrhage, and explain in detail why.

Hypertension

Practice example

A 56-year-old female patient came to the clinic complaining of shoulder pain. When her blood pressure was checked, it surprised us that her blood pressure was 180/120 mmHg, which is classified as severe hypertension. However, she did not realize her blood pressure was so high. We suggested that the patient should go to see her GP for a further medical checkup.

The classification of hypertension is given in Table 15.2. When a patient comes into a clinic, practitioners are strongly recommended to check the patient's blood pressure. If a patient's diastolic pressure is higher than 145 mmHg, practitioners are urged to call an ambulance because when diastolic pressure reaches such a high level, it means the blood vessel can burst at any time. However, first we need to calm the patient down and explain why we need to seek medical help. Ideally, there should be a person looking after the patient when the practitioner or staff member seeks medical help.

Table 15.2 British Hypertension Society classification of blood pressure levels

	Systolic (mmHg)	Diastolic (mmHg)
Optimal	<120	<80
Normal	<130	<85
High-normal	130–139	85–89
Mild hypertension (grade 1)	140–159	90–99
Moderate hypertension (grade 2)	160–179	100–109
Severe hypertension (grade 3)	≥180	≥110
Isolated systolic hypertension (grade 1)	140–159	<90
Isolated systolic hypertension (grade 2)	≥160	<90

Hypertension can be primary (90–95%) or secondary (5–10%). The mechanisms of controlling blood pressure are illustrated in Figure 15.2. Some disorders can cause secondary hypertension, such as kidney disorders and tumour of pituitary gland. Control of blood pressure is also discussed in the urinary system and the endocrine system.

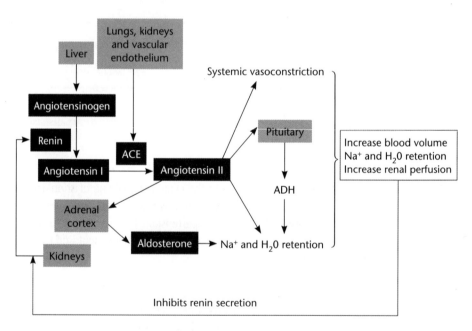

Key: ACE = angiotensin-converting enzyme; ADH = antidiuretic hormone

Figure 15.2 The control of blood pressure

Heart failure

According to the European Society of Cardiology (2005), heart failure is defined as:

The presence of heart failure symptoms (at rest or during exercise), together with objective evidence of cardiac dysfunction (preferably by echocardiography). In cases of doubt a response to treatment is required.

Practice example

A 74-year-old male patient came to the clinic complaining about low back pain. Checking his pulse, I could immediately feel that it was irregularly irregular. We provided the acupuncture treatment for his low back pain, which was unrelated to the irregular pulse, and suggested that he should visit his GP to seek medical advice about the underlying cause of the irregular pulse. An irregular pulse indicates an irregular heartbeat, suggesting there might be a problem in the heart. The GP referred him to a cardiologist and he received treatment for the irregularly irregular pulse.

Practice example

A 67-year-old female patient came to the clinic for the treatment of dystonia (a neurological movement disorder). She had a regular pulse, but it was a pulsus alternans (a pulse with alternating strong and weak pulse waves on consecutive beats – a sign of left ventricle dysfunction).

Having read the above two cases, we need to discuss the causes and clinical features of heart failure so that professional advice and/or appropriate treatment can be provided.

The causes of heart failure can include: ischaemic heart disease, valvular heart disease, dilated cardiomyopathy, cigarette smoking, hypertension, obesity, diabetes, long-term anaemia, myocarditis, and infiltration of amyloidosis.

The clinical features of left heart failure are predominantly fatigue, haemoptysis (coughing up blood), dyspnoea (difficulty in breathing) during exertion, orthopnoea (difficulty in breathing when lying down), and paroxysmal nocturnal dyspnoea. Physical signs are few and not prominent until a later stage. These include central cyanosis, peripheral cyanosis, cardiomegaly (enlarged heart), galloping rhythm during auscultation, and crackles heard at the lung bases.

The clinical features of right heart failure include peripheral oedema (especially pitting oedema), frequent nocturia (urination at night), ascites (fluid accumulated in the abdominal cavity) and coagulopathy (delayed blood clotting). The physical signs can include hepatomegaly (enlarged liver), splenomegaly (enlarged spleen), raised jugular venous pressure and hepatojugular reflex.

Atherosclerosis

Blood vessels have three layers: tunica adventitia (outer layer), tunica media (middle layer) and tunica intima (inner layer). Atherosclerosis (hardening of the blood vessels) is a disease of the tunica intima of the arteries, especially the large arteries, that leads to fatty lesions called atheromatous plaques or atherosclerotic plaques. Atherosclerosis may result in the following complications: calcification of blood vessels, ulcers and thrombosis. Atherosclerosis seriously affects the following three arteries:

1. *coronary artery:* thrombosis leads to coronary heart disease (CHD), which is also known as ischaemic heart disease (IHD) (ischaemia means deficiency of blood supply).
2. *cerebral arteries:* atherosclerosis may result in acute and chronic ischaemia, infarction and stroke.
3. *aorta:* atherosclerosis in the aorta, especially the abdominal aorta, may lead to aneurysm (see below).

Atherosclerosis may also result in gangrene, intracranial haemorrhage, chronic ischaemia of the kidneys and hypertension.

A number of the factors influencing the risk of and susceptibility to atherosclerosis are interrelated. Age, sex and heredity are the three endogenous factors affecting the risk of atherosclerosis and IHD.

Research on epidemiology, according to the Framingham report, has shown that several risk factors are linked to atherosclerosis and IHD. These include hypercholesterolaemia, hypertension, smoking and diabetes mellitus.

Hypercholesterolaemia

Several lines of evidence have demonstrated that hypercholesterolaemia (high cholesterol level in the blood) is related to atherosclerosis. Atherosclerotic plaques normally contain a large amount of cholesterol and cholesterol ester. Diseases prone to hypercholesterolaemia, such as familial hypercholesterolaemia, will result in premature atherosclerosis as well as IHD. The higher the concentration of cholesterol in the plasma, the higher the chances of IHD appear. Two major factors affecting the increase of the concentration of cholesterol in plasma are diet and lipoproteins:

1. A diet high in fat, especially cholesterol and saturated fats: the major organ of cholesterol synthesis in mammals is the liver, although some amounts of cholesterol are also formed by the intestine. About two-thirds of cholesterol in plasma is endogenous and only one-third is exogenous. High cholesterol and saturated fats in the diet will result in an increase in the concentration of cholesterol in plasma.
2. Low-density lipoprotein: cholesterol and triglycerides (also known as triacylglycerols) and other lipids transported in body fluids are lipoproteins. These lipoproteins are classified into six categories: chylomicrons, chylomicron remnants, very low-density lipoproteins (VLDL), low-density lipoproteins (LDL), intermediate-density lipoproteins (IDL) and high-density lipoproteins (HDL). The role of LDL is to transport cholesterol to peripheral tissues and regulate de novo cholesterol synthesis. Cholesterol is a component of all

eukaryotic plasma membranes and is essential for the growth and viability of cells in higher organisms. Several lines of evidence have shown that the higher the amount of LDL in plasma, the higher the risk of ischaemic heart disease occurring. In contrast, the higher the amount of HDL in the plasma, the lower the risk of ischaemic heart disease occurring, because HDL can clear out the cholesterol deposited in the walls of blood vessels.

Hypertension

Hypercholesterolaemia is the main risk factor of atherosclerosis for persons younger than 45 years of age. However, hypertension will be the main factor of atherosclerosis and IHD for people older than 45.

Smoking

Smoking and IHD are strongly related, according to some research data. This relationship culminates between the ages of 35 and 55. When smokers stop smoking for several years, the risk of IHD occurring will be lowered and can be comparable to the risk to non-smokers.

Diabetes mellitus

People suffering from diabetes mellitus are at an increased risk for the formation and development of atherosclerosis, especially women, according to research data.

Besides these four main risk factors, there are some minor risk factors affecting the development of atherosclerosis. They include:

- lack of exercise
- lifestyle
- taking oral contraceptives
- obesity
- too much carbohydrate in diet
- hyperuricaemia
- drinking soft water.

The development of atherosclerosis may lead to ischaemia (lack of oxygen) of local tissues. If atherosclerosis occurs in the coronary arteries, the heart muscle will become ischaemic, resulting in two commonly seen heart disorders: angina pectoris and myocardial infarction.

Angina pectoris

Angina pectoris is chest pain caused by an inadequate supply of blood to the heart. Most patients with angina complain about chest pain, and this kind of pain is described as heavy, tight or gripping. The anginal pain is typically central/retrosternal and may radiate to the back, neck, jaw and/or left shoulder and sometimes to the left arm or left fingers.

Myocardial infarction

Myocardial infarction (MI), also known as heart attack, occurs when the blood supply to the heart or part of the heart is interrupted. This is mostly due to a blockage in the coronary artery as a result of a rupture of an atherosclerotic plaque with a thrombus.

Patients with MI typically present with severe chest pain, similar to angina. The onset is sudden, and often occurs at rest and the chest pain can last constantly for hours. The pain is so severe that the patient is afraid of imminent death. Some patients with MI do not have pain at all. MI is often accompanied with breathlessness, sweating (especially in the forehead), nausea, vomiting and restlessness. However, some patients might not have these symptoms. Here, I would like to share with you the following four cases reported in the health column of the *United Daily News* (a newspaper published in the Republic of China).

Practice example

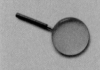

Case One

A 55-year-old taxi driver has been suffering from a stiff neck and shoulder for some time. However, he did not pay any attention to these symptoms because he thought they were because of sitting behind the steering wheel for a long time. He did not seek any medical advice, until one day, he had difficulty in breathing, so he called an ambulance. By the time he arrived at the hospital, he was suffering from crushing pain in the chest, sweat on the forehead, difficulty in talking and could not breathe properly. An ECG and a blood test indicated that he had suffered an MI. He was immediately transferred to the intensive care unit and cardiac catheterization confirmed an MI. After proper medical treatment, he no longer suffers from a stiff neck.

Case Two

A 60-year-old male patient had been suffering from left earache. The earache started not long after he began to walk and stopped after having a rest. He saw an ENT specialist, but no underlying cause of the left earache had been found. He was eventually referred to a cardiologist, and all the medical examinations confirmed MI.

Case Three

A 70-year-old female patient felt pain in the tongue, especially during exercise. Medical examinations showed her pain in the tongue was due to angina pectoris.

Case Four

A 53-year-old male had been suffering toothache (lower left molar). The dentist found nothing wrong with his teeth. Medical investigations confirmed the pain sensation in the lower left molar was due to myocardial ischaemia.

From the above four case studies, we can conclude the following characteristics of MI:

1. Patients suffering from angina or MI will normally have the symptom of chest pain and the pain may radiate to the left shoulder, arm or even fingers.
2. Myocardial infarction may be **asymptomatic** or there may be symptoms other than chest pain, such as toothache, stiff neck, neck pain, pain in the tongue, pain in the jaw, pain in the left arm, left fingers, upper abdomen and so on. However, these symptoms share a common feature: the pain may become worse on exertion and may be alleviated after a rest.
3. The sensory nerve fibres from the heart's connective tissue and blood vessels travel through the cardiac plexus to the dorsal roots and ganglia of T1–T4 spinal nerves. The cutaneous distribution of these spinal nerves goes to the neck, jaw, shoulders, arms and stomach. Therefore, MI may cause pain in different areas, known as 'referred pain'.

Aneurysm

An aneurysm is a blood-filled sac that is localized in a weakened part of a blood vessel. Aneurysms most commonly occur in the arteries, especially arteries in the brain and the aorta. As the size of an aneurysm increases, the risk of rupture of the aneurysm increases. When the rupture occurs, it can cause severe haemorrhage and sudden death may occur. Let's look at the case below.

Practice example

Mrs P, a 53-year-old housewife, had a severe headache and difficulty in breathing after dinner. Shortly after, she collapsed and was rushed to hospital by ambulance. She became unconscious and her right pupil was dilated when she arrived at the hospital. A brain CT scan revealed a haemorrhage in the subarachnoidal layer and intracranial haematoma. Cerebral angiography confirmed the rupture of an aneurysm. An urgent operation was carried out to remove the aneurysm and clear the blood clot, which saved her life.

One year later, Mrs P's 34-year-old son, a computer programmer, suddenly had a severe headache shortly before he left for work. He felt dizzy and briefly lost consciousness. When he arrived at hospital, he complained about a severe headache and stiff neck. A brain CT scan revealed a subarachnoidal haemorrhage, which was confirmed by medical image to be due to the rupture of an aneurysm.

Part V

The symptoms of aneurysm depend on its size, its growth rate and the location. Unfortunately, most of the aneurysm is asymptomatic until it ruptures. The main symptom of the rupture is sudden and severe pain in the local area. So when a patient suffers from sudden severe pain without any known cause, it is strongly suggested that we refer the patient to A&E.

Artery dissection

Artery dissection is a tear in the wall of artery. Most of the dissection occurs in the aorta – aortic dissection. However, artery dissection can occur in other regions as well. Dissection is due to the blood penetrating the tunica intima and entering the tunica media. Most patients with artery dissection present a symptom of severe pain that has a sudden onset. If this dissection occurs in the aorta, some cardiovascular symptoms and signs may become apparent, such as change of blood pressure.

Practice example

During sexual intercourse with his wife, a 29-year-old engineer shouted 'Ouch'. The low back pain came out of the blue. He thought it was just a muscular pain and so did not pay it any attention, and went to work the following morning. The low back pain become more severe and two days later the pain had extended to the upper back. He was rushed to hospital, and medical examinations found that he had suffered from artery dissection. The dissection originated in the lumbar region and had moved up to the thoracic region behind the back.

Respiratory System

Anatomy and physiology

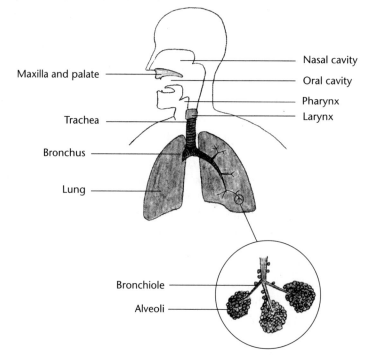

Figure 15.3 The respiratory system

The function of the respiratory system is to provide the body with a constant supply of oxygen and to remove carbon dioxide from the body. The respiratory system (Figure 15.3) can be further divided into the upper and lower respiratory tracts. The upper respiratory tract includes the nose, pharynx, larynx, oesophagus and the vocal cord. The lower respiratory tract consists of the trachea, bronchi and the lungs. The trachea can be divided into left and right bronchi, which further divide into small bronchi, terminal bronchioles and then respiratory bronchioles. The respiratory bronchioles divide further into alveolar ducts, which terminate in alveolar sacs whose chambers open to multiple individual alveoli.

Common Respiratory Conditions

We will now briefly discuss the most common respiratory conditions.

Asthma

Asthma is a chronic inflammatory condition of the lower respiratory tract whose cause is not fully understood. The main symptoms of asthma include cough, wheeze, tightness in the chest, shortness of breath, often worse at night. Asthma has the following characteristics: airflow limitation, hyperresponsiveness to a wide range of stimuli and inflammation of the bronchi.

Two major factors involved in the development of asthma are atopy and allergy, and airway hyperreactivity. There are also other stimuli that can precipitate an asthmatic attack. Atopy is a kind of hypersensitivity that affects parts of the body not in direct contact with allergens, and involves eczema, allergic rhinitis, allergic conjunctivitis and asthma. The **pathophysiology** of asthma is illustrated in Figure 15.4.

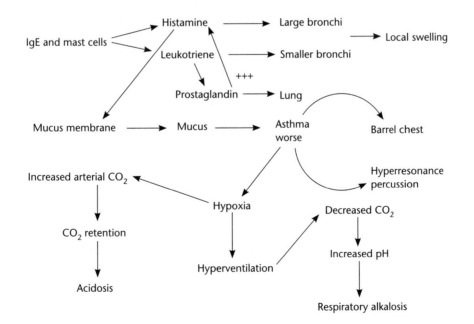

Figure 15.4 Pathophysiology of asthma

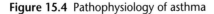

Chronic obstructive pulmonary disease

Chronic obstructive pulmonary disease (COPD) is an umbrella term used to describe patients with chronic bronchitis and emphysema.

Activity

> Mr H, 74 years old, is a retired electrician. He has been suffering from chronic bronchitis for 15 years. The latest medical examinations reveal that he suffers from pitting oedema, hepatomegaly, splenomegaly and cardiomegaly. Use the Further Resources at the end of the chapter, if necessary, to enable you to reflect on how the above symptoms and signs develop as a result of chronic bronchitis.

Chronic bronchitis

The definition of bronchitis is based upon the history, which is described as follows:

> Cough productive of sputum on most days for at least three months of the year for more than one year.

The pathophysiology of chronic bronchitis is shown in Figure 15.5.

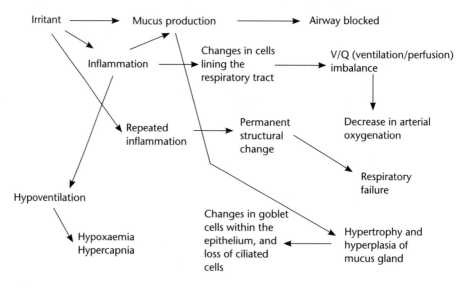

Figure 15.5 Pathophysiology of chronic bronchitis

Emphysema

Emphysema is defined on the basis of the pathological changes of the tissues as:

> Dilatation and destruction of the lung tissues distal to the terminal bronchioles.

Figure 15.6 describes the pathophysiology of emphysema.

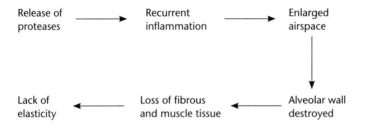

Figure 15.6 Pathophysiology of emphysema

Patients with COPD are classified into type A and type B, according to the clinical observation:

- Type A is the 'pink puffer'. Although the patient is breathless, the level of the arterial oxygen and carbon dioxide is relatively normal, and there is no cor pulmonale. This kind of patient is suffering predominantly from emphysema with little bronchitis.
- Type B is the 'blue bloater'. This type of patient does not suffer from breathlessness, but medical examination shows arterial hypoxia, the retention of carbon dioxide, polycythaemia (or erythrocytosis) and cor pulmonale.

NB: Cor pulmonale (pulmonary heart disease) is a change in the structure and function of the right ventricle of the heart due to a respiratory disorder, and is where right ventricular hypertrophy occurs.

Urinary System

Anatomy and physiology

The urinary system includes two kidneys, two ureters, one urinary bladder and one urethra (Figure 15.7).

The kidneys have numerous biological roles, but the primary one is maintaining the homeostasis of fluids and metabolites. The kidney comprises three parts: the renal cortex, renal medulla and renal pelvis. The nephron is the structural and functional unit of the kidney, which consists of the renal corpuscle and the renal tubule (see Figure 15.8). The renal corpuscle is composed of the glomerulus and Bowman's capsule. The renal tubule can be divided into three segments: the proximal tubule, the loop of Henle and the distal tubule. The glomerulus is a capillary tuft surrounded by Bowman's capsule.

The afferent arteriole carries the blood to the glomerulus and the efferent arteriole carries the blood out of the glomerulus. Because the size of the lumen in the afferent arteriole is bigger than that of the efferent arteriole, it naturally creates a pressure gradient and a process of ultrafiltration, through which fluids and soluble materials in the blood are forced out of the capillaries of the glomerulus and into Bowman's capsule. The fluids and soluble substances then go into the proximal tubule, through the loop of Henle, the distal tubule and finally reach the collecting duct. Glucose as well as varying amounts of water and soluble materials are reabsorbed in the renal tubules. The rest that is not reabsorbed goes into the collecting ducts as urine, into the ureters, and then to the bladder where the urine can be excreted to the exterior through the urethra.

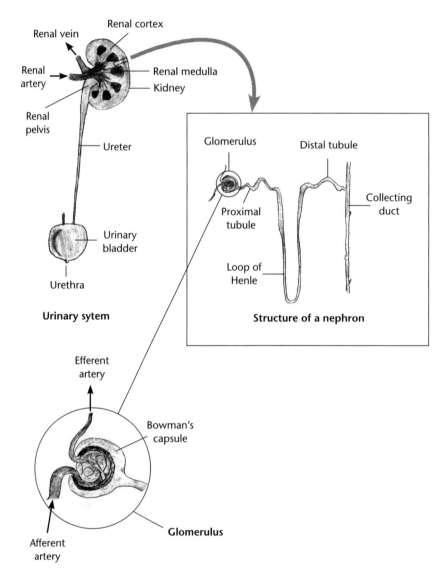

Figure 15.7 The urinary system

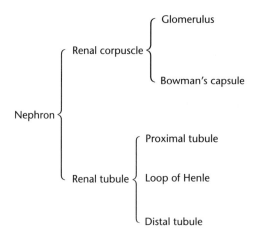

Figure 15.8 The basic structure of the nephron

The juxtaglomerular apparatus is a complex device that regulates the functions of each nephron. This device plays a vital role in controlling the reabsorption of water and electrolytes, especially sodium ions, thereby maintaining blood pressure.

When the blood pressure goes down as a result of a decrease in renal perfusion, this is detected by specific cells in the juxtaglomerular apparatus. The kidney will then secrete an enzyme called renin (sometimes called angiotensinogenase). Renin goes into the blood stream and hydrolyses angiotensinogen secreted by the liver into a polypeptide called angiotensin I. Angiotensin I is further cleaved into angiotensin II by the endothelial bound angiotensin-converting enzyme (ACE). Angiotensin II causes vasoconstriction and an increase of the secretion of antidiuretic hormone (ADH) and aldosterone, resulting in an increase in blood pressure. Aldosterone, a steroid hormone secreted by the adrenal cortex, acts on the distal tubules and the collecting ducts to cause reabsorption of sodium and secretion of potassium and water retention and increases the blood pressure.

Urinary System Disorders

We now move on to discuss some common kidney disorders.

Acute pyelonephritis

Pyelonephritis is an ascending urinary tract infection (UTI), which reaches the renal pelvis (pyelum). Most pyelonephritis is caused by the bacteria in the bowels entering the urinary tract. Female patients with diabetes mellitus or other renal disorders and pregnant women have a higher risk of acute pyelonephritis.

Clinical manifestations include urinary urgency, urinary frequency, burning sensation during urination, nocturia, dysuria, haematuria, cloudy urine, ammonia-like odour, fever, chills, nausea, flank pain, poor appetite, low back pain, fatigue.

Children may have nonspecific abdominal pain, and the elderly may develop other gastrointestinal and/or pulmonary signs and symptoms.

Complications include septic shock, chronic pyelonephritis, and renal insufficiency.

Renal failure

Before discussing renal failure, we have to define the renal failure. Renal failure is based upon the function of the kidney or, more precisely, the glomerular filtration rate (GFR) and creatinine clearance rate (Ccr). The American National Kidney Foundation (Levey et al., 2003) provides a guideline to define the kidney function according to the GFR (Table 15.3).

Table 15.3 Kidney functions and the glomerular filtration rate (GFR)

Stage	Description	GFR
1	Signs of mild kidney disease but with normal or better GFR	>90%
2	Mild kidney disease with reduced GFR	60–89%
3	Moderate chronic renal insufficiency	30–59%
4	Severe chronic renal insufficiency	15–29%
5	End-stage renal failure	<15%

Renal failure can broadly be classified into two categories: acute and chronic renal failure. Acute renal failure implies a rapidly progressive loss of renal function characterized by decreased production of urine (oliguria). Chronic renal failure is stage 5 kidney disease, which develops slowly and shows few symptoms in the beginning.

Acute renal failure

The causes of acute renal failure can be classified into three categories, depending upon the locations of the cause: prerenal failure, intrarenal failure and post-renal failure.

Prerenal failure can be caused by cardiovascular disorders, hypovolaemia (decrease in volume of circulating blood), peripheral vasodilation, and reno-vascular obstruction. Prerenal failure results in hypoperfusion, leading to hypoxaemia and irreversible damage to the kidney. One of major by-products of the metabolism of protein is urea. When kidney function fails, excessive amounts of urea and other nitrogenous wastes accumulate in the blood, leading to azotaemia. Kidney failure also leads to metabolic acidosis as a result of the failure of adequate excretion of various acid anions due to the reduced number of functioning nephrons.

Intrarenal failure can be caused by toxicity, inflammation and ischaemia. Intrarenal failure is also called intrinsic or parenchymal failure as a result of damage to the nephrons. If the damage is caused by nephrotoxicity or inflammation, it will become chronic renal failure. If the damage is due to ischaemia, it results in ischaemic parenchymal damage and renal azotaemia.

Analgesic nephropathy is a special term used to describe the use of NSAIDs (nonsteroid anti-inflammatory drugs) which causes renal toxicity. Acute tubular necrosis (ATN) accounts for 75% of acute renal failure. The cause of ATN can be divided into two groups: ischaemic ATN and nephrotoxic ATN. ATN typically does not produce any specific signs and symptoms.

Obstruction in the urinary bladder, ureters or urethra belongs to postrenal failure.

Chronic renal failure

Causes of chronic renal failure include chronic glomerular disease (for example glomerulonephritis), chronic infection (for example pyelonephritis), vascular disease (for example atherosclerosis), obstruction (for example renal calculi), congenital anomalies (for example polycystic kidney disease), collagen disease (for example Marfan syndrome), nephrotoxic agents (for example NSAIDs, aminoglycoside therapy), and endocrine disease (for example diabetes mellitus).

Chronic renal failure is progressive. The kidneys can still maintain a relatively good function until more than 75% of the nephrons are not functioning. This results in an increased workload for the rest of the 'normal' or 'almost normal' nephrons. Acid-base imbalance, decrease in sodium and water reabsorption and tubular acidosis all increase the burden on the functional nephrons, especially the glomeruli. This eventually causes the glomeruli to become sclerotic and not functional, which results in toxins accumulating in the body, leading to fatal changes to the major organs.

Clinical features of chronic renal failure include hypervolaemia (an increase in volume in circulating blood), hyperkalaemia (an excess of potassium in the blood), hypocalcaemia (deficiency of calcium in the blood), azotaemia, metabolic acidosis, muscle pain, peripheral neuropathy, hypotension, hypertension, irregular heart rate, yellow-bronze skin, dry scaly skin, and muscle cramps.

Possible complications of chronic renal failure can include anaemia, peripheral neuropathy, cardiopulmonary complications, sexual dysfunction, skeletal defects, gastrointestinal complications, and motor nerve dysfunction.

IgA nephritis

IgA nephritis is the most commonly seen glomerulonephritis. It is called IgA nephritis because of the deposition of IgA in the glomerulus. The real cause of IgA nephritis remains unclear. IgA nephritis typically presents with haematuria (red blood cells in the urine), and this may lead to chronic renal failure. IgA nephritis is normally asymptomatic and so the diagnosis of IgA nephritis is made through urinalysis.

Part V

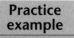

Practice example

Mr T, a 35-year-old engineer, came to the clinic complaining of painful joints, which had been confirmed as gout by his previous medical examination. By chance, we found his blood pressure was 160/105 mmHg. We referred him back to his GP for a proper medical checkup. Urine analysis revealed that he suffered from haematuria and so he was referred to a nephrologist, who later confirmed that Mr T suffered from IgA nephritis, which also resulted in his high blood pressure.

Activity

Mr J, a 39-year-old engineer, suffers from IgA nephritis resulting in hypertension. Explain in detail how IgA nephritis causes this patient's hypertension.

Nephritic syndrome

Nephritic syndrome is a nonspecific kidney disorder characterized by proteinuria (an excess of protein in the urine), hypoalbuminaemia (decrease in albumin in blood), hyperlipidaemia and oedema. The glomerulus is damaged in nephritic syndrome, which causes the leakage of albumin, immunoglobulins and other proteins. More proteins will be produced in the liver, leading to an increase in the level of large proteins. This results in an increase in the amount of lipoproteins, thereby causing the accumulation of fat in the body.

The causes of primary nephritic syndrome include minimal change disease, glumerulosclerosis and membranous nephropathy. Hepatitis B, Sjögren's syndrome, systemic lupus erythematosus, diabetes mellitus, obesity, HIV, and malignant tumour can be the causes of secondary nephritic syndrome.

Chapter Summary

This chapter has examined the main functions of the cardiovascular, respiratory and urinary systems. For more detailed information about these, you should consult the Further Resources below.

REVIEW QUESTIONS

1   What is the main function of the heart and what part do arteries and veins play in this?

2   What is the primary function of the respiratory system?

3   What are acute and chronic renal failure?

**CHAPTER
LINKS**

For further discussion of diagnosis of conditions, see Chapter 18.

**FURTHER
RESOURCES**

Beers, M.H. (2006) *The Merck Manual of Diagnosis and Therapy*, 18th edn, Whitehouse Station, NJ, Merck Research Lab. Provides comprehensive information of different disorders. You can also find it online at www.merck.com/mmpe/index.html.

Bickley, L.S. and Szilagyi, P.G. (2007) *Bates' Guide to Physical Examination and History Taking*, 9th edn, Philadelphia, PA, Lippincott Williams & Wilkins. Essential when you are carrying out physical examinations in the clinic.

Kumar, P. and Clark, M. (2005) *Clinical Medicine*, 6th edn, London, Elsevier Saunders. Gives clear information about symptoms and signs of different disorders. I strongly suggest practitioners/student practitioners read the relevant chapters.

Porth, C.M. (2005) *Pathophysiology: Concepts of Altered Health States*, with disc, London, Lippincott Williams & Wilkins. Gives detailed information regarding pathophysiology.

Tortora, G.J. and Derrickson, B. (2006) *Principles of Anatomy and Physiology*, 11th edn, Danvers, NJ, John Wiley & Sons. Gives clear information about the anatomy and physiology of different body systems. Especially read about the cardiovascular, respiratory and urinary systems.

Web Link

www.nhsdirect.nhs.uk/ – The NHS direct website provides practitioners and patients with some basic information about different disorders; I strongly suggest practitioners read all the relevant information on this website.

Part V

16 Reproductive, Endocrine and Nervous Systems

JASON TSAI

This chapter deals with the reproductive, endocrine and nervous systems. The practice examples illustrate how the complementary practitioner works to understand and respond to the different conditions identified. One purpose of these examples is to indicate where the complementary practitioner would refer cases on to a conventional medical practitioner. It is as important for the complementary practitioner to know when to do this, as it is to know the appropriate circumstances in which to treat the patient.

The Reproductive System

The reproductive system includes external genitalia and some internal organs such as testicles, ovaries, fallopian tubes and uterus (Figure 16.1). The reproductive system is also closely linked to some hormones in the endocrine system. In this section, we focus on the following commonly seen reproductive system disorders: cervical cancer, endometriosis, polycystic ovarian syndrome, fibroids and adenomyosis.

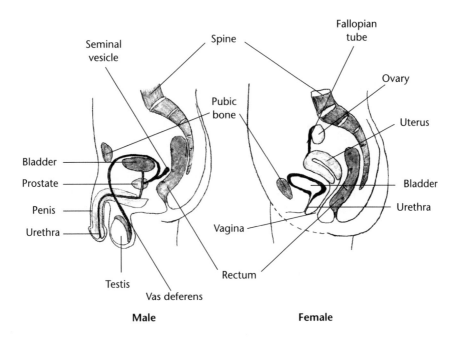

Figure 16.1 The reproductive system

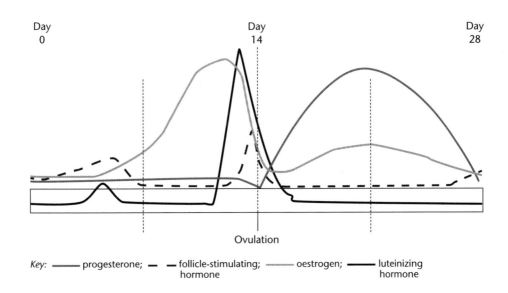

Key: ——— progesterone; — — follicle-stimulating; ——— oestrogen; ——— luteinizing
hormone   hormone

Figure 16.2 The menstrual cycle and the hormones

First we look at the female menstrual cycle, which is shown in Figure 16.2. The main function of follicle-stimulating hormone (FSH) is to promote and sustain the ovarian follicular growth in women and the spermatogenesis in men.

The main functions of luteinizing hormone (LH) include:

1. promoting the androgen synthesis in the thecal cells of the ovaries and in the interstitial cells of the testicles.
2. inducing ovulation – by stimulating the cascade of proteolytic enzymes leading to the rupture of the basement membrane of the follicle.
3. maintaining the corpus luteum during the menstrual cycle.

The principal functions of oestrogen in women are the mitotic effect on the uterine mucosa and on the breast, the feedback (positive and negative) on the pituitary gonadotrophins and its role in bone mineralization.

Progesterone plays many important roles in the development of the foetus.

Cervical Cancer

The causes of cervical cancer include human papilloma virus infection, and other factors, such as smoking, hormonal contraception and HIV infection. The early stage of cervical cancer can be asymptomatic. Symptoms of advanced cervical cancer include loss of appetite, weight loss, fatigue, pelvic pain, back pain, abnormal and heavy vaginal bleeding, and bone fracture.

Endometriosis

Endometriosis occurs when the endometrial cells attach, grow and function outside the uterus, generally in the pelvic region. Endometriosis is one of the commonly seen female diseases, although its cause remains unknown. Several theories have been proposed to explain the **pathogenesis** of endometriosis, retrograde menstruation being the most widely accepted one, which indicates the retrograde reflux of menstrual tissue in the Fallopian tube during menstruation. Although endometriosis generally occurs in the pelvic regions, endometrial tissues can be found in other places, such as the lungs, nose and joints.

Pain is the most common symptom that patients suffer, which can be period pain (dysmenorrhoea), pain during sexual intercourse (dyspareunia), pelvic pain, low back pain, painful joints and ovulation pain. Other symptoms include cyclical abdominal bloating, severe bleeding, diarrhoea, constipation, alternating bouts of diarrhoea and constipation, painful bowel movements, nausea, vomiting, fatigue and infertility.

Practice example

A 25-year-old patient has been suffering heavy periods and period pain for several years. She also suffers from arthritis. Whenever her period comes, her arthritis becomes worse, most especially pain in the hips and the knees. I was wondering whether her period pain might be caused by endometriosis and whether her arthritic pain might be related to endometriosis. I referred her to a gynaecologist for further medical examination. A pelvic ultrasound scan confirmed that she was suffering from endometriosis, and further medical examination revealed endometrial tissues in the hips and the knees.

Polycystic Ovarian Syndrome

Polycystic ovarian syndrome (PCOS) is the most common endocrine disorder affecting women. The pathogenesis of PCOS is poorly understood. In PCOS, an excessive amount of androgen is produced by the ovaries. A patient's fact sheet about PCOS published by the American Society for Reproductive Medicine in 2005 (www.asrm.org/Patients/FactSheets/PCOS.pdf) states:

> The most widely accepted definition of PCOS was based upon the diagnostic criteria recommended in 1990 which classified PCOS as a disorder characterized by chronic hyperandrogenism (elevation of serum testosterone or other androgens) and chronic anovulation (absence of ovulation) in the absence of other specific causes of these problems. More recently, an international consensus in 2003 expanded the definition of PCOS in 1990 to include women who demonstrate two of the following three characteristics: 1) chronic anovulation; 2) chronic hyperandrogenism; and 3) polycystic appearing ovaries (PCO) on ultrasound.

The symptoms of PCOS may include infrequent menstrual periods, no menstrual periods and/or irregular bleeding, infertility or an inability to get pregnant due to no ovulation, increased growth of hair on the face, chest, stomach, back, thumbs and toes, acne, oily skin, dandruff, pelvic pain, weight gain or obesity – usually carrying extra weight around the waist – type 2 diabetes mellitus, cholesterolaemia, hypertension and sleep apnoea.

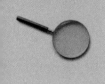

Practice example

A 30-year-old patient has been complaining about the symptoms caused by PCOS. She is very overweight, and she also mentions that she has to shave every single day. It has been normal for her to have only two menstrual periods a year since her menarche. She has been trying to get pregnant over the past few years, but without any success.

Uterine Fibroids

Uterine fibroids are benign tumours that grow from the muscle layers of the uterus. The cause of fibroids is unknown, but there is evidence that oestrogen is required for the growth of fibroids, which may also be affected by other factors, such as progesterone. It is likely that the growth of fibroids is linked to genetics. There is no evidence that lifestyle or nutritional factors influence the development and growth of fibroids.

The symptoms of fibroids may range from none at all to mild or severe, depending on their size and location. The symptoms may include pelvic pain, feeling of pelvic pressure, heavy menstrual bleeding, clots in menstrual flow, long periods, bleeding between periods, increased cramping during periods, dyspareunia, frequent urination, constipation, bloating, enlarged uterus, low back or leg pain, infertility due to blockage of Fallopian tubes, miscarriage and iron-deficiency anaemia.

Part V

Adenomyosis

Adenomyosis is characterized by the presence of ectopic endometrial tissue (the inner lining of the uterus) within the myometrium (the thick, muscular layer of the uterus). The precise **aetiology** and the developmental process of adenomyosis are currently unknown. The most widely held opinion is that adenomyosis develops as a result of inward growth and invagination of the basalis endometrium into the myometrium. What causes the inward growth of the endometrium into the myometrium needs further investigation.

Thirty-five per cent of adenomyosis is asymptomatic. The commonly seen symptoms include menorrhagia, dysmenorrhoea, and metrorrhagia. Dyspareunia is sometimes an additional complaint.

Endocrine System, Hormones and Related Diseases/Disorders

The endocrine system includes endocrine glands, cells and tissues of the body (Figure 16.3). Hormones are chemical messengers (that is, they trigger bodily responses), which are located at distant sites following transportation in the blood (the endocrine effect), or have an effect directly on nearby cells (the paracrine effect). The three main functions of the endocrine system are the control of growth and development, metabolism and reproduction.

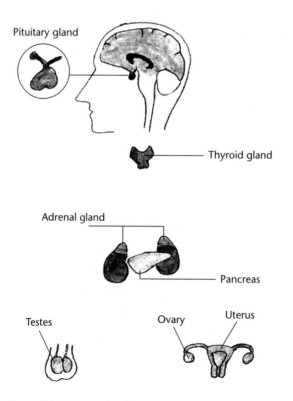

Figure 16.3 The endocrine system

The endocrine glands discussed in this section are the hypothalamus, pituitary gland (anterior and posterior lobes), thyroid gland, adrenal glands (adrenal cortex and medulla). LH and FSH, oestrogen and progesterone were discussed earlier in the reproductive system.

The hypothalamus secretes different hormones including gonadotrophin-releasing hormone (GnRH), dopamine, growth hormone-releasing hormone (GHRH), somatostatin, thyrotrophin-releasing hormone (TRH), corticotrophin-releasing hormone (CRH), antidiuretic hormone (ADH) and oxytocin (Figure 16.4).

Hypothalamus								
	↓	↓	↓	↓	↓	↓	↓	↓
	GnRH	Dopamine	GHRH	Somatostatin	TRH	CRH	ADH	Oxytocin
	↓+	↓+	↓+	−↗↘−	↓+	↓+	↓+	↓+
Pituitary	Anterior						Posterior	
	↓+	↓+	↓+		↓+	↓+	|+	|+
	LH/FSH	Prolactin	GH		TSH	ACTH		
	↓	↓	↓		↓	↓	↓	↓
Target glands/tissues	Gonads	Breast Gonads	Many tissues		Thyroid	Adrenal glands	Renal tubule	Breast Uterus
	↓		↓		↓	↓		
Target hormones	Sex steroids		Insulin-like GH		Thyroxine	Cortisol Adrenaline		

Key: ADH: antidiuretic hormone (also called vasopressin); GnRH: gonadotrophin-releasing hormone; GHRH: growth hormone-releasing hormone; TRH: thyrotrophin-releasing hormone; CRH: corticotrophin-releasing hormone; LH: luteinizing hormone; FSH: follicle-stimulating hormone; TSH: thyroid-stimulating hormone (also known as thyrotrophin); ACTH: adrenocorticotrophic hormone; GH: growth hormone; + = stimulation; − = inhibition

Figure 16.4 The control of secretion of hormones

With the exception of ADH and oxytocin, which are stored in the posterior lobe of the pituitary gland, the other hormones affect the anterior lobe of the pituitary gland:

- GnRH stimulates the pituitary gland to secrete luteinizing hormone (LH) and follicle-stimulating hormone (FSH), both of which then stimulate the gonads (ovary, uterus and testis) to secrete sex steroids, such as oestrogen, progesterone and androgens.
- Dopamine from the hypothalamus stimulates the pituitary gland to secrete prolactin, which stimulates the breast and gonads.
- GHRH stimulates the pituitary gland to secrete growth hormone (GH). GH will then work on many tissues and cells.
- Somatostatin inhibits the pituitary gland from secreting GH and thyroid-stimulating hormone (TSH).

Part V

■ TRH stimulates the pituitary gland to secrete TSH.

■ CRH works on the pituitary gland to secrete adrenocorticotrophic hormone (ACTH), which stimulates the adrenal gland to secrete cortisol and adrenaline.

■ ADH and oxytocin are secreted by the hypothalamus and stored in the posterior lobe of the pituitary gland. ADH affects the functions of the renal tubules. Oxytocin stimulates the breast to secrete breast milk and stimulates the uterus to cause cervical and vaginal constriction.

Thyroid Hormone

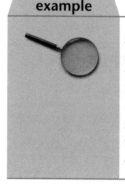

Practice example

A 48-year-old female patient has been suffering from hot flushes since she was 43. Initially she was told that she suffered from early menopause and was given hormone replacement therapy (HRT). Her symptoms responded well for the first month or two. However, the hot flushes started again, but she was still given HRT and has been using HRT for five years until she came to our clinic. When she was examined, we found some irregular lumps around the neck, which suggested that it could be a problem in the thyroid gland. Blood tests confirmed that she suffered from hyperthyroidism, and she has now been given the correct medical treatment.

This case teaches us that we need to collect as much information as possible so that a proper diagnosis can be made, underlying cause(s) found and appropriate treatment can be provided. In this case, the hot flushes occurred as a result of hyperthyroidism.

The clinical features of hyperthyroidism (overactivity of the thyroid gland) and hypothyroidism (underactivity of the thyroid gland) are listed in Table 16.1.

Table 16.1 Clinical features of hyperthyroidism and hypothyroidism

Features	Hyperthyroidism	Hypothyroidism
Heat production	Heat intolerance	Cold intolerance
Skin	Hair loss	Thin brittle hair Dry skin
Eyes	Eye complaints	Puffy eyes
Gastrointestinal system	Increased appetite Nausea Vomiting Diarrhoea	Anorexia
Cardiovascular system	Tachycardia (rapid heartbeat) Palpitations Systolic hypertension	Hypertension (high blood pressure) Hyperthermia (high temperature) Bradycardia (slow heartbeat) Anaemia

Features	Hyperthyroidism	Hypothyroidism
Respiratory	Shortness of breath	
Neuromuscular	Tremor Chorea Myopathy (muscle wasting) Periodic paralysis	Ataxia (inability to coordinate voluntary muscle movement) Psychosis Poverty of movement Arthralgia (painful joints) Myalgia (muscle pain)
Skeletal	Proximal myopathy (disease of the skeletal muscle located towards the centre of the body)	Proximal myopathy
Gynaecological	Loss of libido Oligomenorrhoea (light periods) Gynaecomastia (abnormal development of breasts in males)	Poor libido Menorrhagia (heavy periods) Oligomenorrhoea
Blood features	Low TSH High thyroxine	Hypercholesterolaemia (high cholesterol level in blood) Hyponatraemia (low sodium level in blood)

Growth Hormone

Practice example

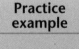

A real story published in the London Underground *Metro* newspaper on 15 February 2008 reported that a GP shook hands with Mr G. The GP immediately felt the 'sponge hand' (big and very soft, like squeezing a big piece of sponge). Sponge hand occurs as a result of a high level of growth hormone, causing a disease called acromegaly. The clinical features of acromegaly may include generalized expansion of the skull, pronounced lower jaw protrusion, soft tissue swelling characterized as enlargement of the hands, feet, nose, lips, ears, and a deep voice and slowing of speech.

Acromegaly is due to the excessive secretion of GH in adults, normally an indication of a tumour in the pituitary gland. However, some other tumours may also cause excessive secretion of GH. Apart from acromegaly, excessive secretion of GH in childhood can cause gigantism, and deficiency of GH will result in dwarfism.

Part V

Corticosteroids

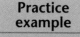

Practice example

When I first saw Ms W in the clinic, my impression was she had a puffy and rounded face (moon face). She also suffered from oedema in her legs. This immediately reminded me of Cushing's syndrome, which was confirmed by medical investigations.

Cushing's syndrome is caused by high levels of corticosteroids as a result of adrenal excess. The clinical features of Cushing's syndrome are listed in Table 16.2. If the level of corticosteroid becomes low due to adrenal insufficiency, the disorder is called Addison's disease. The clinical features of adrenal insufficiency and adrenal excess are listed in Table 16.2.

Table 16.2 Clinical features of adrenal excess and adrenal insufficiency

Features	Adrenal insufficiency (Addison's disease)	Adrenal excess (Cushing's syndrome)
Onset (acute/chronic)	Acute/chronic	Chronic
General body appearance	Fatigue Weight loss Sweating Malaise	Rapid weight gain Central obesity Excessive sweating Oedema
Skin features	Hyperpigmentation (excess pigmentation in bodily parts)	Thin skin Hirsutism (having excessive hair) Poor wound healing
Cardiovascular features	Postural hypotension	Hypertension
Musculoskeletal features	Joint pain Muscle pain Muscle weakness	Buffalo hump Osteoporosis Back pain Muscle weakness Proximal myopathy
Biochemical changes	Hypoglycaemia (low sugar level in blood) Hyponatraemia (low sodium in blood) Hyperkalaemia (high potassium in blood) Eosinophia (high eosinophils in blood) Lymphocytosis (increase in the number of lymphocytes) Metabolic acidosis	Hyperglycaemia (high sugar level in blood) Hypokalaemia (low potassium in the blood)
Gastrointestinal features	Vomiting, diarrhoea	Gastrointestinal disturbance

Features	Adrenal insufficiency (Addison's disease)	Adrenal excess (Cushing's syndrome)
Psychological features	Changes in mood and personality	Euphoria Psychosis Depression Anxiety
Reproductive features		Poor libido Infertility Amenorrhoea (no period) Oligomenorrhoea (light periods) Impotence
Other features	Craving for salt/salty food	Polyuria (excessive urination) Polydipsia (excessive thirst)

Practice example

Diabetes Mellitus

One of my patients has been suffering type II diabetes mellitus (DM) for several years and has been taking insulin for three years. He told me that the other day when he was at home, he had smashed the brand new refrigerator. Actually he did not know what he had done to the fridge and when he regained consciousness, he asked his wife who had smashed the fridge. The reason he had smashed the fridge and did not know what he had done is hypoglycaemia (low blood sugar), one of the complications of DM. This patient was receiving insulin treatment for his type II DM, which is normally given to patients with type I DM, so you might ask why this patient was given insulin (see below).

DM is a syndrome characterized by hyperglycaemia due to insulin deficiency, resistance, or both. DM usually can be classified into two main categories: insulin-dependent DM, also known as type I diabetes mellitus, and non-insulin-dependent DM, also known as type II diabetes mellitus. Although type II DM belongs to the non-insulin-dependent group, patients with type II DM might also need insulin combined with exercise and other medication to control the glucose level. Besides type I and type II, there is another type called gestational diabetes (pregnancy-induced diabetes) and about 20–50% of these patients will develop type II diabetes in their later lives.

The main symptoms of DM are polyuria (excessive urination), polydipsia (excessive thirst) and polyphagia (morbid desire for food), often accompanied with weight loss.

Diabetes can be primary or secondary.

The causes of secondary DM are:

- Liver disease, for example cirrhosis
- Pancreatic diseases, for example cystic fibrosis, chronic pancreatitis, carcinoma
- Endocrine diseases, for example acromegaly, thyrotoxicosis, Cushing's syndrome

- Insulin-receptor abnormalities, for example congenital lipodystrophy
- Genetic syndrome, for example myotonic dystrophy
- Drug-induced diseases, for example thiazide diuretics.

Nervous System

There two major anatomical divisions of nervous systems: the central nervous system and the peripheral nervous system (Figure 16.5).

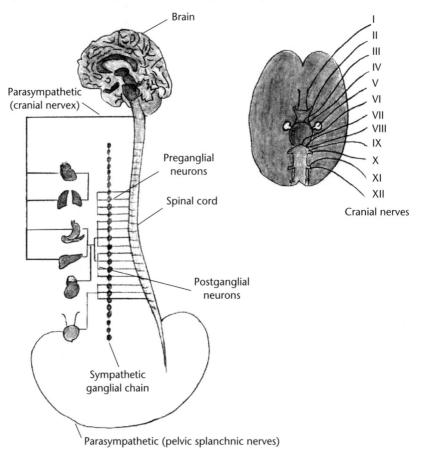

Figure 16.5 The central and peripheral nervous systems

The central nervous system (CNS) consists of the brain and the spinal cord. The CNS is in charge of integrating, processing and coordinating the sensory data and motor commands.

The peripheral nervous system (PNS) includes all the nerves outside the CNS. The PNS conveys sensory information to the CNS and carries the motor commands to the peripheral tissues, organs and systems. Peripheral nerves connected to the brain are called cranial nerves, of which are 12 (Figure 16.5). Their names and main functions are listed in Table 16.3. Peripheral nerves attached to the spinal cord are spinal nerves and there are 31 pairs of spinal nerves.

The PNS is divided into the somatic nervous system (SNS), which controls organs under voluntary control (mainly muscles), and the autonomic nervous system (ANS), which regulates individual organ function and **homeostasis**. The ANS has two divisions, the sympathetic and the parasympathetic. The ANS provides autonomic involuntary control of the cardiac muscle, smooth muscle and secretions.

The ANS is an efferent system that transmits the impulse from the CNS to the peripheral organs:

- The neuron is the structural and functional unit of nerves. It contains a cell body (or soma), dendrites and an axon
- Dendrites receive information from the axons of an upstream neuron. The information is transmitted to the cell body and then the axon. The axon then passes the information to the dendrites of a downstream neuron.

The information is transmitted through two mechanisms: neurotransmitters and electrochemical conduction. Neurotransmitters are released from the axon of the upstream neuron to the downstream neuron or to the CNS (or effectors). Electrochemical conduction is transmitted within the neuron from the dendrites to the terminal end of the axon.

Table 16.3 Names and main functions of the 12 cranial nerves

No.	Name	Main functions
I	Olfactory nerve	Transmits sense of smell
II	Optic nerve	Transmits visual information
III	Oculomotor nerve	Controls eye movements
IV	Trochlear nerve	Controls eye movements
V	Trigeminal nerve	Receives sensation from the face and controls mastication
VI	Abducens nerve	Controls eye movements
VII	Facial nerve	Controls facial expressions Receives the sense of taste from the anterior two-thirds of the tongue
VIII	Vestibulocochlear nerve	Senses sound Senses balance
IX	Glossopharyngeal nerve	Receives sense of taste from the posterior one-third of the tongue Controls pharynx Controls salivary gland
X	Vagus nerve	Controls swallowing Controls nerve fibres in the heart, stomach and lungs
XI	Accessory nerve	Controls muscles of the neck and shoulders Overlaps with functions of the vagus
XII	Hypoglossal nerve	Controls the muscles of the tongue and other glossal muscles

Part V

We now briefly outline five commonly seen neurological disorders in the complementary medicine clinic.

Alzheimer's Disease

Alzheimer's disease is a progressive, degenerative and irreversible disease of the brain that leads to dementia (a decline in brain functions including memory, thinking and reasoning). Although the cause of Alzheimer's disease remains unknown, neurochemical factors, environmental factors and genetics are suggested to be linked to this disorder. The diagnosis of Alzheimer's disease is made by medical exclusion, and can only be confirmed by autopsy.

The most common symptoms and signs of Alzheimer's disease are gradual loss of memory, inability to concentrate, inability to write or speak, loss of coordination, change in personal hygiene, disorientation, difficulty in learning, impaired communication, personality changes, wandering away, loss of eye contact, and fluctuations of mood.

Multiple Sclerosis

Multiple sclerosis (MS) is a disease involving a progressive decline of the central nervous system, characterized by relapses and remissions, where the visual, sensory and motor signs and symptoms vary greatly from person to person. The cause of MS is the demyelination (loss of myelin – white fatty covering) of the axons (nerve fibres), but what causes demyelination is still not clear. However, genetic factors, infectious factors and/or environmental factors may be involved in the development of MS. MS affects the ability of nerve cells in the brain and spinal cord to communicate with each other.

Clinical manifestations of MS may include change in sensation, muscle weakness, abnormal muscle spasm, difficulty in moving, dysarthria (difficulty in speaking), dysphagia (difficulty in swallowing), ataxia (lack of control of movement due to defects in the nervous system), nystagmus (involuntarily rapid movement of the eyes), optic neuritis (inflammation of optic nerve), diplopia (double vision), fatigue, pain syndrome, bowel or bladder difficulty, cognitive impairment, depression, and Lhermitte's sign (shooting pain down the back to the limbs when bending the neck forwards/backwards).

Parkinson's Disease

Parkinson's disease is a chronic, progressive disease affecting the central nervous system. It adversely affects speech and motor control of the body, which is caused by the loss of nerve cells that secrete dopamine in the midbrain.

Clinical features include tremor, rigidity, bradykinesia/akinesia (slow movement/lack of voluntary movement), postural instability, shuffling, turning en bloc, festination (fast and short step walking), stooped forward-flexed posture, gait freezing, hypophonia (abnormal weak voice), monotonic speech, drooling, dysphagia, fatigue, impaired coordination, slowed reaction time, memory loss, insomnia and excessive daytime sleep, urinary incontinence, nocturia, constipation, sexual dysfunction, and weight loss.

Myasthenia Gravis

Myasthenia gravis is an autoimmune disorder, which affects about three people in every 10,000. The acetylcholine receptor in the neuron is destroyed or made unable to bind to acetylcholine, thereby affecting the stimulation of muscle contraction. Clinical features include ptosis (drooping of the upper eyelids), dysphagia, dysarthria, diplopia, waddling gait, shortness of breath, weakness in the limbs, fatigue, and myasthenic crisis.

Dystonia

Dystonia is a disorder that affects the neurological and motor functions of the body and causes involuntary (unintended) movements and sometimes sustained muscular contractions. The exact cause of dystonia is not known or understood. However, based on theories, dystonia can be classified into primary and secondary dystonia. The **pathology** of primary dystonia remains unclear. Secondary dystonia can be caused by trauma or other factors. Clinical features involve abnormal posture especially on movement, continuous pain, cramping, trembling, muscle spasm, involuntary muscle movement and loss of muscle coordination.

Chapter Summary

This chapter has dealt with the main features of the reproductive, endocrine and nervous systems. You should refer to the Further Resources below for more detailed information.

REVIEW QUESTIONS

1 What is the difference between adrenal insufficiency and adrenal excess?
2 What is the difference between endometriosis, uterine fibroids and PCOS?
3 What is the difference between hyperthyroidism and hypothyroidism?
4 How do the kidney, endocrine system and nervous system work together to maintain blood pressure?

CHAPTER LINKS

For further discussion of diagnostic aspects, see Chapter 18.

Part V

FURTHER RESOURCES

Beers, M.H. (2006) *The Merck Manual of Diagnosis and Therapy*, 18th edn, Whitehouse Station, NJ, Merck Research Lab. Provides comprehensive information of different disorders. You can also find it online at www.merck.com/mmpe/index.html.

Bickley, L.S. and Szilagyi, P.G. (2007) *Bates' Guide to Physical Examination and History Taking*, 9th edn, Philadelphia, PA, Lippincott Williams & Wilkins. Essential when you are carrying out a physical examination in the clinic, especially nervous system disorders.

Jameson, J.L., Kasper, D.L., Fauci, A.S. et al. (2006) *Harrison's Endocrinology*, New York, McGraw-Hill. Provides comprehensive information about the endocrine system and different disorders.

Kumar, P. and Clark, M. (2005) *Clinical Medicine*, 6th edn, London, Elsevier Saunders. Provides clear information about symptoms and signs of different disorders. I strongly suggest practitioners/student practitioners read the relevant chapters.

Porth, C.M. (2005) *Pathophysiology: Concepts of Altered Health States*, with disc, London, Lippincott Williams & Wilkins. Gives detailed information regarding pathophysiology.

Tortora, G.J. and Derrickson, B. (2009) *Principles of Anatomy and Physiology*, 12th edn, Danvers, NJ, John Wiley & Sons. Gives clear information about the anatomy and physiology of different body systems. Please read the sections on the reproductive, endocrine and nervous systems.

Web Links

www.nhsdirect.nhs.uk/ – NHS Direct website.

http://health.nih.gov – US National Institutes of Health website, which provides useful information about different disorders.

Immune, Digestive, Musculoskeletal and Integumentary Systems

JASON TSAI

This chapter deals with some of the basic functions of the immune, digestive, musculoskeletal and integumentary systems. It uses practice examples so that you can see how the complementary practitioner works to understand and respond to the different conditions identified. It is important for the complementary practitioner to know the appropriate circumstances, both to refer the case on to a conventional practitioner, and to treat the patient.

Immunology and Infections

The immune system is part of the lymphatic system, although many body systems are involved (Figure 17.1). The immune system is our defence system, which protects us from external pathogenic factors.

Part V

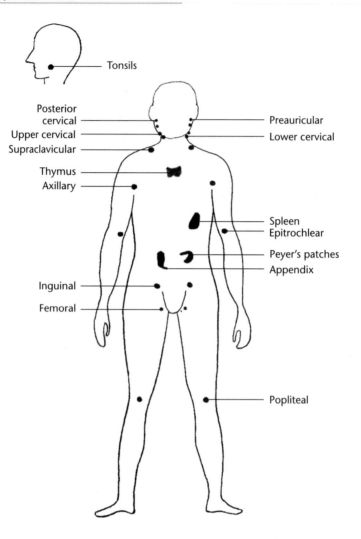

Tonsils

Posterior cervical
Upper cervical
Supraclavicular

Preauricular
Lower cervical

Thymus
Axillary

Spleen
Epitrochlear

Peyer's patches
Appendix

Inguinal

Femoral

Popliteal

Figure 17.1 The locations of lymph nodes and the organs in which lymphoid tissues are found

There are mechanisms in our body that guard us against abnormal substances, which provide us with nonspecific immunity. These systems provide general protection, for example mechanical barriers such as the skin and mucous membranes, tears and mucous; chemical barriers such as the enzymes in tears and the gastric acid in the stomach; and phagocytosis (engulfing and destruction of bacterial cells and foreign bodies by phagocytes) performed by the white blood cells.

We also have specific immunity, which protects us against certain types of agents. Lymphocytes are involved in this specific immunity.

We now tackle the components of the immune system and the antibodies. Antibodies are also called immunoglobulins (Ig), which are Y-shaped molecules (Figure 17.2). There are five different classes of immunoglobulins, listed in Table 17.1. The components involved in the immune response are listed in Table 17.2.

Table 17.1 The classes of immunoglobulins

Name	Description
IgA	Main antibody found in mucous secretions, such as tears, saliva and vaginal fluid
IgD	Acts mainly as a B cells antigen receptor
IgE	Well known for its role in hypersensitivity (allergy), especially type I hypersensitivity (known as anaphylaxis)
IgG	Most abundant antibody in the body, and only antibody that can cross the placenta to give passive immunity to the foetus
IgM	Largest antibody in the body, IgM appears early in a course of infection

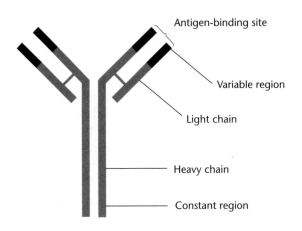

Antigen-binding site

Variable region

Light chain

Heavy chain

Constant region

Figure 17.2 The structure of immunoglobulin (Ig)

Table 17.2 Components of the immune system

Name	Classification	Description
Lymphocytes	B cell/T cell/LGL	B and T cells are small lymphocytes that play an important role in the immune system, like antibody production. Most large granule lymphocytes (LGL) are known as natural killer (NK) cells
Phagocytes	Monocyte/ neutrophil/ eosinophil	Phagocytes ingest and destroy foreign objects, such as microorganisms, through phagocytosis
Others	Basophil/ mast cell	Basophils and mast cells are very close to each other. Mast cells are best known for their role in anaphylaxis and allergies
	Thrombocyte	Also known as a platelet. Interacts with leukocyte during inflammatory process to secrete chemical mediators
	Other cells	Some other cells are involved in immune response, such as tissue dendritic cells

Vertebrates have two levels of defence against foreign objects: innate and adaptive (or acquired) responses. The innate response is a nonspecific immunity. Acute inflammation is an important part of the innate response. The adaptive response is a more highly specific immune response that recognizes and remembers foreign objects.

The Four Hypersensitivities

Type 1 hypersensitivity

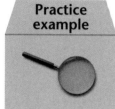

Practice example

A 2-year-old boy was fed a tiny piece of milk chocolate by his mother and five minutes later, he suffered severe abdominal pain, a skin rash and his mouth and eyes were swollen. He was immediately rushed to A&E.

This is a typical type 1 hypersensitivity, known as 'anaphylaxis' (a hypersensitive reaction to a substance). When a patient is first exposed to an antigen, his immune system is sensitized and remembers that antigen. When he is exposed to the antigen again, IgE will bind with the antigen and this antigen-antibody complex will cause the degranulation (a process of losing cytoplasmic granules) of mast cells. Histamine and other chemical mediators will be released, resulting in vasodilation and bronchoconstriction. The symptoms of anaphylaxis include angioedema (a swelling of the deeper layer of the skin), abdominal pain, pulmonary oedema, cramps, diarrhoea, nausea, fever, and other symptoms.

Besides anaphylaxis, there are three other types of hypersensitivities (type II, III and IV), which we now briefly discuss.

Type II hypersensitivity

This type of hypersensitivity is IgG or IgM mediated, and normally needs the involvement of the complement system. The antibody causes cell destruction directly by effectors (for example macrophages, neutrophils, eosinophils, NK cells) or indirectly through the complement system.

The complement system is a biochemical cascade involved in the immune system. There are three pathways in terms of the initiation of the complement system:

1. The classical pathway is activated by the antigen-antibody (Ag-Ab) complex.
2. The alternative pathway occurs when the previously activated complement component binds to the antigen.
3. The mannan-binding pathway is similar to the classical pathway; the mannan-binding lectin binds to the surface of the antigen to initiate the complement cascade.

Type III hypersensitivity

This type of hypersensitivity is mediated by the antigen-antibody complex. The complex will bind, via the complement system, to mast cells to form an antigen-antibody-mast cell complex and trigger the inflammatory process. This hypersensitivity can have a local type reaction (Arthus reaction), or a generalized or systemic reaction.

Type IV hypersensitivity

This is a delayed type of hypersensitivity, which takes some time to develop, and is the only type of hypersensitivity reaction triggered by the antigen-specific T cell.

There are some other immune system disorders not discussed here, but to which attention should still be paid, such as systemic lupus erythematosus (an autoimmune connective tissues disorder that affects any part of the body), rheumatoid arthritis, atopic eczema and urticaria.

Infections

Infectious agents, such as bacteria, virus, parasites, fungi, mycoplasma, Rickettsiae, and Chlamydiae, are everywhere. This means we are exposed to these agents all the time. Among many different infectious diseases, we will briefly discuss tuberculosis and meningitis.

Tuberculosis

Tuberculosis (TB) is caused by *Mycobacterium tuberculosis*, which is regarded as primary tuberculosis. Most TB occurs in the lungs (pulmonary TB), and the symptoms include chest pain, haemoptysis, and a productive prolonged cough for more than three weeks. There are other systemic symptoms including fever, chills, night sweats, loss of appetite, weight loss, pallor and fatigue.

Practice example

A 24-year-old female patient had been suffering from abdominal pain for weeks, but did not seek medical advice until the pain became severe and unbearable. An ultrasound scan revealed serious ascites, and a laparoscopy showed TB in the pelvic cavity, uterus, ovaries, and fallopian tubes, which confirmed TB in the genitourinary system.

A 47-year-old builder had been suffering from weight loss, loss of appetite, fatigue and night sweats for several years. I noticed there were some tiny pearl-like nodules around his neck, and suspected that it could be cutaneous TB and referred him to his GP. Medical tests confirm he was suffering from TB.

Part V

These two cases tell us that TB does not only cause problems in the lungs. TB has been found to affect the bones, joints, lymph nodes, kidneys and gastrointestinal tract. So when a patient presents with symptoms like night sweats, loss of appetite, weight loss, pallor and fatigue, we need to consider the possibility of TB.

Meningitis

Meningitis is inflammation of the meninges that enclose the central nervous system. Meningitis is contagious, and because the early symptoms of meningitis are similar to those of flu, it is often misdiagnosed.

The commonly seen clinical features of meningitis include fever, chills, vomiting, headache, nuchal rigidity (stiffness of the neck), stiff and painful back and joints, a rash that does not fade under pressure, photophobia (dislike of light), and opisthotonos (spasm of the muscles of the back, causing the head and lower limbs to bend backwards and the trunk to arch forwards).

Digestive System

The general features of the digestive system are illustrated in Figure 17.3.

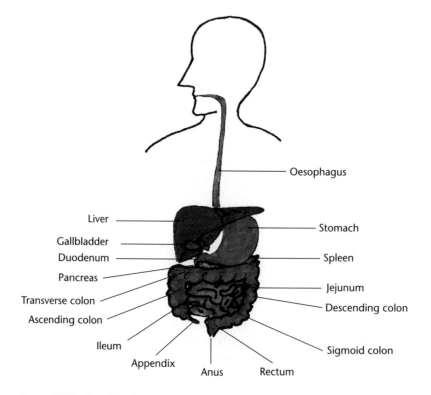

Figure 17.3 The digestive system

We now briefly examine some of the more commonly found diseases of the digestive system.

Gastroesophageal Reflux Disease

A 35-year-old office administrator came to the clinic with the main complaint of having heartburn for several years, which is worse after meals or lying down. With this complaint, it is possibly a chronic gastroesophageal reflux (GER) or gastroesophageal reflux disease (GERD). In order to confirm this, we referred him to his GP for further medical examination, which confirmed gastroesophageal reflux.

Gastroesophageal reflux disease is a more serious form of gastroesophageal reflux. Gastroesophageal reflux means that the gastric acid goes up from the stomach and 'leaks' through the sphincter to the oesophagus causing the discomfort or pain. The causes of gastroesophageal reflux can include:

- Weakened oesophageal sphincter
- Increased abdominal pressure
- Hiatus hernia
- Reduced low oesophageal sphincter
- Medication.

Crohn's Disease and Ulcerative Colitis

A 25-year-old university student came to the clinic complaining of arthritis in his knees. Through proper consultation, we found out that he had been suffering from ulcerative colitis since he was 16. Family history revealed that his father also suffers from ulcerative colitis, and his brother suffers from Crohn's disease. Arthritis is one of the extra-gastrointestinal features of ulcerative colitis and Crohn's disease.

Crohn's disease and ulcerative colitis are classified as inflammatory bowel diseases. The exact cause of both remains unknown; however, it is possible they are closely linked to genetic and environmental factors. The clinical presentations of the two disorders are similar, and are listed in Table 17.3.

Table 17.3 Comparison of ulcerative colitis and Crohn's disease

	Crohn's disease	Ulcerative colitis
Clinical presentations	Cramp-like abdominal pain Inconsistent stool Perianal discomfort Flatus and bloating Faecal incontinence Non-healing sores	Cramp-like abdominal pain Weight loss Diarrhoea Stool mixed with blood and mucus
Other clinical features	Uveitis (inflammation of the uvea of the eyes) Episcleritis (inflammation of the outer layer of the sclera in the eyeball) Arthritis (large joints) Ankylosing spondylitis Weight loss Erythema nodosum (inflammation of the fat cells under the skin) Poor appetite Malabsorption Ulcerating nodules	Aphthosis (formation of ulcers in the mouth) Iritis (inflammation of the iris) Uveitis Episcleritis Arthritis (large joints) Oligoarthritis (inflammation of four or fewer joints) Erythema nodosum Pulmonary embolism Finger clubbing Inflammation of bile duct
Terminal ileum involvement	Usually	Seldom
Colon involvement	Usually	Always
Perianal involvement	Common	Seldom
Sclerosing cholangitis	No	Higher rate
Fistulae	Common	Seldom
Smoking	Higher risk	Lower risk
Distribution of disease	Patchy area of inflammation	Continuous area of inflammation
Depth of inflammation	Deep into tissues	Shallow, mucosal
Affected area	Whole digestive system (from mouth to anus)	Colon only
Cancer risk	Lower	Higher
Stenosis	Common	Seldom
Autoimmune disease	Widely accepted	No consensus

Practice
example

Hepatitis

Ten years ago, Mr L, aged 37, was diagnosed with hepatitis C. He had been a regular blood donor and one day he had been informed that the person who had received his blood was found to suffer from hepatitis C. The blood had been traced back and was found to come from Mr L.

Mr Z, aged 31, has been suffering from tiredness and loss of appetite. He also mentioned that he was suffering flu-like symptoms, such as aching body, fever and vomiting. These symptoms had started several weeks after he had came back from a country where tourists are advised to have a vaccination against hepatitis B. He was advised to have a blood test, which confirmed that he was suffering from hepatitis B.

Hepatitis (liver inflammation) is characterized by the destruction of a number of liver cells and the presence of inflammatory cells in the liver tissue. Most hepatitis is caused by a viral infection, the most commonly known of many hepatitis viruses being A, B and C. Like hepatitis B, hepatitis C will cause damage to the hepatocytes, resulting in scar tissue and fibrous tissue in the liver. This will lead to cirrhosis, which then causes accumulation of the peritoneal fluids (ascites), and acute renal failure (hepatorenal syndrome) develops. Without proper treatment, hepatorenal syndrome is usually fatal.

The commonly seen clinical features of hepatitis include malaise, muscle and joint pain, fever, nausea, diarrhoea, headache, loss of appetite, jaundice, abdominal discomfort, hepatomegaly (enlargement of the liver) and splenomegaly (enlarged spleen).

In the early stage of hepatitis infection, the symptoms are most similar to flu or a cold, so it is not easy to differentiate between them. However, healthcare practitioners are strongly advised to refer patients to medical doctors if hepatitis is suspected.

Practice
example

Irritable Bowel Syndrome

Jane, a 35-year-old fashion designer, came for acupuncture treatment for her irritable bowel syndrome (IBS). The diagnosis of IBS is made by exclusion, meaning that if we cannot find out the underlying causes of the symptoms, it is classified as IBS.

IBS is a blanket term for a variety of diseases causing discomfort in the gastrointestinal tract. The most commonly seen symptom of IBS is abdominal pain, which is usually relieved by defecation. The patient may suffer from constipation, diarrhoea, or inconsistent bowel movement. Bloating and abdominal distension are also very common. An urgency of bowel movement, a feeling of incomplete evacuation or tenesmus (a feeling of the need to pass faeces but unable to do so) may also be present.

Part V

Diverticular Disease

Diverticula (meaning little kinks or irregularities) are frequently found in the colon. Diverticulosis means the presence of diverticula, and diverticulitis is a condition that arises when the diverticula are inflamed. Ninety per cent of diverticular disease is asymptomatic, and they are discovered incidentally on barium enema examination. Diverticular disease can cause alternating diarrhoea and constipation and abdominal pain, symptoms similar to those of IBS, making it difficult to differentiate between the two.

Peptic Ulcer

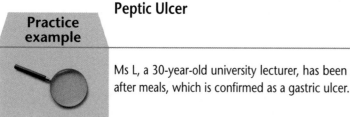

Practice example

Ms L, a 30-year-old university lecturer, has been suffering from stomach pain, especially after meals, which is confirmed as a gastric ulcer.

Peptic ulcers include oesophageal ulcer, gastric ulcer and duodenal ulcers.

The symptoms of peptic ulcers may include abdominal pain, bloating and abdominal fullness, waterbrash (a burning feeling in the stomach and the mouth suddenly fills with acid and excessive saliva), loss of appetite, weight loss, haematemesis (the vomiting of blood), and melaena (black faeces caused by bleeding in the intestine).

More than 80% of peptic ulcers are closely linked to *Helicobacter pylori*. NSAIDs, steroids, smoking and mental stress are factors closely associated with peptic ulcers, and the pathophysiology of these factors linked to the development of a peptic ulcer is illustrated in Figure 17.4.

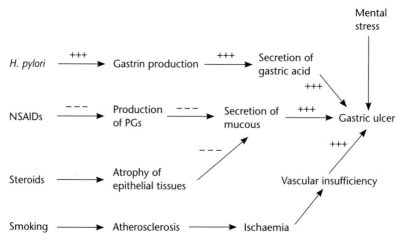

Key: PGs = prostaglandins; + = increase or stimulate; – = decrease or inhibit

Figure 17.4 Pathophysiology of different factors leading to/affecting the development of peptic ulcers

Pain Control and Musculoskeletal System Disorders

Low Back Pain

Jenny, a 55-year-old office administrator, has been off sick for more than three months due to low back pain that radiates to the leg. She cannot walk properly due to the pain. Three months of treatment with painkillers is unsuccessful. When I saw her, I used my elbow to press on her buttock for three seconds. She shouted 'Ouch! The pain has gone.' This is a typical piriformis syndrome.

Piriformis syndrome is a condition in which the piriformis muscle irritates the sciatic nerve, causing pain in the buttocks and referring pain along the course of the sciatic nerve. This referred pain, called 'sciatica', often goes down the back of the thigh and/or into the lower back. The sciatic nerve runs through the piriformis muscle. Therefore, any factors that may cause the piriformis muscle to become tight and compress the nerve can cause this syndrome. Although sciatica can be caused by piriformis syndrome, it is important that the clear spinal cause of sciatica is excluded before the treatment of piriformis syndrome is provided.

Low back pain can be caused by several factors, such as fibrofatty nodules, problems in the spine, sciatica, a strained muscle and muscle tension, and it is important we examine patients carefully. Sciatica is one of commonly seen causes of low back pain, and the pain will normally radiate to various parts of the leg and foot. The causes of sciatica include:

- Spinal disc hernia
- Spinal stenosis
- Spinal tumour
- Infection
- Piriformis syndrome
- Cauda equina syndrome (this is a serious disorder and requires urgent treatment).

It is important to note that the symptoms of Cauda equina syndrome may include low back pain, unilateral or bilateral buttock pain that radiates to the thighs and legs, unilateral or bilateral pain in the saddle area, bowel and bladder disturbances, numbness in the groin, muscle weakness or loss of sensation in the lower extremities.

Osteoarthritis

Osteoarthritis (OA, also known as degenerative arthritis, degenerative joint disease) is a group of diseases and mechanical abnormalities entailing the degradation of joints, including articular cartilage and the subchondral bone next to it. OA is the end result of all kinds of arthritis. The aetiology of OA remains unknown, but it is generally agreed to be multifactorial. A main reason for this is because tissue destruction is already advanced by the time the diagnosis of OA is made. OA results from the gradual degeneration of the cartilage that surrounds and cushions the affected joint. OA may arise as a primary as well as a secondary disorder. Primary osteoarthritis is related to the wear and tear of the cartilage, which can be seen as part of the normal ageing process. Secondary osteoarthritis is a breakdown of cartilage as a result of a particular cause not associated with ageing.

Age, obesity and genetics are responsible for the development of primary OA. A number of processes are involved in the development of secondary OA:

1. Injury to the joint due to repetitive or traumatic injuries
2. Extra stress on joints, mainly overweight
3. Previous inflammation of the joint
4. Biochemical changes of the articular cartilage
5. Hereditary factors.

The pathogenesis of OA is still not fully understood; however, articular cartilage is regarded as the key point of the development of OA. It has been demonstrated that bone metabolism is an important factor in the pathogenesis of OA. The articular cartilage of a diarthrodial joint is composed mainly of collagen and proteoglycans, and it is degradation of the proteoglycans and collagen and changes of hormone concentration that are responsible for the initiation and development of OA.

Rheumatoid Arthritis

Rheumatoid arthritis is a chronic, systemic inflammatory disorder that may affect many tissues and organs, but principally attacks the joints, producing an inflammatory synovitis that often progresses to destruction of the articular cartilage and ankylosis of the joints. The exact cause of rheumatoid arthritis remains unknown.

The clinical features are listed in Table 17.4. Most of the diagnosis of rheumatoid arthritis normally follows the 1987 revised criteria published by the American Rheumatism Society (Arnett et al., 1988).

Table 17.4 The 1987 criteria for the classification of rheumatoid arthritis

	Criterion
1	Morning stiffness lasts at least one hour
2	Arthritis of three or more joint areas
3	At least one area of arthritis in a wrist, metacarpal phalangeal or proximal interphalangeal joint
4	Arthritis on both sides of the body
5	Presence of rheumatoid nodules
6	A positive blood test for rheumatoid factor
7	Radiographic test shows that rheumatoid arthritis affects the joints

Source: Adapted from Arnett et al., 1988

In the criteria (Arnett et al., 1988), it also states:

For classification purposes, a patient shall be said to have rheumatoid arthritis if he/she has satisfied at least 4 of these 7 criteria. Criteria 1 through 4 must have been present for at least 6 weeks. Patients with 2 clinical diagnoses are not excluded. Designation as classic, definite, or probable rheumatoid arthritis is not to be made.

The pathophysiology of rheumatoid arthritis is described in Figure 17.3.

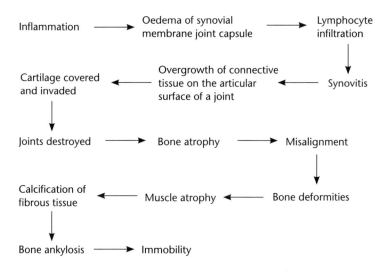

Figure 17.5 The pathophysiology of rheumatoid arthritis

Osteoporosis

Osteoporosis (porous bones) is a silent condition that happens slowly over years, where the skeleton becomes fragile and results in broken bones under normal use.

There is no specific symptom to identify osteoporosis. In most cases, neither a patient nor a medical doctor is aware of osteoporosis until one breaks a bone unexpectedly. A gradual decrease in height due to forward bending of the upper spine is a clinical feature of osteoporosis. Routine X-ray cannot detect osteoporosis until it is quite advanced.

Ankylosing Spondylitis

Ankylosing spondylitis is a chronic inflammatory disease leading to arthritis of the spine and hips. Commonly seen symptoms include stiffness and pain (arthritis) in the lower back sacroiliac joint, and sometimes the pain can radiate down to the leg. Pain is often worse at night, and stiffness is usually worse in the morning. All the symptoms may improve with exercise. Pain and stiffness can sometimes happen to other joints, such as knee, upper back, ribcage, neck and shoulders. When the heart valve or lung is involved, patients may feel chest pain. Fatigue, loss of appetite, fever and numbness are less common.

Fibromyalgia

Fibromyalgia literally means pain in the muscle and fibrous tissues such as ligaments and tendons. Pain can happen anywhere and anytime in the body. Besides pain, fatigue is common and sometimes severe, and in some cases, tiredness can be more distressing than the pain itself. Poor sleep patterns and poor concentration are common. Other symptoms, like headaches, painful periods, diarrhoea, constipation, bloating, depression and anxiety, may also develop.

Myofascial Pain Syndrome

Myofascial pain is a chronic condition that affects the fascia (connective tissue that covers the muscles). Myofascial pain is used to describe a pain caused by a trigger point. This trigger point may be on, close to, or away from the pain area.

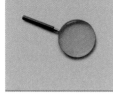

Practice example

Isabelle, a 24-year-old university student, suffered from shoulder pain. After close investigation and palpation, I found a small raised area in the back (the trigger point). Just a gentle touch can immediately make her feel the extreme pain on the trigger point and the shoulder.

Integumentary System and Skin Disorders

Skin is the largest organ in the body – the interface between our body and the exterior environment – and comprises the following layers: epidermis, dermis and the subcutaneous layer. The epidermis is composed of five more layers. The dermis lies under the epidermis layer and is basically connective tissues in which a variety of structures can be found, such as sweat glands, sebaceous glands, hair follicles, collagen and elastic fibres. Underneath the dermis lies the subcutaneous layer, which is made up of loose connective tissue, including adipose tissue.

The following are a few disorders of the skin.

Psoriasis

Psoriasis is a papulosquamous disorder characterized by red scaly plaques. The exact aetiology remains unknown, but increasing evidence shows that it is a T lymphocyte-driven disorder. About 5% of patients develop psoriatic arthritis.

Eczema

Eczema means boiling, which describes acute, inflamed, weeping skin. It is sometimes called dermatitis. The typical eczema presentation is itchy erythematous scaly patches, especially in front of the elbows, behind the knees and around the ankles. In infants, eczema often appears from three months old and starts on the face. Broken skin commonly becomes infected by bacteria, such as *Streptococci* or *Staphylococcus aureus*. Eczema is also linked to genetics.

Fungal Infections

Fungal infections have a high prevalence in humans, the most commonly seen being thrush and athlete's foot.

Viral Infections

Herpes simplex, herpes zoster and human papilloma virus are the most commonly known viruses that cause skin disorders.

Practice example

A 67-year-old retired bricklayer came to the clinic complaining about pain in the left leg. After close investigation, we found some crusts over the skin, the pattern of the crust being distributed along the sciatic nerve. The severe pain was due to herpes zoster infection (postherpetic neuralgia).

A 21-year-old university student came to the clinic for treatment of insomnia. He also mentioned a little mole growing on his left middle finger. The mole looked like a tiny colourful flower, which was later confirmed as a wart caused by human papilloma viral infection.

A 62-year-old female patient came to the clinic for acupuncture treatment for a slight deviation of her mouth, which, according to her, was caused by herpetic infection. However, for this kind of treatment, acupuncture needles would need to be inserted in her face and we could not be sure that acupuncture was suitable, as we did not want to cause any further infection. She was advised to contact her GP to confirm she could be treated with acupuncture.

A 31-year-old male came to the clinic for the treatment of blisters in his mouth. When I looked at the mouth, I could see a lot of small blisters. I then asked whether there were also some blisters in any other, private, area. He hesitated, but nodded. He then said it was an infection of herpes simplex type II, which was confirmed by medical investigation and laboratory tests. This case shows us that when we see blisters in the mouth, we also need to check whether there are blisters in other areas, which can provide us with more information.

Skin Cancer

Some skin tumours are benign, but some are malignant. The three common skin cancers are melanoma, squamous cell carcinoma and basal cell carcinoma.

Practice example

Having finished washing, Mr L, a 43-year-old legal adviser, discovered a tiny dark spot in the left infraorbital region (under the eye orbit). He paid it no attention until several months later when he found the dark spot had grown into a small mole. He sought medical advice, and medical investigations confirmed that the small mole was a melanoma.

Chapter Summary

This chapter has discussed some of the main features of the immune and digestive systems, with brief reference to the musculoskeletal and integumentary systems. For more information about these systems, please refer to the Further Resources below.

REVIEW QUESTIONS

1 What is the difference between osteoarthritis and rheumatoid arthritis?

2 What is the difference between eczema and psoriasis?

3 In terms of pathophysiology, what are the major factors associated with the development of peptic ulcers?

4 What is the difference between the four hypersensitivities?

CHAPTER LINKS

For further discussion of the musculoskeletal and integumentary systems, see Chapter 14.

FURTHER RESOURCES

Beers, M.H. (2006) *The Merck Manual of Diagnosis and Therapy*, 18th edn, Whitehouse Station, NJ, Merck Research Lab. Provides comprehensive information of different disorders. You can also find it online at www.merck.com/mmpe/index.html.

Bickley, L.S. and Szilagyi, P.G. (2007) *Bates' Guide to Physical Examination and History Taking*, 9th edn, Philadelphia, PA, Lippincott Williams & Wilkins. Essential when you are carrying out a physical examination in the clinic.

Kumar, P. and Clark, M. (2005) *Clinical Medicine*, 6th edn, London, Elsevier Saunders. Gives clear information about symptoms and signs of different disorders. I strongly suggest practitioners/student practitioners read the relevant chapters.

Porth, C.M. (2006) *Essentials of Pathophysiology: Concepts of Altered Health States*, London, Lippincott Williams & Wilkins. Gives detailed information regarding pathophysiology.

Tortora, G.J. and Derrickson, B. (2009) *Principles of Anatomy and Physiology*, 12th edn, Danvers, NJ, John Wiley & Sons. Gives clear information about the anatomy and physiology of different body systems. Please read the sections on the immune, digestive, musculosketal and integumentary systems.

Web Link

www.nhsdirect.nhs.uk/ – NHS Direct

Differential Diagnosis 18

JASON TSAI

Learning outcomes

By the end of this chapter, you should be able to:

■ list different underlying causes of commonly seen symptoms (main complaints) in complementary medicine clinics

■ identify the 'red alert' symptoms

■ exercise your professional judgement to decide when to send a patient to hospital for urgent treatment or back to their GP

This chapter explores the use of differential diagnosis in the work of complementary practice. It illustrates how the complementary practitioner integrates knowledge of anatomy, physiology and some of the commonly encountered symptoms of illnesses and conditions. It uses examples so you can see how the complementary practitioner works to understand and respond to the different conditions identified. Practitioners are strongly recommended to update their knowledge through all possible mechanisms, such as reading articles published in medical journals, visiting websites of medical associations/societies, professional bodies, and attending conferences to share knowledge and clinical experience with colleagues.

Practice example

Noel, a 44-year-old university lecturer, suffered from chest pain at night. He was taken to hospital by ambulance. Medical examinations confirmed he had suffered from a heart attack, and he stayed in the cardiology ward for two weeks.

Craig, a middle-aged university lecturer, suffered from pain in the chest and shortness of breath at night. He was rushed to A&E. Medical checkups revealed that it was indigestion.

The above two patients suffered from chest pain. Was it indigestion or a heart attack? This is a life and death situation. Just imagine if a patient suffers from chest pain caused by a heart attack, and our diagnosis is indigestion or heartburn. What will happen to this patient? The two examples above demonstrate why differential diagnosis is such an important subject for all healthcare practitioners. Differential diagnosis is used to differentiate between one or more disorders through careful comparison and contrast of the clinical manifestations of different disorders to achieve accuracy in diagnosis.

Chest Pain

The causes of chest pain may include:

1. Ischaemic (deficiency in supply of blood) heart disease, for example angina pectoris (chest pain due to an insufficient supply of blood to the heart muscles) and myocardial infarction (heart attack) (see Chapter 15)
2. Inflammation, for example pericarditis (inflammation of the pericardium), endocarditis (inflammation of the endocardium)
3. Aortic dissection (a tear in the wall of the aorta; see Chapter 15)
4. Pulmonary thromboembolism (blockage of a blood vessel by a particle that has broken away from a blood clot at its site of formation)
5. Pneumothorax (a condition in which air is present in the pleural cavity)
6. Gastrointestinal conditions, for example heartburn
7. Psychogenic pain (a pain condition that is caused, increased or prolonged by psychological factors, for example anxiety)
8. Disorders of muscles, for example a pulled muscle
9. Bones and joints, for example costochondritis (inflammation of the cartilage connecting the inner end of the ribs to the sternum).

When a patient complains of chest pain, we will need to ask some questions about the pain, which should cover: onset, pattern, frequency, duration, severity, location, radiation, nature of pain, pain on exertion, aggravating factors, family history, shortness of breath, sweats, nausea, pain or stiffness in the shoulder, neck and jaw. Questions should also be asked about medication and past medical history.

The following tests can be used:

- Physical examinations include blood pressure, ECG (electrocardiogram), pulse, heart sound and breath sounds.
- Imaging tests include chest X-ray, echocardiography (heart ultrasound scan) and lung VQ scan (V = ventilation and Q = perfusion; this test measures the air and blood flow in the lungs).
- Laboratory tests include blood tests and exercise tolerance tests.

Red alert: Some of the causes of chest pain can be life-threatening. So if a patient comes to the clinic with a chest pain, complementary medicine practitioners, if unsure about the cause, are strongly advised to send the patient to A&E.

Headache

Causes of headache can be classified into four categories based upon the International Headache Society Classification (http://ihs-classification.org/en/):

1 *Primary headaches:* Migraine, tension-type headache, cluster headache, and other primary headaches.
2 *Secondary headaches:* Head/neck trauma, cranial/cervical vascular disorder (headache linked to the vascular condition, such as ischaemic or haemorrhagic stroke), non-vascular intracranial disorder (headache caused by a change in intracranial pressure, such as an increase or decrease in cerebrospinal fluid pressure), a substance or its withdrawal, infection, disorder of homeostasis (maintenance of relatively stable internal physiological conditions, such as temperature, water metabolism and pH of the blood), disorder of cranium, neck, eyes, ears, nose, sinuses, teeth, mouth or other facial or cranial structures, and psychiatric disorders.
3 *Cranial neuralgias, central and primary facial pain:* Trigeminal neuralgia (episodes of intense paroxysmal pain radiating along the course of the trigeminal nerve), occipital neuralgia (episodes of pain occurring in the back of the head and upper neck due to tenderness or inflammation of the nerves supplying this area, such as occipital nerves), ophthalmoplegic migraine (a headache felt around the eyes due to abnormality of the nerves supplying the area, particularly the oculomotor nerve, the third cranial nerve), and central causes of facial pain.
4 *Other headaches:* Headaches not classified elsewhere and unspecified headaches.

The most commonly seen causes of headache are tension headache, frontal sinusitis, migraine and cervical spondylosis (a degenerative disease of the intervertebral joints and discs of the neck) (Table 18.1).

Table 18.1 Comparison of commonly seen headaches

	Tension headache	Frontal sinusitis	Migraine	Cervical spondylosis
Worse on lying down	No	Yes	No	Possible
Worse on neck movement	No	No	Possible	Yes
With congested nose	No	Yes	Possible	No
Unilateral	No	Possible	Possible	No

When a patient is complaining of a headache, we will need to ask some questions about the headache, which should cover: onset, pattern, frequency, duration,

Part V

severity, location, radiation, nature of pain, associated symptoms, premonitory symptoms, neurological symptoms, activity during headache, effect of headache on daily activity, aggravating/relieving factors, intermittent/cluster, diurnal/nocturnal (diurnal means occurring in the day, nocturnal means occurring at night), and family history. Questions should also be asked about medication and past medical history.

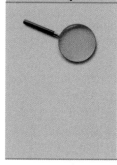

Practice example

Simon, a young university student, has been complaining about migraine for several days. Painkiller treatment was not successful. The patient then remembered he started using air freshener several days ago. Two days after the removal of the air freshener, his migraine was completely relieved. It was later confirmed that this patient was allergic to the freshener.

James, a postgraduate student in his twenties, has been suffering from migraine for two weeks. Lack of sleep was eventually identified as the cause of migraine.

My clinical experience with patients suggests that any changes in environment and lifestyle should be questioned and closely investigated.

Physical examinations of headaches include checking blood pressure, fundoscopy (a medical examination using a fundoscope to check the eyes), sinus tenderness, neck movement, cranial (of or related to the skull) nerve assessment, and jaw movement. Investigations include CT (computed tomography) scan, MRI (magnetic resonance imaging) scan, erythrocyte sedimentation rate (erythrocytes are red blood cells; erythrocyte sedimentation rate is a test for nonspecific inflammation), and other blood tests.

Red alert: Patients complaining of headache accompanied with the following clinical features should be taken seriously. If in doubt, seek medical advice or send the patient to A&E:

1 *Sudden severe headache without any forewarning; patients might describe this kind of pain like a blow to the head*
2 *If temporal arteritis (inflammation of the temporal artery) is suspected*
3 *Pregnant woman complaining of headache in the third trimester (weeks 27–42 of the pregnancy); it is essential to check blood pressure, ankles and urinalysis. Remember to check if there is any visual disturbance*
4 *Elderly patients with a new complaint of migraine*
5 *Patients with a new complaint of headache, who also present with a stooping or straining gait.*

Back Pain and Low Back Pain

The causes of low back pain (LBP) may include:

1. Lumbar disc herniation (slipped disc of the lumbar region; hernia/herniation is a protrusion of an organ or part of the body, such as a spinal disc)
2. Peripheral neuropathies (disease or degenerative disorder of the peripheral nerves)
3. Cauda equina syndrome (a serious condition that causes acute loss of function of the nerves in the lower portion of the spinal canal, and if untreated, can cause permanent damage to these nerves)
4. Fracture
5. Spinal cord tumour
6. Vascular disease (related to the blood vessels)
7. Primary or metastatic carcinoma (primary or change of the position of malignant tumours)
8. Rheumatoid disorders
9. Infection
10. Mechanical origin
11. Visceral disease (related to the internal organs)
12. Unknown reason (nonspecific LBP).

When a patient complains of LBP, we will need to ask about the onset, pattern, frequency, duration, location, radiation, nature of pain, and aggravating factors. Questions should also be asked about medication and past medical history, especially any injury to the spine. Do not forget that it can also be a referred pain. (Referred pain is pain felt in a part of the body other than the site of the original pain. For example, pelvic/abdominal diseases can cause LBP, which is a kind of referred pain.)

Physical examinations include observation, palpation (a medical diagnosis by touching or feeling the surface of the body) and other physical tests. Imaging tests include X-ray or an MRI scan.

Red alert: Patients complaining of LBP and with the following three conditions should be referred to a specialist:

1   Pain with major or minor trauma
2   Pain with a history of cancer, unexplained weight loss, night sweats, or pain worse when lying down
3   Pain radiating to the saddle area, or numbness in the saddle area (perineum, buttocks and inner side of the thigh), and with bowel/bladder dysfunction.

Abdominal Pain

Abdominal pain can be acute or chronic. The commonly seen causes of abdominal pain include peptic ulcer, biliary colic, appendicitis, gastroenteritis, and renal colic. Other causes include cholecystitis (inflammation of the gallbladder), irritable bowel syndrome, diverticulitis, pancreatitis, abdominal muscle pain, hepatitis,

Part V

ulcerative colitis, Crohn's disease, tuberculosis, abdominal aorta aneurysm and ischaemic bowel disease.

From these different disorders, we can conclude that abdominal pain can be caused by three mechanisms and will have different clinical patterns: visceral pain, parietal pain and referred pain:

- *Visceral pain:* This occurs when internal organs contract forcefully or are stretched. Internal organs can be classified into hollow organs, such as the stomach and the intestines, and solid organs, such as the liver. Visceral pain varies in quality, such as burning or cramping, and when it becomes severe, it can cause sweating, vomiting, restlessness, pallor of complexion. Because most visceral pain occurs near the midline of the body between the xiphoid process and the suprapubic area, it can be difficult to localize it. However, we can still have an idea about which organs the pain is in (Figure 18.1).
- *Somatic pain:* This occurs in the parietal peritoneum (the smooth transparent serous membrane that lines the abdominal cavity) due to inflammation. This type of pain is normally aching; however, the quality of pain can be worse than visceral pain. The area of the peritoneum can be precisely localized. This kind of pain can be aggravated by movement, taking a deep breath and coughing.
- *Referred pain:* Because of innervation (the distribution of nerves to or in a part of the body), referred pain can be felt at the same spinal level as the pathological area. This type of pain can also be localized deeply or superficially. Pain can also be referred to the abdominal area from the chest, spine or pelvis, which makes the assessment of abdominal pain more complicated.

Because the localization and quality of abdominal pain provide practitioners with information about its possible pathology, it is important that practitioners assess the severity, aggravating factors, time of the pain, and type of pain when seeing a patient.

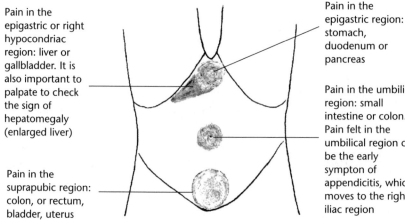

Pain in the epigastric or right hypocondriac region: liver or gallbladder. It is also important to palpate to check the sign of hepatomegaly (enlarged liver)

Pain in the suprapubic region: colon, or rectum, bladder, uterus

Pain in the epigastric region: stomach, duodenum or pancreas

Pain in the umbilical region: small intestine or colon. Pain felt in the umbilical region can be the early sympton of appendicitis, which moves to the right iliac region

Figure 18.1 Areas of visceral pain

Laboratory tests include blood tests including full blood count, urea (a nitrogen metabolic waste product), electrolytes (substances containing free ions in solution, such as sodium, calcium, potassium, chlorides and so on), amylase, *Helicobacter pylori* antibody (checks the existence of *Helicobacter pylori*, a bacterium accounting for most cases of peptic ulcer), liver function, and erythrocyte sedimentation rate. Imaging tests include X-ray, ultrasound, CT scan and endoscopy (internal examination using an endoscope).

Practice example

An elderly male patient suffered from abdominal pain. He was seen by a gastroenterologist (specialist in the treatment of disorders of the gastrointestinal tract), who could not find anything causing the abdominal pain and so referred him to a cardiologist (specialist in disorders of the heart). It was later confirmed that his abdominal pain was caused by an abdominal aorta aneurysm. An emergency operation was carried out.

Red alert: Patients suffering from abdominal pain with the following symptoms should be referred to a specialist:

1 *Anorexia/weight loss*
2 *Severe and persistent back pain*
3 *Changes in bowel habits*
4 *Iron-deficiency anaemia*
5 *Haematemesis (the vomiting of blood), melaena (black tarry stools, an indication of gastrointestinal haemorrhage)*
6 *Acute pain with signs of shock.*

Fatigue

Fatigue is a feeling of lethargy or weariness, often stress or anxiety-related, and 50% of patients have a physical disease. Fatigue is a common symptom of an underlying chronic disease. The symptoms of fatigue can include constant tiredness or sleepiness, lack of energy, headaches, muscular pain and pain in the joints, muscle weakness, slow response rates, poor judgement, low mood, changes in appetite, lowered immune system functioning, poor concentration, and low motivation.

The causes of fatigue can be classified as follows:

■ *Systemic metabolic diseases* (diseases/disorders that disrupt the metabolism, which affects the body generally): hypothyroidism (low thyroid hormone; also refer to Chapter 16), cancer/chemotherapy, anaemia, cardiac conditions (for example coronary heart disease and heart failure), diabetes mellitus, chronic infections, kidney disease, thyroid disease, liver disease (for example hepatitis A, B or C).
■ *Ventilatory dysfunction* (not enough air reaches the lungs due to respiratory system disorders): sleep apnoea (cessation of airflow during sleep preventing

air entering the lungs), chronic alveolar hypoventilation (insufficient ventilation leading to an increase of CO_2 concentration in the body), and hypoxaemia (low oxygen concentration in the blood).

■ *Psychological disturbances*: depression and anxiety. Several lines of evidence link chemical compounds to the pathophysiology of anxiety and depression, one of which is serotonin (5-hydroxytryptamine or 5-HT). It is possible that depression and anxiety are partly caused by overactivity of the hypothalamus-pituitary-adrenal axis (HPA axis), which is similar to the neuroendocrine response to stress. There is evidence showing that the HPA axis is linked to sleep and the genesis of chronic fatigue syndrome, hence it is possible that depression and anxiety can cause fatigue.

Questions to ask in the differential diagnosis of fatigue should cover: all previous history, recent viral infections, depression or other psychiatric illness, major surgery, chronic disease, medication (past and present), alcohol intake, family history, and social history. Other areas to explore include a constant feeling of tiredness, insomnia, nervousness, irritability, anything related to work, and relationships. Physical symptoms such as muscle pain, shortness of breath, palpitations, tremors, bowel movements, sleep pattern, thirst, urination and appetite need to be investigated.

Physical examination of the patient includes pallor of complexion, cyanosis (blue colouration of lips, mucous membrane and skin due to oxygen deficiency), oedema, eye contact, joint swelling/deformity, blood pressure, pulse, heart sound, lymph nodes, abdomen and chest.

Laboratory tests include full blood count, blood gas test, thyroid function test, blood sugar test, electrolytes, and erythrocyte sedimentation rate. Imaging tests include chest X-ray, ECG and echocardiogram (heart ultrasound scan).

The differential diagnosis of fatigue includes: anaemia, infection, depression, thyroid disorders, rheumatological disorders, TB, coeliac disease, surgery, fibromyalgia (a chronic disorder characterized by widespread pain in the body, accompanied by sleep disturbance, fatigue and headache), raised intracranial pressure, chronic fatigue, heart failure, kidney failure, cancer and cancer treatments, diabetes and hepatitis.

Red alert: Patients complaining about tiredness accompanied by the following signs or symptoms should be taken seriously. If necessary, seek medical advice or refer the patient to a specialist:

1 *Weight loss*
2 *Enlarged lymph nodes*
3 *Depressive illness.*

Nocturia

The causes of nocturia (the need to get up at night to urinate) can be:

Fluid balance factors:

■ Excessive evening fluid intake

■ Diuretics (chemical drugs that promote urination)

■ Disruption of normal ADH (antidiuretic hormone) secretion

■ Nocturnal redistribution of fluid

■ Sleep apnoea.

Neurological factors:

■ Cord compression (also known as spinal cord compression, where the spinal cord is compressed by bone fragments of the vertebra, tumours, abscesses or other lesions)

■ Tethered spinal cord syndrome

■ Parkinson's disease

■ Multiple sclerosis

■ Diabetic cystopathy (impairment of bladder sensation and bladder contractility, which causes increased bladder capacity and residual urine in the bladder).

Low urinary tract factors:

■ Bladder outflow obstruction

■ Prostate disease

■ Urethral disease

■ Bladder overactivity

■ Sensory urgency

■ Urinary tract infection

■ Inflammation

■ Malignancy

■ Pregnancy.

Besides nocturia, patients might suffer from polyuria (excessive urination). The causes of polyuria can be:

■ Excess fluid intake

■ Diabetes mellitus

■ Diabetes insipidus (excessive thirst and excessive urination, which cannot be stopped by reduced fluid intake). The regulation of urination is controlled by the hypothalamus, which produces ADH. ADH works on the collecting ducts and distal tubules of the kidneys to increase the reabsorption of water and condense the urine. Diabetes insipidus occurs when there is a deficiency of ADH or when the kidneys fail to respond to ADH

■ Hypercalcaemia (excess calcium in the blood). The reabsorption of calcium in the renal tubules is linked to sodium and water reabsorption in the renal tubules. Hypercalcaemia impairs the sodium and water reabsorption, thereby causing polyuria

■ Renal failure – it is more likely to be chronic renal failure.

Dizziness

The term 'dizziness' sometimes makes practitioners feel frustrated or confused because it may mean different things to different people. Some people may use other terms, such as giddiness, unsteadiness or light-headedness.

The causes of dizziness can be:

- Drugs, for example anticonvulsants (chemical drugs for seizures and epilepsy)
- Anaemia
- Hypotension
- Cardiac arrhythmia (may cause low blood pressure, thereby leading to fainting or dizziness)
- Endocrine disorder, for example hypothyroidism
- Infective, systemic infection
- Psychological factors, for example anxiety and depression.

Vertigo

Vertigo means dizziness with a feeling of movement inside the head. The causes of vertigo include:

Peripheral disorders:
- Vestibular neuritis (inflammation due to infection of the eighth cranial nerve connecting the inner ear and the brain). It may cause vertigo, dizziness, difficulty in balance and hearing
- Vascular problems
- Benign positional vertigo (simple vertigo caused by a disorder of the inner ear)
- Ménière's disease
- Post-traumatic stress
- Local infections
- Drugs, for example aminoglycosides, which are ototoxic (can damage the hearing or balance functions of the ear) and cause vertigo.

Central disorders:
- Brainstem pathology, for example ischaemia and infarction. Vertigo is an early sign of brainstem ischaemia or brainstem stroke, a neurological clinical feature due to lack of blood supply to the brainstem.

Menstrual Disorders

An office worker in her thirties had her period as she expected because her menstrual cycle is always regular. But this time the period came and only lasted one day. She thought it was because she had a cold. In fact, she was pregnant.

The first 12 weeks of pregnancy are the most critical, as 1 in 5 pregnancies abort during this stage.

When we see a female patient aged 11 or over, do not forget to ask questions related to menstruation. The questions may cover menarche, last period, menstrual cycle (how long, how often), intermenstrual bleeding, sexual urge, use of contraceptives, postcoital bleeding, and dysmenorrhoea (painful menstruation).

I overheard the following conversation between a practitioner (A) and a patient (B) in the clinic:

A: Let's move on to your periods. Are your periods regular?
B: Yes.
A: How many days?
B: Every 28 days.
A: Are they heavy or light?
B: How much is heavy?
A: The normal range is between 60–80 ml.
B: Oh, I don't know.

We should not be surprised that the patient cannot answer the question when put in such a way, because no one measures the volume of blood during menstruation. However, if we put the question another way, we would probably get the answer. For example, if we ask the patient how many tampons/sanitary towels they use per day/per cycle, hopefully they will be able to give us a clear answer, from which we can deduce whether the period is heavy or light.

Here is another conversation conducted between a practitioner (A) and a patient (B) in the clinic:

A: I would now like to ask you about your periods.
B: My periods are normal.
A: That's good. Can you tell me how long your periods last?
B: It depends. They are irregular.
A: Oh right. In that case, what makes you think your periods are normal?
B: Because my mother's periods are irregular, and my grandmother's periods were irregular, so I think irregular periods are normal.
A: Are there ever any blood clots?
B: I don't know. I don't pay any attention to the blood.
A: Is the colour dark, dull or bright red?
B: I don't know because no one told me to look at the colour.

It is important that we also pay attention to some related symptoms, such as weight, acne, hirsutism (excessive growth of facial or body hair in women), sweats/hot flushes, fatigue, nausea/vomiting, emotional change, pain in abdomen/pelvic, and vaginal discharge.

We also need to investigate what causes amenorrhoea (abnormal absence of menstrual flow). Amenorrhoea can be primary or, in most cases, secondary. The causes of amenorrhoea include mental stress, pregnancy, weight loss, hormonal imbalance, and polycystic ovarian syndrome.

The opposite is menorrhagia (abnormally profuse menstrual flow), the causes of which include fibroids, pelvic inflammation/infection, cancer, polyps, hyperthyroidism (excess of thyroid hormone; also refer to Chapter 16), dysfunctional uterine bleeding, and endometriosis (endometrial cells deposited outside the uterus; also refer to Chapter 16).

Red alert: Patients with the following symptoms should be referred to a specialist:

1   *Intermenstrual bleeding*
2   *Postcoital bleeding*
3   *Anaemia*
4   *Weight loss*
5   *Abdominal distension*
6   *Postmenopausal bleeding*
7   *Nausea/anorexia without pregnancy.*

Chapter Summary

This chapter has shown how differential diagnosis may be used to develop an understanding of the patient's condition. It is not possible to give a simplistic route to diagnosis, but the complementary practitioner needs to be aware of the possible routes that may need to be followed when a patient presents with particular symptoms. None of the information supplied here is a substitute for detailed examination and it is provided as indicative of possible avenues to explore, rather than as a definitive route to diagnosis. There will be an absolute requirement for referral by the complementary practitioner to a medical practitioner in appropriate cases.

REVIEW QUESTIONS

1   What are the possible causes of low back pain? What are the main similarities and differences between these causes?

2   What are the possible causes of chest pain? What are the main similarities and differences between these causes?

3   What key questions would you need to ask when a patient comes to your clinic with abdominal pain?

4   What are the main causes of fatigue? What red flag symptoms would you watch for, which would require you to refer the patient to a medical doctor or a specialist?

CHAPTER LINKS

For further discussion of particular aspects of anatomy and physiology referred to here, see Chapters 14, 15, 16 and 17.

FURTHER RESOURCES

Beck, E.R., Souhami, R.I., Hanna, M.G. and Holdright, D.R. (2003) *Tutorials in Differential Diagnosis*, 4th edn, Edinburgh, Churchill Livingstone. Covers the most likely causes and symptoms of different clinical features.

Beers, M.H. (2006) *The Merck Manual of Diagnosis and Therapy*, 18th edn, Whitehouse Station, NJ, Merck Research Laboratory. Useful reference book, providing medical and healthcare professionals with necessary information about medical examinations, diagnosis and treatment. You can access it online at www.merck.com/mmpe/index.html.

Bickley, L.S. and Szilagyi, P.G. (2007) *Bates' Guide to Physical Examination and History Taking*, 9th edn, Philadelphia, PA, Lippincott, Williams & Wilkins. Provides comprehensive clinical skills: observation, consultation and palpation, useful for medical and healthcare professionals.

Seller, R.H. (2007) *Differential Diagnosis of Common Complaints*, 5th edn, Philadelphia, WB Saunders. Covers the most commonly seen complaints patients may present with and practitioners may see in their daily practice.

Part V

Resource file

The Roots of Practice

The Context of Ideas

Ideas about complementary therapies and alternative medicine challenge conventional medicine based on orthodox medical science. The ideas and assumptions of these challenging approaches remain largely excluded from conventional medical practice. On the whole – and this is a generalization, so there are exceptions – conventional practice is based on a biomedical idea of the body, rather than adopting a holistic approach to understanding the person as body, mind and spirit. This statement is made in recognition that spirituality remains a somewhat marginal item on the curriculum of many professional qualifying programmes for practitioners with people. The reality, however, is that many communities in developing and developed countries have a faith dimension and incorporate ideas about spirituality in the culture of their everyday life and, correspondingly perhaps, the literature on spirituality and various areas of the practice of working with people is expanding.

Historical Shifts and Key People

It is often said that a particular person founded a particular complementary approach. It is important, however, to appreciate three key points:

1. Many seeming modern approaches have their roots in prehistory.
2. History is not solely the product of the works of 'great men', for two main reasons:
   - Women have made a substantial contribution as well as men.
   - A combination of historical – economic, social, cultural, religious, political, as well as personal – factors have contributed to the growth of traditional medicine in India, China and the Mediterranean regions in particular, over the millennia and, more recently, to the spread of complementary and alternative approaches throughout the world.
3. Healing and medicine have not always been led by the male-dominated professions of surgery and medicine. For centuries before the creation of professionalized Western doctoring and surgery, women were the traditional healers and midwives in many societies.

The following table provides a thumbnail guide to some of the main features of these developments.

Table RF5.1 Timeline of complementary and traditional practice

Name/Approach	Key developments
Hippocrates (*c.* 460–377 BCE) (**Ancient Greece**)	Hippocrates and his followers, the Hippocratics, are generally regarded as responsible for advancing medicine beyond the pursuit of health through using magic and religion. The founders of naturotherapy – the use of natural products to heal people. Their approach focuses on the physical, that is, separating medicine from philosophy and concentrating on curing the body, by restoring the balance between the humours – essential fluids
Galen (*c.* 130–200 CE) (**Ancient Rome**)	Galen of Pergamum studied anatomy – superimposing on the notion of the humours the development of dietary means of improving wellbeing and drug treatments directed at body functions
Traditional Chinese medicine (TCM)	The Chinese traditional form of medicine, at least 3,000 years old. Huangdi's *Canon of Medicine* was collected and written down more than 2,000 years ago

Name/Approach	Key developments
Ayurveda	The Indian tradition of medicine, gradually gathered from folklore and written down by scholars from almost 2,000 years ago
Unani	The traditional Persian system of medicine, drawn from roots in Greek and Arabic medicine, and still practised in India by nearly 30,000 practitioners in about 100 Unani hospitals
Aromatherapy	A form of therapy popular in the twenty-first century, rooted in the ancient practice of aromatics and encountered in Indian, Egyptian and Arab traditional medicine
Avicenna (980–1037) (Persia – now Iran)	'The Arab Galen'. Developed studies of epidemiology – the study of the control and treatment of disease. Studied emotions as well as the body. Examined smells and bodily excretions in order to shed light on health. Used massage and other therapies. Emphasized health-giving properties of diet, for example liquids such as water, tea and fruit juices
The Renaissance (14th–17th century)	Led to a move away from the notion of bodily harmony, towards scientifically based medicine
Paracelsus (1493–1541)	Identified some external causes of disease such as dirty water and food. Argued that plants and metals could cure diseases. Argued against alchemy – a medieval philosophic system of chemistry based on magic rather than science. Developed some modern medicines using, for example, sulphur, arsenic and opium
Nicholas Culpeper (1616–54)	Herbalist and author of influential book, *The English Physitian* (1652)
Samuel Hahnemann (1755–1843)	German doctor who criticized extreme medical treatments. Argued that people's living conditions – nutrition, housing and fresh air – should be improved as a route to better health. Founded the idea of homeopathy in 1796
Samuel Thompson (1769–1843)	Developed a system of medicine based on botanical principles
Dr Coffin (1790–1866)	Founded the National Association of Medical Herbalists in 1864, now the National Institute of Medical Herbalists
James Compton Burnett (1840–1901)	A leading thinker and practitioner of homeopathy, who published *Vaccinosis* (1884), a study of how vaccination can bring about illness
F. Matthias Alexander (1869–1955)	An Australian actor who developed the educational Alexander technique
Mikao Usui (1865–1926)	A thinker and practitioner who developed reiki, a form of spiritual practice, in the early 1920s
Maharishi Mahesh Yogi (1918–2008)	A thinker who became well known for bringing the practice of transcendental meditation to Western countries from the late 1950s

Part V

Approaches to Practice

Part VI
Approaches to Practice

Introduction

This part of the book consists of chapters illustrating some of the main approaches to practice. It is important to note that Part VI is directly rooted in practice. The authors of these chapters have been commissioned to write from their experience as practitioners and each writes as authoritative advocate for the particular approach.

The approaches covered in Part VI are grouped as follows.

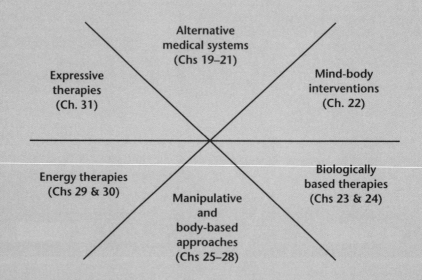

To provide a comprehensive picture of all the different approaches under these six headings would require a shelf of books. Hence just a selection of approaches from each group of approaches has been chosen, to provide a thorough overview. To complement this selection, a resource file at the end of each of the six groups of chapters is provided, which summarizes information about other major approaches of relevance in the group and includes further reading for each. The reader can use the chapters and these resource files as different forms of stimulus to critical reflection and further study, since they approach the same subject matter from different vantage points.

Homeopathy 19

SUE ARMSTRONG

Learning outcomes

By the end of this chapter, you should be able to:

■ understand the underlying principles and philosophy of homeopathy

■ grasp the essentials of how the method is applied in practice

■ appreciate the evidence base supporting the use of homeopathy and the need for further study

What is Homeopathy?

Homeopathy is a therapeutic method using preparations of substances to treat disease according to the 'similia' principle or 'like cures like', that is, the substance used to treat the symptoms of disease in a sick individual will have a direct correspondence with the symptoms the substance will produce when administered to a healthy individual over time. The method, which incorporates a comprehensive understanding of health and disease using clear principles and laws to govern the administration of preparations to sick individuals, was developed by Samuel Hahnemann (1755–1843). He coined the word 'homeopathy' from the Greek words *homos* (same) and *pathos* (suffering). The complete clinical picture of the patient including mental, general and local (particular) symptoms plus signs and diagnostic test results if appropriate are taken into account to provide what is known as the 'totality of symptoms' specific to the individual patient. Homeopathy is more than the giving of remedies to treat the patient, it also focuses on the identification and removal of the 'obstacles to cure' for patients and offers the path to health. Obstacles to cure include obvious blocks such as excessive alcohol, drugs and environmental factors but also the continued use of suppressive medications.

Knowledge about the Remedies

The medicinal properties of remedies are determined in three ways – toxicology reports, cured case evidence and, most importantly, results of testing the substances in material dose, mother tincture or potency by administration to healthy volunteers. The tests, known as 'provings' or homeopathic pathogenetic trials, are carried out under strict conditions and all the symptoms of the provers are recorded and collated, for example physical symptoms, modalities (factors modifying a symptom), sensations, emotions, dreams. The information about the therapeutic potential for each remedy is collated into materia medica. Repertories then provide a cross-reference of symptoms and disorders to the homeopathic remedies in whose materia medica they occur. Repertories are available in both written and electronic form; however, with the vast amount of information to be cross-referenced, computer versions are now extremely important tools for the homeopath.

The remedies are made from any substance that can alter the health of an individual and may be used as a 'mother tincture' or a 'potency'. The raw substances used in the manufacture of potentized remedies are all first put into solution (insoluble substances undergo a procedure known as 'trituration' to render them soluble) and then made into the recognized potencies through a series of dilutions and 'successions' (vigorous shaking with impact or 'elastic collision'), following a homeopathic manufacturing procedure described in the approved pharmacopoeia of the country involved. Three scales of dilution and succussion are used:

1. Decimal scale – 1:10
2. Centesimal scale – 1:100
3. LM (50 millesimal) potency – 1:50,000.

Potencies are initially produced in a liquid form, which is usually via a water-alcohol vehicle, and either used in a liquid form or this is used to medicate a solid dosage form, for example soft pillules, granules, powders or hard tablets.

Values and Principles Guiding Practice

Homeopathy is a truly holistic system of medicine that deals with the individuality of the patient on the mental, emotional and physical level, with prescribing being based on the totality of symptoms expressed by the individual on all levels and on the factors that modify these symptoms for the individual. Homeopathy recognizes the non-material/chemical life force or 'dynamis' that in modern language is often described as the patient's vitality, wellbeing or immunity. This intangible realm of the living organism is recognized in many other therapeutic modalities, for example traditional Chinese medicine. It is the 'mistunement' of this 'dynamis' in the living body that is ideally matched by the dynamic nature of the similar individual homeopathic remedy to affect cure.

In his final work *Organon of the Medical Art* (first published in 1810 and revised five times, the sixth edition being published in 1921), Hahnemann stated that the highest ideal of cure is the 'gentle, rapid and permanent restoration of health' in the 'shortest, most reliable and least disadvantageous way, according to clearly realisable principles' (Hahnemann, 1995). Not only does the homeopathic medical system respect the concept that the body has the ability to heal itself but it also honours the need to treat the body without violence, suppression or by replacing one set of symptoms with another, for example those belonging to the realm of drug side effects. Quality of life for the patient is paramount throughout the journey from birth through to death. The primary focus of the homeopathic process is on the restoration of health, allowing the patient to fulfil their life purpose rather than the maintenance of chronic ill health through a long-term commitment to palliative drugs that have no curative potential.

What Practice Entails

The skill and art of the good homeopath is in being the unprejudiced observer of each of their patients and to receive rather than take the patient's case. Good practice requires that the homeopath provides a safe space for their patients, which includes not only the physical environment of the consultation room but also the space and time to allow the patient to openly tell their story without prejudice or judgement. It is essential to provide a clear contract to help manage both patient and practitioner expectation, particularly in the case of chronic case management.

The totality of symptoms is used as the basis to treat both acute and chronic disease presentations; however, in chronic disease cases, this totality includes the past disease profile within the current totality in a three-dimensional way. In chronic cases, there is also the concept of the return of old symptoms and the removal of symptoms in the reverse order of their coming in successive diseases, with the direction of cure being from the most important organs, such as the heart, to the least important, which often ultimately ends in a skin eruption, however fleeting.

The homeopathic world has developed a number of different case-taking, analysis and prescribing methodologies, for example causation or trigger events, totality of symptoms, essence, for example a 'miasm' or trait making the individual susceptible to a certain pattern of morbidity, kingdoms and families of remedies and so on.

There are two distinct pathways for those wishing to practise homeopathy in the UK. The first route is that of the medical or veterinary professional who undergoes training by an accredited organization, and then, having passed the examinations set by the Faculty of Homeopathy, becomes a member of the Faculty of Homeopathy. The practitioner is then subject to its code of conduct and ethics. This is currently the only route available for those wishing to treat animals other than their own, as under the Veterinary Surgeons Act 1966, it is illegal for anyone other than a Royal College of Veterinary Surgeons-registered veterinary surgeon to treat animals in the UK. The second route is for the non-medically trained who can undergo training and examination that is accredited by one of the UK's associations of homeopaths. The Society of Homeopaths is currently Britain's largest professional association of homeopaths and was the first to form a register of members, with professional standards, a code of ethics and practice and fitness to practise procedures.

Practice example

Miss J is a 20-year-old woman who presents with headaches that tend to be one-sided and she feels as if her head will burst. The pain tends to be frontal but can also travel into the face and teeth. The headaches started at puberty and are variable in intensity; she reports that the headaches are worse if she has a lot of college work to do. They are better if she walks in the open air.

From this information, the homeopath has details of the particulars of the local problem and will then go on to ask questions about the patient in general, including their previous illnesses and incidents in their lives as well as observing the nature of the patient and their reactions in the consulting room.

This patient dislikes being too hot or too cold and has a great dislike of fatty food, which also disagrees with her, although she likes butter. She has a very low thirst, occasionally liking sharp rather than sweet lemonade. She was prone to colds when younger and would produce a lot of bland catarrh, which could also be produced as expectoration from the lung.

As a child, she would talk in her sleep and would prefer to sleep with her mother. She presented as mild and did not answer the homeopath freely without questioning, so this had to be done with great sensitivity as she easily became tearful.

This is a typical presentation for a patient needing the remedy pulsatilla, which is being expressed not only at the local level of the headache symptoms but by the totality of symptoms on the mental, emotional and physical level.

Activity

Spend time reflecting and making notes on your own general modalities, for example your thirst, your preference for warmth or cool, your response to noise, your need for company and consolation, the time of day when you have higher and lower energy, the quality of your sleep and if you regularly wake during the night, the time that you do. Listen for modalities being offered by other people in conversation. Reflect upon how easy it is to filter out this information when listening to other people talking of their illnesses.

It is easy to filter out this information when listening to people, largely because in conventional medicine this information is mostly irrelevant and will not alter the selection of medication. When in company, try to become conscious of actively listening to what people are saying, how they are moving, what preferences they are showing, how they dress, how they respond to others. Becoming conscious of the way the body expresses itself in the form of symptoms and in the art of receiving information without prejudice is the first step to receiving the case from a client as a homeopath.

What Research Tells us about the Effectiveness of Homeopathy

It is often cited that there is no proof that homeopathy works and that homeopathic research at best provides weak positive evidence with a tendency towards both bias and flawed methodology. Problems with the quality of research are a major issue in all medical paradigms including our current conventional medical model. A review published in *The Lancet* in 2005, which again concluded that the effectiveness of homeopathy was seriously flawed, has now, in two published studies, been shown to be equally flawed in its own methodology. There are, in fact, a significant number of high-quality trials showing that for certain conditions, for example allergies, upper respiratory tract infections, childhood diarrhoea, influenza, postoperative ileus, rheumatic disease and vertigo, homeopathy is not just placebo, that is, there is a positive effect over and above placebo (Table 19.1).

Table 19.1 Research contributing to evidence base for homeopathy

■ Barnes J, Resch K-L, Ernst E. Homeopathy for postoperative ileus? A meta-analysis. *J Clin Gastroenterol* 1997; 25: 628–33	■ Bornhöft G, Wolf U, Ammon K, et al. Effectiveness, safety and cost-effectiveness of homeopathy in general practice: summarized health technology assessment. *Forsch Komplementärmed* 2006; 13 Suppl 2: 19–29
■ Bell I, Lewis D, Brooks A, et al. Improved clinical status in fibromyalgia patients treated with individualized homeopathic remedies versus placebo *Rheumatology* 2004; 43: 577–82.	■ Colin P. Homeopathy and respiratory allergies: a series of 147 cases. *Homeopathy* 2006; 95, 68–72.
■ Bell IR, Lewis DA, Brooks AJ, et al. Gas discharge visualisation evaluation of ultramolecular doses of homeopathic medicines under blinded, controlled conditions. *J Altern Complement Med* 2003; 9: 25–38	■ Cucherat M, Haugh MC, Gooch M, Boissel JP. Evidence of clinical efficacy of homeopathy: a meta-analysis of clinical trials. *Eur J Clin Pharmacol* 2000; 56: 27–33
■ Bellavite P, Ortolani R, Pontarollo F, et al. Immunology and homeopathy. 4. Clinical studies – Part 2. eCAM 2006; 3: 397–409	■ Diefenbach M, Schilken J, Steiner G, Becker HJ. Homeopathic therapy in respiratory tract diseases: evaluation of a clinical study in 258 patients. *Z Allgemeinmed* 1997; 73: 308–14
■ Belon P, Cumps J, Ennis M, et al. Histamine dilutions modulate basophil activation. *Inflamm Res* 2004; 53: 181–8	■ Elia V and Niccoli M. Thermodynamics of extremely diluted aqueous solutions. *Ann N Y Acad Sci* 1999; 879: 241–8

■ Fisher P. An experimental double-blind clinical trial method in homoeopathy: use of a limited range of remedies to treat fibrositis. *BrHomeopath J* 1986; 75: 142–7

■ Friese K-H and Zabalotnyi DI. Homeopathy in acute rhinosinusitis: a double-blind, placebo controlled study shows the effectiveness and tolerability of a homeopathic combination remedy. *HNO* 2007; 55: 271–7

■ Jacobs J, Jonas WB, Jimenez-Perez M, Crothers D. Homeopathy for childhood diarrhea: combined results and metaanalysis from three randomized, controlled clinical trials. *Pediatr Infect Dis J* 2003; 22: 229–34

■ Jacobs J, Springer DA, Crothers D. Homeopathic treatment of acute otitis media in children: a preliminary randomized placebo-controlled trial. *Pediatr Infect Dis J* 2001; 20: 177–83

■ Jonas WB, Linde K, Ramirez G. Homeopathy and rheumatic disease: complementary and alternative therapies for rheumatic diseases II. *Rheum Dis Clin North Am* 2000; 26: 117–23

■ Kleijnen J, Knipschild P, ter Riet G. Clinical trials of homeopathy. *Br Med J* 1991; 302: 316–23

■ Linde K, Clausius N, Ramirez G, et al. Are the clinical effects of homoeopathy placebo effects? A meta-analysis of placebo-controlled trials. *Lancet* 1997; 350: 834–43

■ Linde K, Scholz M, Ramirez G, et al. Impact of study quality on outcome in placebo controlled trials of homeopathy. *J Clin Epidemiol* 1999; 52: 631–6

■ Linde K, Jonas WB, Melchart D, et al. Critical review and meta-analysis of serial agitated dilutions in experimental toxicology. *Hum Exp Toxicol* 1994; 13: 481–92

■ Ludtke R and Rutten A. The conclusions on the effectiveness of homeopathy highly depend on the set of analyzed trials. *Journal of Clinical Epidemiology* 2008; 61, 12: 1197–204

■ Sevar R. Audit of outcome in 829 consecutive patients treated with homeopathic medicine. *British Homeopathic Journal* 2000; 89: 4

■ Shang A, Huwiler-Muntener K, Nartey L, et al. Are the clinical effects of homoeopathy placebo effects? Comparative study of placebo-controlled trials of homoeopathy and allopathy. *Lancet* 2005; 366: 726–32

■ Sharples F, van Haselen R, Fisher P. NHS patients' perspective on complementary medicine. *Complement Ther Med* 2003; 11: 243–8

■ Shealy CN, Thomlinson RP, Cox RH, Borgmeyer RN. Osteoarthritic pain: a comparison of homeopathy and acetaminophen. *Am J Pain Manage* 1998; 8: 89–91

■ Spence D, Thompson E, Barron S. Homeopathic treatment for chronic disease: a 6-year university hospital based outpatient observational study. *J Altern Complement Med* 2005; 5: 793–8

■ Taylor MA, Reilly D, Llewellyn-Jones RH, et al. Randomised controlled trials of homoeopathy versus placebo in perennial allergic rhinitis with overview of four trial series. *Br Med J* 2000; 321: 471–6

■ Trichard M, Chaufferin G Nicoloyannis N. Pharmacoeconomic comparison between homeopathic and antibiotic treatment strategies in recurrent acute rhinopharyngitis in children. *Homeopathy* 2005; 94: 3–9

■ van Haselen RA and Fisher PAG. A randomized controlled trial comparing topical piroxicam gel with a homeopathic gel in osteoarthritis of the knee. *Rheumatology* 2000; 39: 714–19

■ Vickers A, Smith C. *Homoeopathic Oscillococcinum for preventing and treating influenza and influenza-like syndromes* (Cochrane Review). In Cochrane Library, Chichester, John Wiley & Sons, 2006

■ Weatherley-Jones E, Nicholl JP, Thomas KJ, et al. A randomized, controlled, triple-blind trial of the efficacy of homeopathic treatment for chronic fatigue syndrome. *J Psychosom Res* 2004; 56: 189–97

■ Wiesenauer M, Lüdtke R. A meta-analysis of the homeopathic treatment of pollinosis with Galphimia glauca. *Forsch Komplementärmed Klass Naturheilkd* 1996; 3: 230–6

■ Witt C, Keil T, Selim D, et al. Outcome and costs of homeopathic and conventional treatment strategies: a comparative cohort study in patients with chronic disorders. *Complement Ther Med* 2005; 13: 79–86

■ Witt CM, Lüdtke R, Baur R, Willich SN. Homeopathic medical practice: long-term results of a cohort study with 3,981 patients. *BMC Public Health* 2005; 5: 115

■ Witt CM, Bluth M, Albrecht H, et al. The in vitro evidence for an effect of high homeopathic potencies: a systematic review of the literature. *Complement Ther Med* 2007; 15: 128–38

■ Yakir M, Kreitler S, Brzezinski A, et al. Effects of homeopathic treatment in women with premenstrual syndrome: a pilot study. *Br Homeopath J* 2001; 90: 148–53

■ Zabolotnyi DI, Kneis KC, Richardson A, et al. Efficacy of a complex homeopathic medication (Sinfrontal) in patients with acute maxillary sinusitis: a prospective, randomized, double-blind, placebo-controlled, multicenter clinical trial. *Explore* (NY) 2007; 3: 98–109

■ Zell J, Connert WD, Mau J, Feuerstake G. Treatment of acute sprains of the ankle: controlled double-blind trial to test the effectiveness of a homeopathic ointment. *Fortschr Med* 1988; 106: 96–100

The biggest issue facing any homeopath is that there is uncertainty as to the underlying mechanism of homeopathy. High dilution research is now being produced by a variety of disciplines, for example material science and physics as well as homeopathy, and it will be the results of high-quality studies with full methodological rigour, which aim to demonstrate the 'similia' principle and the effects of high dilutions, that will ultimately change the future for homeopathy. This lack of understanding of the underlying mechanism has in part been responsible for the great diversity in the way that homeopathy is practised globally as methodology is largely varied according to which teaching practice has been followed.

The evidence base for practice includes four types of research:

1. randomized controlled trials (RCTs) of homeopathy
2. systematic reviews of RCTs of homeopathy
3. clinical observational studies
4. basic science looking at high dilutions and the properties of water.

Any paradigm that has a basis in individuality has an issue with time, funding and clinical study modelling. To receive and work up a chronic case takes time – a first consultation for a chronic patient would require a minimum of one hour, plus time for case analysis after the consultation to select the initial treatment protocol. The long-term costs both in time and money may in fact be highly favourable towards homeopathy, but there is a tendency to compare the time of a single appointment with a GP rather than the overall time and money spent over the duration of a patient's chronic illness. Individuality means that there is no given remedy for a named disease, hence there is no incentive for research and development within the pharmaceutical industry sector for homeopathy. This makes the funding of homeopathic research a major issue, plus the fact that there are a relatively small number of suitably qualified homeopaths who are willing to participate in research. Research models that cater for the needs of individualizing patients have also proved difficult in the clinical setting, as the standard RCT is based on the conventional model of 'one drug fits all'.

Chapter Summary

This chapter has explored the origins and nature of homeopathy, shown how its holistic principles are applied in practice and given illustrations of the evidence base for practice.

REVIEW QUESTIONS

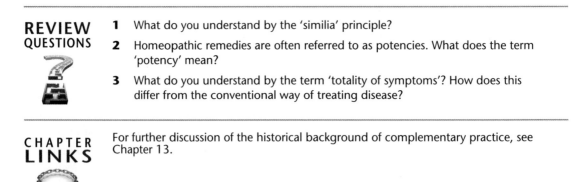

1   What do you understand by the 'similia' principle?

2   Homeopathic remedies are often referred to as potencies. What does the term 'potency' mean?

3   What do you understand by the term 'totality of symptoms'? How does this differ from the conventional way of treating disease?

CHAPTER LINKS

For further discussion of the historical background of complementary practice, see Chapter 13.

FURTHER RESOURCES

Bonamin, L.V. (ed.) (2008) *Signals and Images: Contributions and Contradictions about High Dilution Research*, London, Springer. Third volume published by Groupe International de Recherche sur l'Infinitésimal. Presents peer-reviewed multidisciplinary contributions on the issues of high dilution research.

Boyd, H. (1989) *Introduction to Homeopathic Medicine*, 2nd edn, Beaconsfield, Beaconsfield Publishers. Easy to read introductory book that acts as a handy reference guide containing a small materia medica useful in differentiating between remedies in acute conditions.

Hahnemann, S. (1995) *Organon of the Medical Art*, 6th edn, trans. S. Decker, ed. and annotated by W. Brewster O'Reilly, Washington, Birdcage Books. All serious students of homeopathy should read this book as it holds within its pages the bedrock understanding of homeopathy, as relevant today as it was when the work was finally completed in 1842.

Kaplan, B. (2001) *The Homeopathic Conversation: The Art of Taking the Case*, Natural Medicine Press, London. Excellent book for students and practitioners alike that includes specific chapters on children, nonverbal clues, learning and teaching case-taking skills, and Rogerian psychology/counselling.

Kayne, S. (2006) *Homeopathic Pharmacy: Theory and Practice*, New York, Elsevier Churchill Livingstone. Good text, which not only acts as a reference for pharmacists but also contains comprehensive material on all aspects of basic homeopathic principles and practice.

Owen, D. (2007) *Principles and Practice of Homeopathy: The Therapeutic and Healing Process*, London, Churchill Livingstone. Most comprehensive book currently available for providing homeopathic students with a practical and thorough basis for understanding the application of the homeopathic process.

Vithoulkas, G. (2008) *Homeopathy: Medicine for the New Millennium,* 27th edn, Alonissos, Greece, International Academy of Classical Homeopathy. Presents the historical scientific basis for homeopathy in simple terms and addresses the health of the whole person and how homeopathy can be used to treat many chronic conditions.

Web Links

www.trusthomeopathy.org – The British Homeopathic Association, a charity founded in 1902, exists to promote homeopathy practised by doctors and other healthcare professionals. It believes that patients should be able to choose homeopathy as part of a healthcare system, which recognizes the benefits of conventional and complementary medicine, and works to provide high-quality information about homeopathy for the public and healthcare professionals.

www.homeopathy-soh.org – The Society of Homeopaths is the largest organization registering professional homeopaths in Europe. This site gives basic information about homeopathy, training, funding and research as well as providing a valuable resource for registered members.

www.hpathy.com – Homeopathy 4 Everyone is an excellent e-journal on homeopathy. This site provides extensive information about homeopathy, cured cases, materia medica, homeopathic philosophy and carries articles written by leading contemporary homeopaths.

www.facultyofhomeopathy.org – The Faculty of Homeopathy promotes the academic and scientific development of homeopathy. It sets the standards for and regulates the education, training and practice of homeopathy by dentists, doctors, nurses, midwives, osteopaths, pharmacists, podiatrists, veterinary surgeons and other statutorily registered healthcare professionals.

20 Life, Spirituality and Chinese Medicine

FANYI MENG

Distinctive Beliefs Associated with Chinese Medicine

In Chinese medicine, the concept of patient is essentially the same as that of Western medicine, but the real meaning is different in some ways. When a patient is mentioned, it becomes a subject of the human being, rather than the body. A human being is the whole of the life object, including the spiritual or mental and physical aspects, and these aspects are the varying faces of the human being.

Chinese medicine deals with the quality of life as a whole, rather than just trying to correct visible health problems. It emphasizes the quality of life experienced by the patient, and the importance of maintaining a harmonized life to fend off diseases. The physical side of human beings is understood as a functioning model, the unique Zang Fu and meridian systems, which are at the centre of

Chinese medicine theories. They are not solid organs or structural units, but rather functional/managing centres, considered to be where many vital life functions take place. Although the terms, when translated into English, appear to be like terms used in conventional medicine, they are different. This will be discussed in Chapter 21.

In this chapter, I discuss the traditional Chinese view of life and the main beliefs encountered within Taoism and Buddhism. This chapter is written by a practitioner from within the beliefs associated with traditional Chinese medicine, rather than about them.

Traditional Chinese View of Life

It is widely accepted that Chinese medicine is one of the oldest branches of knowledge in ancient China. Its origin is thought to be from two main sources: people's daily observation and experience and mythology. According to this mythology, when knowledge was accumulated, it was collected and recorded, and therefore mastered by the Wisdom Man (Wu 巫), who knew everything the ancient Chinese societies possessed, from astronomy to seasonal changes, from agricultural skills to war and human beings. So, early knowledge about life was a mixed picture of mysterious legends and knowledge obtained from observation of humans, animals and plants, and birth and death. Although humankind was thought to be unique and the most precious creatures in the world, most people believed that humans were part of the animal kingdom. So knowledge gained from dissecting animals should apply to humans as well. The knowledge of the internal structures of the human body was widely accepted as the result of comparing human bodies with animal bodies.

About the origin of life, the idea that God created humankind was widespread. According to an ancient Chinese legend, humankind was created by a god called Nu-Wa (女娲). He/she shaped the figures of humans out of mud according to his/her own shape and blew air into the figures, so humans received life and started to act. From this legend, it is believed that human life is blessed by the god, the heaven and the earth, all the most powerful forces in the world and therefore human life is the most powerful and important life. Knowledge, including that of human life and health, accumulated during the period from 6,000 BC to 1,000 BC. Around 800 BC, medical doctors (Yi, 医), who were in charge of health issues, were formally separated from the general role played by the Wisdom Man in the community. These doctors carried out healing as part of their service to society as a whole. Medical officers were responsible for looking after the health of royal families. At that time, doctors and the Wisdom Man in the community shared the healthcare services among ordinary people of all social classes. Later, when Confucian beliefs predominated, medical practice was established as the sole preserve of doctors (黄帝内经·素问》中所说，'拘于鬼神者不可与言至德'。都是医学摆脱巫术，确立自身价值的标志). (The Chinese characters used here and at the end of paragraphs in the rest of this chapter are from the Chinese classics and identify the source of the information referred to.)

So Chinese medicine originated as a natural way of understanding the world and human life. The knowledge and skills used in medicine were those from practice and observation, rather than simply from thinking. The notion of what life is and how it started was always considered to be important. The origin of human life was thought to be the combination of the essences from heaven and earth. In other words, the combination of the best parts of the world gives life to human beings. According to this view, the best part of heaven is named as yang, heaven qi, while the best part of the earth is named as yin, earth qi. Both have their role in human life.

Life is considered to consist of the interaction and unity of qi in the environment, the heaven qi and the earth qi:

> Qi from Heaven and Earth merges, and then the six dimensions of movement are created, and all creatures are formed and created. (the Plain Question, part of the *Yellow Emperor's Internal Classic*) (天地合气, 六节分而万物化生矣, 素问.宝命全形论)

Qi is considered to be the finest particle in the world and invisible. It is also the source of energy. It releases energy for all kinds of movements and changes. With the energy from qi, there is wind and stars, growth and decay. Qi forms everything in the world, including human beings. The differences found in all the kinds of materials and objects come from the different combinations of qi. There are numerous possible combinations, therefore there are endless forms of lives. In the environment, the exchange of qi maintains life. Human life has the most complicated combinations of qi, and is therefore the most precious form of qi. The *Yellow Emperor's Internal Classic* stated:

> Heaven covers and earth bearing, then all things could take place. When all creatures are produced, then the human being is created. Among all things, nothing is more precious than the human being. The human being is generated by the Qi of Heaven and Qi of Earth, and complies with the law which changes the four seasons. '天复地载, 万物悉备, 莫贵于人. 人以天地之气生, 四时之法成.' (素问. 宝命全形论)

Chinese medicine is deeply rooted in natural philosophy, and believes in the unity of spirit and body. This is different from the Western model of medicine, which puts the emphasis on the physical study of the body.

The creation of individual life is the combining of the two kinds of essence, the **yin** essence from the mother and the **yang** essence from the father, which reflect the heaven qi and earth qi. This is another example of the holism in Chinese medicine. The masculine force, in the father, represents the force from heaven and the sky, which is active; while the feminine force, in the body of the mother, represents the force of earth, the solid foundation and the stability of the universe. Humankind lives between the two forces of heaven and earth, and is generated by the interaction of them, in the special form of the interaction of the father and mother. Since individual life is generated in the special form of interaction, the new individual life is then heavily influenced by the interaction and the bearing force of the father and mother, especially the mother.

The development of the body is the constant developing of spiral balance and imbalance between the yin and yang in the new body. In childhood, it is the yang, which has the power of starting movement and changes, that causes the growth. The new body alternates between very active and relatively less active build-ups. When it is very active, the yang takes the power and lifts the activity level to a new height. The body then gains its materials to build up its structure, which is the foundation and belongs to yin. The building of the physical structure is the function of yin, giving more stability and bearing power. When the building up reaches a certain level, a new balance is then reached at the new height. The yang is always the dominating power in childhood. In adulthood, the yang and yin maintain a dynamic balance, and always return within the balancing range. The body is no longer growing. When the body is ageing, the system change is driven by the declining force of yin. The declining of yin dominates the change. The active force has to lower its activity level since the support from the structure and materials is drying out.

The maintenance of life lies in the dynamic balance between the body and the spirit. It is part of the balance of yin and yang, but is more complicated than this. The spiritual condition is not simply decided by the exchange of qi between a human and the environment, but can also be altered by internal developments inside the body and between the body and the social environment.

The intake of qi from the environment and the discharge of qi into the environment remain in a stable condition. In childhood, the exchange of qi between the human body and environment is always positive, the body keeps putting on weight, and activity level is high. In adulthood, this reaches a dynamic balance, body weight and height are maintained in a certain range, and the energy level is flat. In old age, the body's intake of qi from the environment is negative, the body is weak and its structure is shrinking.

Qi: Life and Nature

Qi is considered to be the basic building block of all materials of the world. It is the finest particle existing in the world. Qi has energy in it. This energy could be used for physical movement, the flowing of itself, or to combine qi into more complicated forms of materials, like water, air, metal and rock.

The inspiration behind the establishment of qi is mainly through the observation of natural phenomena. The ancient people found that some materials could disappear, and when they are disappearing, they will change into another form as they go. For example, the water in a container will dry up in open air. In the early days, people did not know how the water disappeared. But when they noticed that when water is heated, it evaporates into steam, they understood that water could become steam and disappear. They also noticed that in the early morning, when the sun is shining, the mist in the fields will rise into the air and disappear. Similarly, they noticed that when wood is lit, it produces not only heat and flames, but also smoke. And afterwards, most of the wood has disappeared and left only a little ash. It was suggested that the flames and the smoke are the forms of materials that disappear.

So, the ancient people realized that water, wood, grass can all become some kind of gas, like mist, steam, flames and smoke, and disappear into the air. And then people gradually realized that mist and clouds are the same thing and they can become water again in the form of dew and rain. Eventually, they realized that the gas-like material is the medium of changes. One material can change into it and then change back or into another form of material or object. It was considered that all materials could take changes in the ways of changing into this gas-like material and disappear into somewhere, and could also be produced by the changes of some of the gas-like materials. This gas-like material is named as qi (气). Qi in different forms means different materials. We can see the ancient Chinese character above showing the flowing line of the air. We now discuss some of the most important concepts of qi.

Natural qi is also called the 'one qi' or 'yuan qi', which refers to the single source of the world, the building material of all kinds of other combined forms of qi, the other basic materials. The qi could combine into any form and show features of all nature of characters. This concept is the cornerstone of Chinese natural philosophy. It is the hypothesis of the origin and development of the world.

Genuine qi is the qi that belongs to the human body and exists in each individual. It is also called 'original qi' (yuan qi). When an individual life starts, there is a life force belonging to this life. This genuine qi will stay inside the body from the beginning to the end. It is not transferable. When it leaves the body, the life is finished. It always stays in a very deep level of the body to be appropriately protected. One cannot borrow genuine qi from another. The strengthening of the genuine qi can only be achieved by the smooth supply of surplus body essence, which can be produced by a healthy body in balanced yin and yang. Genuine qi does not carry out the functions of maintaining daily activities. It is the root of all life functions and provides the support for all the human functions.

An individual human body must maintain its stability, staying as it is, otherwise life cannot continue. To maintain life, the living body must take in from the environment and give out to it as well. But, free exchange means genuine qi could easily run out of the body, or something could easily take over the body, then life is no longer the same. To maintain life, good things are needed, while bad things should be avoided:

- Good source of qi: food and nutrition can easily be assimilated into the body and utilized by the life. When this kind of material enters the body, the body can build up or maintain normal function. This intake should be encouraged.
- Bad source of qi: toxins or poisons are those materials in the natural world containing qi not compatible to human life. When they enter the body, disturbance or disruption will happen, which weakens the genuine qi of life, or threatens death.

Maintaining appropriate discharge is also important. Without discharge, the body would hold everything it took and would quickly burst. Ideally, for an adult, the body should discharge the same amount of intake, to maintain a balance.

Body and Spirit

In Chinese medicine, the spirit is part of genuine qi with its activities. The spirit is named as Shen (神) in Chinese medicine. It is defined as the collective term of all mental activities, including the thinking, memory, perception, planning, reasoning, emotions, and controlling and coordinating power of the whole body.

The spirit is produced when a new life is started, which is initialized by the combination of the two essential materials for new life, the yang essence from the father and the yin essence from the mother. Because it is a kind of collective activity of the special form of qi, it is the most active part of the life, and should never stop. The spirit is constantly working, even during sleep, so it needs to be constantly supplied with supportive material for its activities. It never works when it is separated from the body.

Death

Death in Chinese medicine is defined as the separation of yin and yang, which means that yang (the spirit or genuine qi) leaves the body, and the structural body (yin) is not controlled by the spirit. Because the spirit will run out of energy shortly after the separation, it will dissipate itself immediately, and become part of the natural qi again. Without the spirit, the body has no driving force and will remain inert. The body structure will slowly run out of maintaining force and decay. The cause of death could be anything that destroys the body or depletes the genuine qi.

Holism

Since the natural environment, the social environment and humankind are all derived from the same source of qi, they share the same features of the universe, and therefore are closely brought into the unity.

The natural laws governing the natural world will also apply to humanity. Humanity keeps exchanging with the environment, so the environment has a great effect over the human body and spirit. Our human activities affect the environment as well. These mutual interactions make the whole system dynamically balanced.

Mental activities must be based on the body's support, and mental activity decides the action of the body. The spirit and the body are actually two sides of a coin. The spirit greatly affects the condition of the body. Appropriate mental control will benefit the body and maintain it in good condition.

The different parts of the body serve the same purpose, to maintain a normal life. All the organs and systems in the body must work together under the control of the spirit. No organ can work separately, or survive the body. The function of life is not the sum of individual organs put together. There is a fundamental difference regarding the function of the body as a whole compared with those functions performed in each individual organ or system.

Changing Time and Space: *Yi Jing (I Ching)*

About 3,000 years ago, a legendary figure, the first king of the Zhou dynasty of central China, was put in prison due to his rebellion against the government. This gave him time to think about the fundamental questions about the natural law. These thoughts were recorded as the *Yi Jing (I Ching)*, the *The Book of Changes*. Actually, this account is a legend, and most scholars would recognize that it is the collective efforts of all intellectuals at that time who made such break-through thought possible.

The *I Ching* provided the foundation of Chinese natural philosophy. It emphasizes five principles:

1. The world is always changing, and the changes take place in all directions when not linked to time
2. Time moves forwards and never backwards
3. The changes follow the natural law, rather than human will
4. The changes can be understood, therefore they can be predicted
5. It is possible to select a good way of living from all those changes.

The *I Ching* tried to answer why there are so many changes in the world and how to understand the changes, which provides the chance of living with good changes and avoiding bad changes. The principles in it also apply to humankind and health. In history, many famous Chinese medicine scholars started their study of Chinese medicine with the *I Ching*. The influence of the *I Ching* is apparent throughout the theory and practice of Chinese medicine.

The Natural Way of Life: Taoism

The word Taoism here refers to the school of philosophy, rather than the religion of Taoism/Daoism. There are fundamental differences between the two. Chinese medicine is hugely influenced by the philosophic idea of the Taoists, but had very little to do with the religion.

The philosophic aspect of Taoism has a long history of more than 3,000 years and is one of the oldest philosophies developed. It tried to answer the eternal questions of the origin of the world and humankind, and also tried to find a way of understanding the changing world. It was put forward by LaoZi (Lao Tzu) and further developed by ZhuangZi and other scholars. The main document collecting all the doctrines is the *DaoDeJing (Tao Te Ching)*.

According to Taoism, the Tao is the supreme law of nature, and the Tao is the supreme origin and the law of the natural world. The Tao generates the taiji, taiji splits into yin and yang, and the yin and yang interact with each other to produce numerous objects and materials in the world, including human bodies. The natural world and humankind follow the same natural law, the Tao.

Tao is to Follow the Natural Way

The Tao is not created by humans. It stands there eternally. Humankind has the intelligence to understand it, but not to create it or revise it. To understand the Tao, we can observe nature, we can do Qigong, and we have to follow the rule of 'Dao is in the Nature'.

From the basic of the Tao, we know the world is formed by the constant dividing of the Tao. And the world is constantly moving in all directions. Nothing stays the same for ever. So, the law we understand is changing from time to time. The truth is that we will get closer to it, but never be there, since we can only observe the change and when change happens, then we can see it (Dao Ke Dao, Fei Chang Dao).

Tao is not created. Tao is there when the universe is there. It is not created by humankind, but could be understood. Only when we see ourselves as part of the world and integrate ourselves into it, can we see it.

When we get rid of the human's own desire, there is nothing that can stop us. The intention of any individual must comply with the law of the universe. If the intention is in line with the natural law, and allowed by it, then we can achieve it. But if the wish is not what the natural law allowed, then no way can lead to success. When you totally melt down into nature (no personal desire of personal benefit), the world is yours and you are the world (Wu Wei Er Wu Bu Wei).

Tao applies to the human body and life, and humans can achieve the natural limit (天年) of life by following the principle of Tao. There are two different domains in this field:

1. the Tao in philosophy, which emphasizes that humans can reach the natural limit of life by living a healthy way and practising Qigong
2. the religion of Tao, which emphasizes that longevity can be achieved by following the discipline and sticking to the practice of some approaches.

In Taoism's view of health, there are very many traps in the world, which will upset the life course, cause health problems and mental confusion, and then shorten life. So to live longer, we have rid ourselves of unrealistic desires and not take too much enjoyment.

Life and Tao

A life integrated into nature is a real life. In Tao, human beings are not only social beings, but are also part of nature. We need human life and natural life. To understand the real meaning of life, the only way is to get inspiration and realization by getting rid of the disturbances and obstructions created by daily issues. We need to sit down and clear the mind, to purify the mind, and then the natural mind will be revitalized, and the real world can be seen clearly. This will happen relatively easily in a natural peaceful environment. So, meditation in a peaceful environment is considered to be essential for keeping a healthy body and mind.

Every life is a natural phenomenon and life should reach its natural limit. Human beings should not chase longevity beyond the natural limit, nor should they simply enjoy life without caring. Chasing immortality is disrespectful of the natural law, while shortening life is an offence against nature, since every life is unique and should be treasured.

Good health is the achievement of harmony and balance. The balance between the mental and physical is the most important. A peaceful mind is more important than any therapeutic measure. Material temptation is contrary to the goal of health, both mental and physical. Material things obscure the true meaning of life, and pull people into a dead circle of more and more. There is no end to this chasing, since nature is so big, and nobody will have a chance to own it all. The balance of give and take is then totally lost.

The Positive Way of Life: Confucianism

The centre of Confucianism is 'ren'. Ren is harmony and trust in relationships. Following the thought of ren, we should respect elderly people, keep our promises to our friends, love our elders and our children. Ren also means respect, knowledge and intelligence, and attention to the principles of correct behaviour.

Ren is self-restraint. We must maintain order and keep social rules, even when there is nobody else with us. This self-restraint is not imposed by other people or the government. It is the principle of leading a harmonized life.

Confucianism considers humankind and society, rather than being a philosophy seeking to answer the basic questions of the world. The world is there and we live in it. How to make life better is the central concern. So, humankind is the centre of discussion.

The Heaven Way is Positive (Tian Xing Jian)

We cannot rely on gods or other powers to improve our life, including health. What we should rely on is what we can do. Only by doing our best is it possible to have a better life. We try our best, but our power is limited. So we still have many uncertainties in our life. The opinion of Confucianism is 'The planning and intention is upon ours, while the success is laid on the harmony of the nature.'

Human effort will be rewarded

According to Confucianism, only when we try is it possible to achieve. If we do not try, there will be no reward waiting for us. The natural way is that only the diligent will be rewarded for their effort, since they have more chance to succeed.

To succeed, one must have all three major aspects in a harmonized support, the heaven and timing, the earth and the environment, the people surrounding and social relationships. We cannot control heaven and earth, but we can work hard to make the environment and social relationships better and changing towards our favoured direction.

Humans cannot change the natural law, but can choose their way of living. We cannot change the heavenly and earthly condition and their law, but by studying the natural law, we can choose when and where to act, and select the best combination of these.

The heavenly and earthly conditions keep constantly changing. This changing could be in line with our favoured activities, or hamper our activities. When the time is wrong, no matter how hard we work, it seems to fail. In this situation, what we can do is to wait for the good time to come. But while waiting, we have to work hard to prepare for the time to come. When the good time comes, the person who is well prepared will find it easier to achieve something.

Life is matter of our own

Life is unique and given by parents. It is the most precious gift. So self-harming and suicide are condemned. We must treasure life and do our best to ensure the body will go back to earth integrated with dignity. This is the respect we owe to ourselves and our parents.

A healthy life must be a meaningful life with a positive attitude towards health. Exercising and avoiding bad habits are important to us. Our body must be exercised regularly.

Do not simply wait

Time is like river, flowing forwards and never flowing backwards. And our life is limited by time. Anything that can be done now should be done now, because if it is done later, it may not be needed or may be too late. The world changes and what is needed changes. So, do the thing at the time. Waiting will only make for a waste of time and chances, and life itself.

Beating the difficulty

Life is deemed not to be easy. There are numerous difficulties waiting for us to overcome. Commitment, determination and confidence are all key virtues that will help us to overcome difficulties.

The Influence of Buddhism

Buddhism in ancient China was mainly dominated by two schools, the Pure Land school (Jing Tu Zong) and the Zen school (Chan). The name Zen is the popular word originally spread from the Japanese pronunciation. There were fundamental differences between the two schools regarding their approaches to achieving enlightenment. However, the basic concepts are shared across the world, the Four Noble Truths (concepts about human suffering) and the Eightfold Path (the ways leading to the right destination), and the view of the world and life.

Life is an endless circle. The life we live is the result of something that happened previously. And after death, life will continue in another form. Everything has its reason.

In Buddhism, human life is one of the states of all life, among the heavenly form, human form, other spiritual ways, animal, ghost and hell form. Except for the heavenly form, all other forms have to bear all kinds of suffering. It is possible to reach heaven by following Buddhist ideas, in human, spiritual or animal form.

There are three stages of existence: past, present and future. Our behaviour in our current life will decide what kind of life form we adopt in a future stage. All is empty – nothing is real, except the spiritual world and heavenly form. All material ownership and social achievements are phantoms and may tempt us to do wrong. Being lured into evil will lead to endless suffering due to the endless chasing of fortune and fame. Since fortune is not attached to human life, and fame is just a perception, they both lead to wrongdoing, and indulgence in them will lead to suffering in the next life.

To get rid of suffering, the only way is to jump out of the circle, and move into a state of utmost peace and wisdom. This is the spiritual form of life, in which it is possible to progress into the heavenly form, the eternal life with real happiness. To achieve the spiritual form and then the heavenly form of life, Buddhist practice is the only way. However, the practice could be carried out through many routes, the following two of which – Pure Land and Zen – are the most influential in Chinese medicine.

Pure Land

What matters is what we do every day. The best ordinary people can achieve is Buddhahood, which means an eternal life without the circle of suffering. Buddhahood is a lifelong target, and can only be achieved by doing good all the time and after the current life judgement by gods will decide if the person has attained Buddhahood. There are many requirements for the behaviour of a believer. Among the disciplines of daily activities are: no killing (animals), not being indulgent in sex, not being indulgent in money, daily praising (could be at home), worshipping and reading Buddhist classics, not eating meat and being honest. Donating is also essential. The reward for these lies in the future.

Zen

The Zen school of Buddhism emphasizes the true beliefs of Buddha, and the real understanding of the world is the spiritual existence. According to this, what matters is what you believe and realize. Zen emphasizes the result of practising Buddhism, rather than the details. Whenever one sees the real picture of life, knowing the phantom nature of the material world, focusing the mind on following Buddha and keeping a serene mind, then the life of that person transforms into Buddha's life and any troubles cease to matter.

The reward could come in the next second of apprehension, not necessarily in the future life. To achieve a Buddha life in Zen, one must learn, read, reflect and meditate. All these are mentally purifying. What the Zen achieved is a freedom of spirit. When realizing that any material part of life is not relevant to the meaning of life, even the body, then what can bother a person? In Zen, the form of practice is less important. One does not need to stay in the temple, or worship in formal rituals. The worship is showing respect to the Buddha who tells the truth and points to the way of liberation.

Both schools lead to a peaceful mind and a lifestyle free of material traps. There are several more major schools practising worldwide, but they are less influential in China, and have very little to do with Chinese medicine.

Chapter Summary

This chapter has introduced some of the main beliefs associated with the philosophies associated with Chinese medicine. I have only indicated the bare outlines of these different beliefs, but the Further Resources below provide more in-depth information about the aspects covered here.

REVIEW QUESTIONS

1 What is qi?

2 What are yang and yin and what is the relationship between them?

3 What three aspects of unity are identified as part of the principle of holism?

CHAPTER LINKS

For further discussion of the past and present of traditional Chinese medicine, see Chapters 13 and 21.

FURTHER RESOURCES

Birch, S.J. and Felt, R.L. (1999) *Understanding Acupuncture*, Edinburgh, Churchill Livingstone. A good introduction to acupuncture.

Cassidy, C. (2002) *Contemporary Chinese Medicine and Acupuncture*, Edinburgh, Churchill Livingstone. A helpful survey of theories and approaches.

Cheng, X. (2003) *Chinese Acupuncture and Moxibustion*, rev. edn, Beijing, Foreign Languages Press. A simple, concise introduction, written in the Chinese style.

Deadman, P. (2000) Yin and yang revisited, *Journal of Chinese Medicine*, 63: 34–6. Focused discussion on yin yang theory. Good preparation for the serious learner.

Deadman, P., Al-Khafaji, M. and Baker, K. (2007) *A Manual of Acupuncture*, 2nd edn, London, Journal of Chinese Medical Publications. Reference book for all key knowledge related to qi flowing in the body, and everything needed for practice.

Flaws, B. (2000) *Imperial Secrets of Health and Longevity*, Boulder, CO, Blue Poppy Press. In-depth study of the attitude of life and the philosophy behind it. Life, health and diseases are the main concern.

Kaptchuk, T. (2000) *Chinese Medicine: The Web That Has No Weaver*, London, Rider Press. An easy overall introduction to Chinese medicine, covering most aspects.

Liu, Y. (1998) *Fundamental Theories of Traditional Chinese Medicine*, Beijing, Academy Press. Textbook that defines and discusses the major concepts and ideas. For the serious reader.

Maciocia, G. (2005) *The Foundations of Chinese Medicine*, Edinburgh, Churchill Livingstone. Covers all the basic concepts, theories and philosophies, with plenty of original information translated from original Chinese books.

Zhang, Y. and Rose, K. (2000) *Who Can Ride The Dragon?*, Brookline, MA, Paradigm. Easy introduction to Chinese medicine.

Traditional Chinese Medicine: Acupuncture, Herbalism and Massage

R MIKE CHAN

Learning outcomes

By the end of this chapter, you should be able to:

■ identify the historical aspects of traditional Chinese medicine (TCM)

■ understand the principles of TCM

■ know how TCM is practised

■ appreciate the different TCM practices of acupuncture, herbalism and massage

■ distinguish between Chinese and Western acupuncture.

Traditional Chinese medicine is a complete system of medicine, rooted in ancient traditions extending over thousands of years and containing three facets in one:

1. Acupuncture
2. Herbalism
3. Massage (T'ui Na'ar).

It is important to appreciate that these and their variants referred to in this chapter are not separate techniques but are all part of the holistic system of TCM. I shall deal with all three in this chapter, but first I shall put modern TCM in its historical context.

Historical Aspects of TCM

The written history of TCM can be traced back to 2,000 BC, but the history before records began could, arguably, be backdated another 1,000 years or so.

Part VI

The first 'master' of TCM was a man called Shen Nong who lived in China *c.* 2500 BC, before written records. From traditional tales and folklore, a book was compiled a few thousand years later in honour of him. In the book, the writer(s) honoured him as an emperor, a spirit and even a god. One interesting point is that he was a farmer, a cultivator and, arguably, the first researcher who worked in the fields and tested all the herbs he prescribed, in his so-called 'glass' stomach (because of his resilience in taking these treatments). Therefore, we can say that herbalism is, chronologically, the first of the three facets of TCM.

Up until the 1970s, the teaching method lay only in the master–apprentice relationship, usually from the father to the first-born son. Traditionally, hardly any females have been able to learn from their families, because of the 'traditional' thinking that they do not carry the family name. Due to this traditional approach to recruiting and training practitioners, there are many thousands of 'secret family formulae' that no one else except the family can learn, or are even privileged to have heard of.

Principles of TCM

For the above-mentioned reason, there are quite a few schools of thoughts in TCM. Fortunately, all traditional TCM practitioners agree with the ancient medical books, such as *Huang Di Nei Jing* (*Yellow Emperor's Inner Canon*). TCM believes that a person's health is like a circle of dominoes that are all interlinked. If one falls down, it will take the others down with it. Pain/illness is only a sign or symptom of a bigger problem. The practitioner needs to find the root of the problem and not just treat the sign/symptom. This is why the practitioner will sometimes ignore the sign or symptom on the basis that this is less important and will treat the more important underlying problem, and in turn, the sign or symptom will be eliminated. Some may say this is not acceptable.

There are five principles of TCM, as follows:

1. *The five elements* (五行): all things on earth are made from metal(金), wood(木), water(水), fire(火) and earth(土). From this, the seasons, the directions, feelings, internal organs in humans, secretions, tastes, features on the face and colours are all formed.
2. *I Ching* (易经) (pronounced yee ching): everything is either positive (yang)(阳) or negative (yin)(阴), inside or outside, hot or cold and so on. Basically, things are located in pairs of opposites.
3. *Zang Fu* (脏腑): the internal organs are divided into two groups. The five Zang organs are the heart, the liver, the spleen, the lungs and the kidneys. They belong to yin (negative). They store and do not pass on. The six Fu organs are the gall bladder, the stomach, the large and small intestine, the bladder and the three burners. They belong to yang (positive). They pass on and do not store.
4. *Meridians* (经络): there are 12 main meridians, plus the centre one in the front and the centre one at the back, making 14. There are three positive and three

negative meridians in the arms and legs. The centre one in the front is negative and the one on the back is positive.

5. *Balance*: underlying the other four principles is the main principle of balance; that if any of the organs/meridians/five elements or yin and yang are not balanced, the person will be or is ill (Figure 21.1).

Although TCM is most influenced by the teaching of Taoism (道学) and Buddhism (佛学), it also works for people who do not believe in these religions.

Practice of TCM

At the outset, it is important to clarify with patients the basis on which they are treated. In some countries, the spouse invariably accompanies the patient throughout the treatments. In the UK, it is recommended that male practitioners suggest that the male partner also attends and observes the treatments of female patients.

The process of TCM begins with the diagnosis and continues with the treatment. The diagnosis uses four main techniques: observation (望诊), the sense of smell (闻诊), interview (问诊) and the sense of touch/palpation (切诊). One of the significant goals is to identify the extent to which the patient's system is in balance and, if not, where the imbalance lies. Figure 21.1 shows the two key dimensions used to assess the degree of balance.

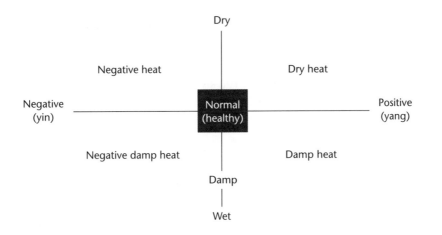

Figure 21.1 Dimensions used to assess extent of balance

Treatment commonly involves bringing the system back into healthy balance, that is, Jing Qi Tong – Jing (正) = central, balanced, Qi (气) = energy, Tong (堂) = place, that is, the place that will balance your energy. It is important to bear in mind that the condition of health, or illness, varies from patient to patient. Some people can display a higher degree of negative or positive dryness or damp, for example.

Observation (望诊)

The practitioner is concerned to gather the 'aura' or spirit of the patient, for example through the manner, the posture. Is the person alert, positive and making eye contact with the practitioner, or are they depressed, looking down at the floor?

Looking at a patient is important in TCM, particularly the skin tone of the face and the colour of the whites of the eyes. Is the face dry or oily? Is the person unshaven, with unkempt hair, or smartly presented?

The eyes are the windows of organs such as the liver and gall bladder. If the whites of the eyes are yellow, this could indicate problems with one or both of these. If they are bloodshot, it could indicate a lack of sleep, or a problem with the heart.

The practitioner asks the patient to open the mouth, so that the tongue can be observed (Figure 21.2).

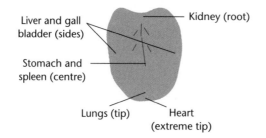

Figure 21.2 The tongue

The tongue is believed to be a mirror of the alimentary canal, as well. The colour, the fur, the shape, the thickness and the movement (tremor) all need to be observed. Different illnesses have different indications on the tongue.

The Use of Smell (闻诊)

The practitioner may place the patient's chair close enough so that any 'natural' smell will be noted. The use of perfume by the patient may make this less easy. Sometimes the practitioner may smell the patient's sweat and although this could simply be due to not having washed recently, it may also be a clue to problems in the patient's respiratory system. Bad breath may indicate digestive problems and smelly feet may indicate damp heat (see Figure 21.1), which again points to possible problems in the digestive system.

The Interview (问诊)

The interview is the centre of the diagnosis. The practitioner may take more than an hour at the diagnostic meeting with the patient, which is usually the second meeting, after the first meeting at which the patient first comes with the request for treatment.

The practitioner works like a detective, using a range of techniques to gather a holistic picture of the patient. The practitioner asks about daily habits, both parents, upbringing, any hereditary factors as well as previous conditions, injuries or operations. Table 21.1 gives an idea of some of the areas covered as an indication of the scope of the interview.

Table 21.1 Checklist of areas for assessment

Name	
Date of birth	
Address – for the practitioner to understand the patient's environment	
Childhood	
Education	
Work	
Diet	
Sleep patterns	
Smoking	
Exercise	
Elimination	
Sweat	
Children	
Allergies	
Endocrine	
Skeletal	
Nervous	
Senses	
History of illnesses	
Respiratory	
Gynaecological	

As Table 21.1 shows, information is sought about allergies, the endocrine and nervous system, the senses and the functioning of the major systems of the body. Questions may be asked that also give clues to the condition of the major organs, the 'powerhouse' of the body, such as the lungs, stomach, liver and heart. While the environment in which the person lives is important, questions about eating and drinking habits are used to find out, for example, whether the person eats breakfast, eats spicy food such as chilli, uses vinegar, drinks alcohol regularly or excessively, or sufficient daily water.

Part VI

The Use of Touch/Palpation (切诊)

Touch plays an important part in diagnosis and treatment, for example through massage. One of the main uses of touch is in feeling the pulse of the patient. The nature of the pulse provides clues to the condition of the patient. The practitioner can also, if he suspects there is imbalance, touch certain acupuncture points to confirm the suspicion. If the respective point(s) are sensitive/painful to touch or pressure, this confirms that the particular organ is deficient or imbalanced. According to traditional Chinese medical practice, there are 8 main pulses and 28 subpulses. However, at least 64 types of pulse have also been identified, usually taken as the radial pulse.

Radial pulse

The radial pulse is divided into three parts (from the fingers towards the elbow): inch, gate and ruler. The pulse in the left wrist differs from the right:

- The left hand inch indicates the heart and the sternum.
- The right hand inch indicates the lungs and the front ribcage.
- The left hand gate indicates the liver and the gall bladder.
- The right hand gate indicates the stomach and the spleen.
- The left hand ruler indicates the bladder, left kidney and the small intestine.
- The right hand ruler indicates the life gate, the right kidney and the large intestine.

Some indication of the power and accuracy of the pulse as a diagnostic tool can be gathered by the fact that TCM practitioners are able to diagnose medical conditions simply through the pulse. A practitioner known to the author was able to identify through the pulse whether a non-drinker had returned to alcohol use since the previous treatment.

While one hand takes the pulse, the other hand can touch the fingers and the hand. It is possible to find out if the skin is sweaty, which may be a clue to the condition of the lungs. Again, while putting needles into the leg with one hand, the other can feel the condition of the leg and the skin.

Practice example

Mr A came to see me at my clinic, complaining of stomach ache. After seeing his red face, smelling acetone on his breath, a few quick questions and feeling his pulses, I sent him to his GP as an emergency case. He was diagnosed with early stage angina. Without the observation, smell, interview and touch diagnostic procedure, it would have been impossible to know that this was not a simple case. The diagnostic interview led to me suggest a course of treatment and to prepare a herbal prescription to accompany the acupuncture.

Practice example

Mrs B came to see me about her recurrent fainting episodes. I noticed the pale colour of her skin, despite the fact that she works part time (22 hours per week) outdoors. I could smell the odour from her hair, which she said she was afraid of washing too often because she loses some more hair every time she washes it. I checked her pulse and there was a distinctive problem in the gynaecological department. During the diagnostic interview, I found that she has been suffering extremely heavy menstrual cycles for over 20 years. I prescribed a course of herbs and acupuncture.

Acupuncture (针灸)

Acupuncture is a holistic part of TCM that involves regarding the person's overall condition and devising appropriate treatments, involving the use of needles to treat the patient's condition. These are inserted as groups/sets selected from more than 670 acupoints (穴位) on the body. All areas are sterilized before the insertion of a needle and all needles are used only once and then discarded as clinical waste. Regarding the patient holistically leads to focusing on how the different parts of the body – in particular the major organs such as the heart, liver and systems such as the digestive system – are functioning, the overall level of energy (qi气) the patient has and the extent to which this is negative (yin阴) or positive (yang阳). Many conditions arise in these areas and often it is impossible to specify one particular 'cause', although the practitioner is guided by experience of how they relate to each other. For example, the heart looks after the mind/psychological wellbeing.

Treatment with needles commonly engages with the major organs and systems referred to above, such as heart, liver and digestion, as well as the level of energy, which leads to perhaps as many as five needles being inserted for each of these four aspects.

Needles may be inserted into parts of the body close to the problem, a painful knee for example, or into one of the four parts of the body that is a miniature 'map' of the body as a whole – the ear (which resembles a curled, upside down embryo), the top of the head (commonly used in the East, although in the UK, I avoid this area when sterilizing the hair before the treatment is not easy) and the palm and back of the hand.

The Five Elements (五行)

Taoism, on which TCM is mostly based, believes that there are five basic elements (Figure 21.3):

■ Water (水): Water begets wood and governs fire. The kidneys beget/look after the liver and govern the heart.

- Metal (金): Metal begets water and governs wood. The lungs beget/look after the kidneys and govern the liver.
- Earth (土): Earth begets metal and governs water. The spleen begets/looks after the lungs and governs the liver.
- Fire (火): Fire begets earth and governs metal. The heart begets/looks after the spleen and governs the lungs.
- Wood (木): Wood begets fire and governs earth. The liver begets/looks after the heart and governs the spleen.

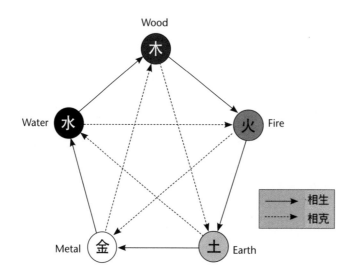

Figure 21.3 The five elements

Meridians (经络)

TCM is based on the assumption that the invisible energy – qi – travels throughout the body in channels called **meridians**. The meridians in the body can be described as a system of brooks, streams and rivers for the qi to travel from one internal organ to another part of the body. Sometimes the qi will stay at a certain point, like ponds, lakes and seas. Sometimes one or more of the ponds or brooks are blocked and the qi cannot travel around the body, thus making the person ill. The principle of acupuncture is to use needles to unblock the blocked ponds or brooks and let the qi flow again.

Alternatives to Needles

There are methods other than needles that can be used to achieve the same effect:

- A low powered laser (under 1.5 watts) is the latest effective painless alternative. An electronic pulse machine can achieve the same result.

- Smouldering moxa (艾灸) can be used to warm the acupoints (known as moxibustion).
- Magnetized ball bearings (耳磁珠) can be attached to the ear by miniature skin-tone plasters.
- A magnetized probe (磁针) can be placed over the acupoints. The Chan family invented a qu'un needle (辊针) or smooth probe, which they have used for more than seven generations.
- Herbal plasters (中药膏布) are used in healing muscular and skin conditions.
- Cupping (拔罐) is an effective way to heal respiratory and yang illnesses.

Cupping uses a purpose-made cup. Cotton wool is dipped in surgical spirit, placed in the cup and lit so that it dries and expands the air in the cup. It is quickly placed on the back of the patient when the flame extinguishes, so that a vacuum is created. In some cases, this is used as an alternative to needles, although caution needs to be exercised as it can bruise delicate or aged skin. Its usefulness may lie in healing and treating respiratory problems, such as colds, coughs and influenza. There are new inventions to replace the flame by using a pump to create the vacuum.

Chinese and Western Acupuncture

Acupuncture is an aspect of TCM that has travelled from China and is now a well-established complementary practice in Western countries, in particular. Western acupuncture seems to look after the signs and symptoms more than seeing the root of the problems, that is, it is

- not practised as a system of medicine
- not holistic
- not based on traditional Chinese philosophy, for example Taoism.

Partly for these reasons, the number of needles used is generally less than TCM acupuncture. The effect, in most cases, is less long-lasting than TCM acupuncture.

Also, Western acupuncturists tends not to twist the needles because they do not believe in the yin yang principle, that is, by putting the needle in while twisting clockwise, the practitioner introduces yin in the patient; and twisting anti-clockwise, the practitioner introduces yang.

Herbalism (中草药)

The basis of the contribution of herbal preparations to health and wellbeing in TCM is the balancing of the five elements of metal, wood, water, fire and earth. Traditional practitioners prepare their own herbal prescriptions from among several hundred original herbs and plant sources and this is held by them to be superior to commercial preparations, in which the vitality of the source plant is not known at the time of prescription. Herbs are dried and made into a decoction or broth, or they are ground into powder and put into a capsule, or mixed with honey or rice and pressed into tablet form.

As a practitioner following this traditional method of herbalism, I spend about half of my working time with patients and the other half in the preparation of herbal prescriptions tailored specifically to each person's needs.

Massage (T'ui Na'ar)(推拿)

In massage, the TCM practitioner uses the fingers, knuckles, fists and elbows on the different acupressure points. Massage can be used when adults are afraid of needles, when muscular injuries are present, or when babies or young children are being treated, for example for asthma, where it is particularly effective.

In adults, massage is particularly used in sports injuries. Normally, the treatment of an athletic person turns out to be more straightforward, where the injury is local and the person does not have other conditions requiring treatment.

I find that massage is only possible when I am not tired. So, because of the physical exertion involved, I usually set 20 minutes as the limit of a massage session.

T'ui Na'ar (推拿) is an ancient form of massotherapy, involving the practitioner pressing with fingers or palms on acupoints to heal, a technique that is particularly useful when treating infants and children.

Practice example

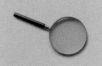

Ms C was an English teacher in Italy. After about five months in the job, she started to need to defecate two to three times a day; when she needed the toilet over ten times a day, she consulted a doctor. She was diagnosed with irritable bowel syndrome (IBS), and prescribed drugs to counter the condition, but then suffered from constipation. Her condition seesawed for over a year. Finally, she was too weak to sign on for another contract and decided to come home. In the consultation, I found that the IBS was not the main problem. She did not get used to the food in Italy because she had not eaten cheese since she was a young child. Her job was very demanding and, combined with the school politics, caused her to suffer from insomnia. On top of all this, she suffered from hereditary menorrhagia, for which I had already successfully treated her mother and her three sisters. I prescribed acupuncture and some herbs. After three courses of acupuncture, she had improved enough to become a supply teacher.

Practice example

Mr D is a professional body builder. He had heard that acupuncture can look after skin and hair and so tried a course of five treatments to enhance his chances in competitions. He went on to win three competitions and has been a regular 'patient' ever since. He says that since the treatment, he has been eating less but is absorbing more nutrients. He is sleeping better and therefore spending fewer hours in bed. He can focus his mind a lot better and, most importantly, his hair and skin actually look more shiny and natural.

Practice example

Master E was a child of eight when I first treated him for asthma. I was dubious about using needles on him because of his age and I decided to use T'ui Na'ar instead. I also prescribed some herbs as part of the package. He responded well to the treatment and within 18 months, he was cured of the condition.

Practice example

Mrs F was diagnosed with endometriosis and was told that the only solution was to have a hysterectomy. She came for Jing Qi Tong as a last resort, but without much hope of a cure. Under my late uncle's watchful eye, I have successfully treated this condition in Hong Kong at least three times, so I was able to reassure her that I had experience of this illness. I prescribed five courses of acupuncture with herbs. The first MRI scan showed that the cyst had stayed the same size, but her menstrual pain was less. A year later, the scan showed that her condition had improved, and another year later, she was given the all clear.

Practice example

Miss G was diagnosed as suffering from clinical depression. She was sectioned under the Mental Health Act because she was suicidal, and prescribed a heavy antidepressant. Six months later she was discharged home. Every time the medical team reduced the dosage, she lapsed into cutting herself. Her brother suggested she sought help with Jing Qi Tong. I prescribed two courses of acupuncture with some herbs to wean her off the antidepressant. After three weeks, she was just using the herbs, with no desire to self-harm. Six and a half months later, she was working in a café, drug and herbs free and living a normal, peaceful life.

Note: The point made above about practitioners only being able to give massage for a short period of time applies more broadly across TCM, in that I was taught not to practise if feeling ill. This is because an out-of-condition practitioner can pass on negative qi to the patient.

Chapter Summary

This chapter has introduced the basic principles of traditional Chinese medicine in practice. It has illustrated acupuncture and other aspects of TCM, using examples from practice.

REVIEW QUESTIONS

1   In TCM, what are the five elements from which all things on earth are made?

2   What is the main principle of the *I Ching*?

3   What does the principle of balance refer to?

CHAPTER LINKS

For more relevant material on the roots of TCM, see Chapters 13 and 20.

FURTHER RESOURCES

Kaptchuk, T.J. (2000) *The Web That Has No Weaver: Understanding Chinese Medicine*, London, Weaver. A basic book, providing authoritative information for the practitioner.

Ni, M. (1995) *The Yellow Emperor's Classic of Medicine: A New Translation of the Neijing Suwen with Commentary*, Boston, MA, Shambhala Publications. A history-based book, with a lot of information but easy to understand. Covers a number of theories.

Qiao, Y. (2008) *Traditional Chinese Medicine Diagnosis Study Guide*, Seattle, Eastland Press. Detailed book about how the practitioner does his detective work on finding out what is the base of the illness.

Yanfu, Z. (2002) *Science of Prescriptions (Library of Traditional Chinese Medicine: Chinese/English edition)*, Shanghai College of Traditional Chinese Medicine. One of a series of books published by Shanghai and Nanjing Universities, arguably the top two TCM universities in modern China. I use this series as my daily reference. The committee members boast combined bedside experience of nearly 5,000 years.

Resource file

Alternative Medical Systems

This resource file gives supplementary information on alternative medical systems, over and above the individual areas of practice referred to in the three preceding chapters, and offers suggestions for further reading.

Let us remind ourselves at the start of this section of two things:

- the great antiquity of many alternative medical systems
- the breadth and depth of the ideas embodied in them.

In Greek mythology, followers of Asclepius (god of medicine) believed that the first duty of physicians was to treat disease, while the supporters of Hygieia (goddess of health, daughter of Asclepius) believed that health is the positive state that people maintain naturally if they live wisely by following the natural laws of health. All alternative medical systems follow one of these two sets of beliefs, and although most pursue the holistic principles of Hygieia, some also incorporate the assumptions of Asclepius, which approximates nowadays to the term 'biomedical model'. Distinct from each of these, there is the biopsychosocial view, which is explained below.

The category of 'alternative medical systems' is a general umbrella category, intended to include approaches that meet two criteria:

1. They are based on a philosophical, theoretical or conceptual framework.
2. They attempt to tackle the health and wellbeing concerns of people holistically and across the range of human experience, rather than focusing on one category of problem or adopting one kind of response.

So 'alternative medical systems' is a somewhat imprecise category, but it does enable us to recognize the scope of systems, such as traditional Indian medicine (TIM) and traditional Chinese medicine (TCM), and to give these and other less generic but no less complete 'systems' of medicine their proper due for being equivalent to Western medicine, even though some of them – homeopathy, for example – are not equal in terms of size and comprehensiveness. It may seem odd at first reading, but I have included a number of approaches – for example shiatsu and yoga – which, in Western terms, might seem to be more techniques than systems of medicine. However, I have included them because they embody philosophies and theories that give them a wholeness, which qualifies them as systems, as well as techniques.

- *Acupressure* is a technique derived from acupuncture based on the application of pressure to stimulate the flow of energy, using the finger, thumb, fist, elbow, or devices such as acuballs or rollers, which have protuberances for use on the spine or the feet. Acupuncture and acupressure, as approaches, are rooted in traditional Chinese, Korean and Japanese medicine, but as techniques are used in many parts of the world.

Further Resources

Beresford-Cooke, C. and Albright, P. (1996) *Acupressure: (Naturally Better)*, New York, Quarto.

Kenyon, J. (1987) *Acupressure Techniques*, London, Thorsons.

- *Acupuncture* is a technique that uses needles applied to specific parts of the body, known as acupuncture points or meridians, as a means of affecting energy levels and improving health and wellbeing.

Further Resources

Birch, S. (2001) An overview of acupuncture in the treatment of stroke, addiction, and other health problems, in G. Stux and R. Hammerschlag (eds) *Clinical Acupuncture: Scientific Basis*, Berlin, Springer-Verlag.

Part VI

Birch, S. (2002) Treatment of pain by acupuncture, in C.M. Cassidy (ed.) *Contemporary Chinese Medicine and Acupuncture*, Edinburgh, Churchill Livingstone.

MacPherson, H., Thomas, K., Walters, S. and Fitter, M.A. (2001) Prospective survey of adverse events and treatment reactions following 34,000 consultations with professional acupuncturists, *Acupuncture in Medicine*, **19**(2): 93–102.

MacPherson, H., Scullion, A., Thomas, K.J. and Walters, S. (2004) Patient reports of adverse reports associated with acupuncture treatment: a prospective national survey, *Quality and Safety in Health Care*, 13: 349–55.

So Tin Yau, J. (1985) *The Book of Acupuncture Points*, Brookline, MA., Paradigm Publications.

White, A., Hayhoe, S., Hart, A. et al. (2001) Survey of adverse events following acupuncture (SAFA): a prospective study of 32,000 consultations, *Acupuncture in Medicine*, **19**(2): 84–92.

■ *Ayurvedic medicine* is the term used to refer to TIM. TIM (Ayurveda) is a natural healing system whose roots lie in ancient (more than 6,000 year old) Vedic science, which is an integrated way of understanding the physical, mental and spiritual universe. Ayurvedic medicine uses the Vedic assumptions of three basic cosmic forces of energy of life (Prana), light (Jyoti) and cohesion manifested in harmony and love (Prema). The body has three primary life forces and related humours, given here in brackets: air (vata), fire (pitta), and water (kapha). When these humours are out of balance, illness occurs and the physician works to restore this balance.

Further Resources

Frawley, D. (2003) *Ayurvedic Healing: A Comprehensive Guide*, 2nd edn, Delhi, Motilal Barnarsidass.

Morrison, J.H. (1995) *The Book of Ayurveda: A Holistic Approach to Health and Longevity*, New York, Fireside.

■ *Biopsychosocial* medicine is an alternative to the biomedical approach to ill health, which emphasizes not just the social context of the patient but also the role of the system of healthcare in creating and relieving conditions and illnesses. The biomedical approach does not simply assert that professionals need to take into account the social factors relevant to the patient's condition. It argues that the health of people with illnesses and chronic conditions will improve where the healthcare settings are taken into account and where professionals critically examine their own assumptions and beliefs about illness and communication with their patients (White, 2005: 225).

Further Resource

White, P. (ed.) (2005) *Biopsychosocial Medicine*, Oxford, Oxford University Press.

■ *Chinese herbal medicine* is an aspect of TCM that is used in conjunction with other components, such as acupuncture.

Further Resources

Craze, R. and Tang, S. (1995) *Chinese Herbal Medicine*, London, Piatkus.

Fratkin, J. (1986) *Chinese Herbal Patent Remedies: A Practical Guide*, Long Beach, CA, Oriental Healing Arts Institute.

Hyatt, R. (1978) *Chinese Herbal Medicine: Ancient Art and Modern Science*, Aldershot, Wildwood House

Rogans, E. (1997) *In a Nutshell: Chinese Herbalism*, Rockport, MA, Element Books.

■ *Colour therapy* (also known as chromotherapy or colorology) is sometimes claimed to originate in Ayurvedic medicine and sometimes in research on the therapeutic powers of colours, applied to particular acupoints on the body. In this way, colour therapy is used holistically to balance emotional, physical, mental and spiritual energy in the person. Colour therapy may be used in conjunction with aromatherapy and hydrotherapy.

Further Resource

Lilly, S. (2001) *Modern Colour Therapy*, London, Caxton Publishing.

■ *Holistic medicine* is the general label for a wide variety of holistic approaches, which can fall into many or all of the six categories set out in Table 3.6. Holism was developed by Fritz Perls (1893–1970) and others, the principles of which are expressed in Gestalt therapy, itself derived from Gestalt psychology (see resource file at end of Chapter 22).

As an example of the breadth of application of holistic principles, holistic dentistry was boosted by the publication of a book by Ziff (1984) on the dangers of mercury and amalgam dental fillings, known about since the introduction of amalgam in the early nineteenth century. Holistic dentistry draws on the mouth as a source of diagnostic insight into a person's health and wellbeing. Holistic dentists may use homeopathic and herbal approaches as well as recommending nutritional and dietary supplements, as an accompaniment to major treatments that involve introducing substances such as metallic compounds in the process of repairing and replacing teeth.

Further Resources

Cousins, N. (1991) *Anatomy of an Illness, as Perceived by the Patient*, New York, Bantam Books.

Gould, F. (2006) *Holistic Therapy: A Practical Approach*, Cheltenham, Nelson Thornes.

McGuinness, H. (2000) *Holistic Therapies: An Introductory Guide*, London, Hodder & Stoughton.

■ *Naturopathic medicine* is a general term for approaches that rely on the ability of the body 'naturally' to heal itself, using holistic principles and the minimum of intrusive treatments such as drugs. Holistic approaches commonly focus on the individual, but there is an interface with social perspectives on health promotion and environmental medicine, which is a conventional medical approach to identifying risk factors in the environment that contribute to illness, health and wellbeing.

Further Resources

Hoffer, A. and Prousky, J. (2008) *Naturopathic Nutrition: A Guide to Healthy Food and Nutrition Supplements*, Toronto, Canadian College of Naturopathic Medicine Press.

Thiel, R. (2001) *Combining Old and New: Naturopathy for the Twenty First Century*, Morton Grove, IL, Whitman.

Turner, R.N. (1984) *Naturopathic Medicine: Treating the Whole Person*, London, Thorsons.

■ *Pilates* is a system of exercise, developed by Joseph Pilates (1880–1967), based on ancient Greek approaches to mental and physical conditioning (Robinson and Thomson, 2004: 2).

Further Resources

Bass, M. (2004) *The Complete Classic Pilates Method*, London, Pan Macmillan.

Robinson, L., Fisher, H., Knox, J. and Thompson, G. (2002) *Official Body Control Pilates Manual*, London, Pan.

Robinson, L., Thompson, G. and Thomas, G. (1999) *Pilates: The Way Forward*, London, Pan.

■ *Psionic medicine* was developed in the 1960s by Dr George Lawrence. It uses principles similar to homeopathy to induce symptoms in the body in order to promote self-healing.

Further Resource

Reyner, J., Laurence, G. and Upton, C. (2001) *Psionic Medicine: Study and Treatment of the Causative Factors in Illness*, revised by Dr Keith Souter, Saffron Waldon, C.W. Daniel.

■ *Shiatsu* is a form of massage using such techniques as acupressure to release energy in the body. The term shiatsu has roots in Japan, where the word *shi* means 'finger' and *atsu* means 'pressure'. The terms 'jitsu' and 'kyo' are applied in Zen

Part VI

shiatsu, in a similar way to the use of yin and yang in TCM. The application of pressure – employing the fingers, palms, elbows and feet – to parts of the body, such as the meridian points of the soles of the feet, aims to improve the passage of natural energy, known as qi.

Further Resources

Cowmeadow, O. (1992) *The Art of Shiatsu*, Rockport, MA, Element Books.

Oschman, J. (2000) *Energy Medicine: The Scientific Basis*, 8th edn, Edinburgh, Churchill Livingstone.

Ohashi, W. (1977) *Do-it-yourself Shiatsu*, London, Mandala Books.

■ *Tai chi* is an ancient Chinese approach that uses slow, smooth movements to develop mental as well as physical wellbeing.

Further Resources

Crompton, P. (1993) *The Art of T'ai Chi*, Rockport, MA, Element Books.

Crompton, P. (1987) *The T'ai Chi Workbook*, Boston, Shambhala.

■ *Traditional Japanese medicine* is an ancient medical system that has been revitalized since the nineteenth century. It uses some techniques inherited from traditional practice in the Indian subcontinent, Korea and China, and since the twentieth century, meridian therapy has become widespread, using herbal medicine (kampo) and such techniques as acupuncture to treat the zones, or meridians, of the body.

Further Resource

Chin, R. (1995) *The Energy Within: The Science behind every Oriental Therapy from Acupuncture to Yoga*, New York, Marlowe.

■ *Traditional Korean medicine* is based on both ancient Korean practice and influences from other countries such as India and China. It relies on traditional methods such as herbal prescriptions and acupuncture.

Further Resource

Oegungmung, C. (1963) *Fresh Achievements in Korean Medicine*, Potonggang, Pyongyang, North Korea, Foreign Languages Publishing House.

■ *T'ui Na'ar* (tui na) is a form of Chinese massage that focuses on acupoints so as to improve the flow of energy throughout the body.

Further Resource

Mercati, M. (1997) *The Handbook of Chinese Massage: Tui Na Techniques to Awaken Body and Mind*, Rochester, VT, Healing Arts Press.

■ *Yoga* is a Sanskrit word meaning different things, including 'to join' and 'to control'. It has its origins in the ancient history of the Indian subcontinent, is a part of Ayurvedic practice and employs meditation, physical movement and postures, sometimes as ways of reaching higher states of consciousness, and invariably as a way of developing mental and bodily health and wellbeing. Yoga is widely practised, in many different forms, in Eastern and Western countries. There are six main types of yoga: karma yoga, jnana yoga, hatha yoga, raja yoga and bhakti yoga.

Further Resources

Flood, G. (1996) *An Introduction to Hinduism*, Cambridge, Cambridge University Press.

Fraser, T. (2003) *The Easy Yoga Workbook: The Perfect Introduction to Yoga*, Edinburgh, Duncan Baird.

Pattabhi, S.K. (2000) *Ashtanga Yoga*, London, Gaia Books.

Vishnudevananda S. (1980) *The Complete Illustrated Book of Yoga*, New York, Harmony Books.

■ *Zhong yi xue* – a form of TCM – relies on a range of approaches, including diet, massage, physical exercise and detoxification.

Further Resource

Wisemann, N. and Ellis, A. (1997) *Fundamentals of Chinese Medicine*, Herndon, VA, Paradigm.

Meditation

LAMA RABSANG

Learning outcomes

By the end of this chapter, you should be able to:

■ understand the nature of meditation

■ know what meditating entails

■ understand the main uses of meditation

■ appreciate how meditation may help people with problems

This chapter explores the nature of meditation and in the process discusses the importance of mindfulness. It examines how Buddhism relates to meditation and what Buddhist meditation entails. It explores how to meditate in practice.

What is Meditation?

Let us examine the mind for a moment. Look at your mind. Where is it? Where is it coming from? What colour does it have? What is the shape of your mind? Is your mind in the head or in the heart? If you can say that you found your mind somewhere, look closer – can you pinpoint the place where the mind is? Can you put a needle somewhere and say 'Here is my mind'? If you can, it is your thought that pinpoints somewhere. When you look deeper into your thoughts and your mind, you can see that it is empty in the same way that a space is. The quality of the mind is like space. We can say that the mind is empty. Emptiness does not, however, mean that nothing exists. We see, taste and hear things and it means that our mind also has the quality of clarity. Emptiness means that things are basically empty of independent existence. We simply see them as solid, material and permanent of nature at the moment, which can be called 'illusion'. These two qualities – clarity and emptiness – are present at the same time.

Problems such as suffering and dissatisfaction arise when we grasp at the phenomena as real and solid. Let us briefly examine the grasping at ourselves. Take our hand – where is this hand? We have given names to different parts of the hand but we cannot find any independently existing hand. Everything consists of parts and we give names to these entities. Everything is born from the mind. Also 'I' is a name that we give. We say 'I am good, bad, I want this, why has this happened to me?' But look deeply and you cannot find 'me'. When we look closer and examine that deeply, we can only find emptiness and impermanence.

The reason why we so easily become distracted from this present moment is because we are not aware of the basic nature of our mind, we live in an illusion. Distraction then causes negative emotions and actions. Ignorance means not being aware of the nature of our mind, and it causes us to evaluate things as good, bad or indifferent. When our mind evaluates and makes judgements about things, it starts wanting and rejecting. We develop attachment towards the things we want and grasp at them. On the other hand, we want to avoid some objects and run away from them. Our evaluating and judging the object is mind-made. The object itself is neither good nor bad. Some people like coffee and some do not but the coffee is the same. When we recognize the mind's habit of judging, many things become easier. If we do not like something, it is our own problem, not the quality of the object.

At the moment, we naturally have negative emotions (anger, jealousy, pride and so on). They arise from grasping and attachment. Every day we can see our mind's way of working. One day everything goes well and we are happy; the next moment things change and we have problems. Desire gives rise to jealousy and then to anger and this usually causes more problems and suffering. All this, however, originated in our own mind and from the habit of evaluating. We are grasping at our own views of what is good and bad and this serves as a basis for wanting and rejecting. Because of this grasping and rejecting, our mind is like a crazy monkey running everywhere uncontrollably. Our mind is constantly commenting on what we are doing and making judgements. This habit of mind makes us restless and tense.

What is the answer to calming the mind? When you start meditating, you become more aware of what your mind is actually doing all the time. We can think of the mind as being like a bird in a cage. When you keep it in a closed cage, it wants to be out. Then you take the bird in the cage and go on a ship to the middle of the sea where there is no land and let the bird out. At first the bird is happy to be out and flies over the sea. After while, however, it cannot find any land and so it returns to the ship. This is what our mind does; it wants many things and if we try to control it, it does not succeed. However, if we free it but give it no place to land, that is, grasp, it calms naturally. The mind relaxes and returns to the present moment.

That is what meditation is about. You are consciously in the present moment without grasping at yesterday or tomorrow, not even in this moment. It is easy to relax when you are not grasping, you are just in the here and now. In this moment, there is space, clarity and emptiness. In the present moment, when you open your heart and just be there, you may get a flash of the nature of your mind, the wisdom of your mind, which, in Buddhism, we call 'Buddha nature'. Usually, however, our mind is so restless and busy running around that we do not recognize it, but even these flashes of insight are important experiences.

Meditation is too simple and that is why it is so difficult for us. We do not trust ourselves. We think that meditation is something special and we expect some complicated answer to the question as to what meditation is. Meditation, however, is our natural state, which you do not have to buy anywhere and it cannot be made. We can say that the mind is like sand and water mixed together. If you stir it, you cannot see through it, but if you just let it be, it becomes clear naturally. This means that when you relax in the present moment, your mind is naturally clear. The mind can also be compared to an ocean, where the thoughts and feelings are the waves. It is all about the same ocean; waves are simply the movement on the surface. Being is completely natural, but we have forgotten it, we have lost it. We have lost the ability to be in the present moment and we do not see that happiness is already here and now in this moment. Let us take an example. You are thirsty and you want a drink. When you finally find something to drink, for a moment you are happy and relaxed. This happened naturally, you did not have to make the feeling of happiness. All the time we have these kinds of moments but we just don't recognize them. When we investigate our mind, we will find our true nature and its quality. If you find meditation boring, it means that you do not recognize the nature of your mind.

In meditation, mindfulness is a crucial thing. Mindfulness means that you are conscious of what you are doing, it is being conscious of the present moment. For example, when you are writing with mindfulness, you do not make mistakes. If your mind is somewhere else, thinking, you are not aware of the present moment. Mindfulness, however, is a little different from concentration. If you are too focused and concentrated, you lose other things around you and your mind becomes tense. Then you are easily bothered and distracted. Mindfulness and relaxing go hand in hand. When you really relax, there is mindfulness. If your mind is tight and tense, you cannot be mindful, if you are relaxed, it is easy to stay mindful. You could compare relaxing and mindfulness to making tea. You need both water and tea leaves. Mindfulness is also openness. If your mind is relaxed, you can be aware of many things around you.

Sometimes, even though meditation is supposed to help us, calm our mind, make us happier and more joyful, we start becoming more tense and tight-minded, probably because we have been grasping at how meditation is supposed to be. Perhaps, during the meditation, we are continually judging ourselves as good or bad. We may have some goal in our mind and we are pushing ourselves towards that. When we do not reach it, we are disappointed. If this happens, meditation begins to bring us more problems rather than vice versa. In this case, meditation does not help to calm our mind.

It also might happen that we try to run away from our problems and emotions with meditation. Meditation is then just another way of trying to avoid facing this present moment and our life as it is, which is the opposite of the meaning of meditation. Meditation is being here and now. At this very moment, we have opportunity to influence things; at this moment, we have the opportunity to be happy with what we have. If you find it difficult to feel happy, you can just try to deal with whatever feelings you have by being in the present moment. You can try to be content with your life and do the best you can. Of course we will encounter difficult situations and suffering, but when we learn to take things as they are, not judging them as good or bad, our mind calms down and we find contentment and also happiness.

It is important to notice that meditation does not just consist of what we think about; it is not meditating in our head. If we just meditate in our head, it is not really changing us in the best way. Meditation happens in the heart, it is a heartfelt experience and only then it starts revealing all the good qualities we already have in our heart.

There is a saying that with meditation there is no distraction. Actually there is no meditation, there is only a state of mind where the mind does not become distracted and you do not lose awareness of what is going on. You are in the present moment and keep the mindfulness.

Meditation in Buddhism

Buddhists believe that we are born over and over again. In this life, you can see the results of previous lives, which is the law of karma. Karma means that our deeds have consequences. This rebirth is caused by grasping at samsara, the cycle of rebirth that leads to moksha, the Buddhist heaven. We are ignorant of the nature of our mind and thus are living an illusion – we see things as permanent and solid. We are grasping at ourselves and this gives rise to many negative emotions. We do not have control over our emotions and we are not conscious of our own actions. This is why we commit unwholesome actions and cause suffering for ourselves and others as well. In Buddhism, meditation is seen as the only way to freedom from suffering and samsara. Meditation develops the insight of our true nature and compassion towards all living beings and thus decreases the grasping and our belief in illusion.

Meditation brings us freedom from suffering, which is also called 'enlightenment'. Enlightenment does not mean that we disappear somewhere in space. The focus is on the quality of the enlightened mind, which has the quality and capability of spontaneously benefiting others. At this moment, we cannot help many beings but the enlightened mind has the blessing of benefiting millions of beings in just one moment.

Enlightenment involves not evaluating or judging things. However, you cannot create enlightenment. By meditating you learn to understand your mind, and impermanence and emptiness. This way you will understand that there is no need to grasp because there is actually nothing you can grasp at. Enlightenment happens naturally even though you do not think about becoming enlightened. It is like work that you do without thinking all the time of the results – you just do it and some day the work is finished. When you concentrate more on doing than on the outcome, you grasp less at enlightenment. You just are naturally wise and happy, you do not have to think about whether you are good or bad. This prevents pride increasing. Without this kind of practice, you cannot reach enlightenment. In Buddhism, good motivation is crucial; when you act out of a good and pure heart and motivation, this brings the best outcomes. Good motivation accumulates positive karma, which is needed for enlightenment.

Buddhist teachings recommend that you study and check thoroughly the Buddha's teachings yourself, not just unquestioningly believing what he said. Your own practice is important. If you find these teachings good and beneficial and your aim is enlightenment for all beings, you usually take refuge in Buddha, Dharma and Sangha because these elements, called the Three Jewels, are needed on the path to that aim, in the same way that every day we resort to eating food because we do not want to die of hunger. The role of the teacher is also important as a guide to us on that path. The teacher who shows us the nature of our mind is called the 'root guru' or root teacher. Through prayers to the root guru who is connected to the Three Jewels comes the blessing that helps us on the path. Important things are our own motivation, faith and trust in the teachings and also feelings of respect and devotion to the teacher. These help to get the most benefit out of the teachings. Practising then accumulates positive merit and karma, which is dedicated to enlightenment for all beings not just our own benefit. If our motivation, faith and trust are strong, if we are diligent and committed to the practice from our heart, if we investigate impermanence and let go of the grasping at samsara, it is possible to reach enlightenment in one lifetime.

How Do We Practise Meditation?

We can practise meditation in day-to-day life. At first we have to recognize and appreciate that we have this precious human life. We have in us great potential for wisdom. Also, this moment is important and special. We can lose it so easily because our mind is busy thinking and always somewhere else. At this moment we are free but we don't recognize it. When we begin to exercise our mind, the moments of mindfulness increase.

You can practise wherever, whenever and with whatever situation occurs. Conscious awareness is with you every moment. It is not doing. Just keep your mind and heart open to this moment and to what is going on. When you practise awareness or mindfulness in everyday life, it slowly becomes easier. It is like learning the alphabet: at first it seems to be so difficult and you need to think of what you are doing, but sooner or later you will read fluently even without thinking about the alphabet.

Our mind continuously comments on how we meditate. Perhaps you think that you cannot meditate because you have such a busy mind. You may think that you want to be like that. If you have a thought that you cannot think, actually more thoughts will come. When you begin to meditate, thoughts start arising. Do not follow the thoughts or push them away; just notice them and let go; don't make a story out of them. Whether good or bad thoughts, they are just thoughts – you don't have to be bothered by them or grasp at them. You can leave the thoughts in their natural state. This way you will relax naturally.

There are different methods of meditation. You can try them according to your own feelings and at different times. It is as though you were in the supermarket trying to choose crisps from the range available. Although they are a little bit different, they are all made from potatoes. At first when we start meditating, our mind is restless and we need a change. The more you practise, the more stable your mind becomes and you can stay longer with the same technique without getting bored.

The posture for meditation is better straight, so that the energy winds flow freely. Then our mind stays free from dullness or tensions more easily. You can imagine these energy channels as a water pipe – if there is a fold, the water cannot flow freely. Keep the posture, however, as natural as possible. You can keep your eyes open or closed. Keeping your eyes open is better because then it is easier to stay in the present moment. When we close our eyes, we usually start having pictures in our mind and we can become lost in them.

When you begin to meditate, you may become excited and may want to meditate for two hours continuously. That may work for few days but soon your mind begins to become more tense and even the thought of the meditation makes you feel sick. So it is recommended that you start with shorter sessions, 5–10 minutes, and slowly increase the duration.

You can choose between object meditation and objectless meditation. Objectless meditation is the best. It is being open and mindful in the moment – just open your mind and heart to everything that exists. Relax, look and you see your mind everywhere.

Objectless meditation might, however, be too difficult at first, and object meditation might be an easier starting place. Here you can take any object to help you in your meditation. The object is like an anchor that helps to keep your mind in the present moment. Let your mind rest in the recognition and awareness of the object. Recognizing happens when your consciousness is with the object you are recognizing. If you look at a flower, you don't recognize it even though you look at it as if your consciousness is not there. So if your mind is somewhere else and not with the object, there will be no recognition. Your mind might come and go but don't judge that. Sometimes you'll get distracted and start following your thoughts. When you see your mind wandering and you become aware of the object again – that moment your mind is there with you, you don't especially have to 'bring it back'. You shouldn't concentrate too tightly on the object either because it tightens your mind and body and might thus create aches and pains. You can also take your thoughts as the objects of your meditation. Become aware of the thought you have and stay there with it. When the thought naturally changes after a while, you can take that new thought as the object and again stay there.

You can use many methods and objects as a focus for meditation: breathing, a visual object, pain, sound, walking and sitting, eating or sleeping, or practice during the day:

- *Breathing as an object:* Do not try to control your breathing, let it flow freely. Keep your awareness in your breathing. You can also count your breath. At first you might find it difficult to breathe naturally, but it will get easier in time as you learn to relax.
- *Visual object:* Let your awareness rest in the recognition of the object. Do not tighten your eyes, you could have visual problems, such as seeing some lights or one object as many.
- *Pain as an object:* If you naturally have pain somewhere in your body, you can use that as an object. Also, sometimes during the meditation, you may start having pains. Instead of fighting back, let your mind rest in the feeling of the pain. When you are not fighting, your mind relaxes naturally. The pain may then go away or at least decrease. Some of the pain is in the mind, some is in the body. If you have lots of pain and you cannot keep your awareness there, then you can meditate on the feeling that the pain causes to you, for example becoming depressed.
- *Sound as an object:* You can take whatever sound you like as the object of your awareness. Let your mind rest there, do not make stories about it. If you use music, it is recommended that it does not have vocals.
- *Walking and sitting meditation:* Your mind is not somewhere else but there with you in the motion or in the posture. Keep your awareness in what you are doing.
- *Eating meditation:* At the beginning, you can start finding the feeling of gratefulness of the food you have. Eat, then quietly taste the food, keeping the awareness in the experience. Stay conscious of what you are doing.
- *Sleeping meditation:* You can also meditate during sleep. You relax and keep awareness when falling asleep. If you maintain the awareness, you will stay conscious of your surroundings all night and then your sleep becomes meditation. That is not easy but is possible with practice.
- *Practice during the day:* In the morning before getting up, you can start the day meditating in your bed for 5–10 minutes. Sit up and relax there, be aware of the feelings you have at the moment. During the day, keep awareness of what you are doing. You can see how your mind is working – judging and evaluating all the time. All this gives us an opportunity to practise. When we encounter problems, we can relax, let go and use the compassion that we all have naturally. It is important to recognize and contemplate the impermanence of things – every second things change naturally. You cannot change what has already happened and you do not know about the future. Time goes fast and it makes you more satisfied if you can appreciate what you have here in this moment and be contented with that.

The Main Uses of Meditation

Meditation can help us in our everyday life. The purpose is to learn how to deal with our emotions in more beneficial ways so that we don't create more problems for us and others. We may try to escape our problems but actually we cannot run away from our own mind. Life always brings us difficult situations and the best way is to learn how to deal with them. We may lose something we would not want to lose and gain something we do not want to gain. Qualities like compassion, love, kindness, self-knowledge, self-confidence, peacefulness, wisdom and mindfulness, which develop though meditation and mind practice, usually improve the quality of our relationships with other beings as well as with ourselves. Meditation teaches us to deeply relax our mind and our body. When we learn to relax and let go of useless worries, we create less stress for us, so meditation is a good way of controlling stress. Meditation also may help us with pain, by relieving it through relaxing and having a less grasping attitude. Through meditation, we also finally find our own inner wisdom mind, the nature of mind.

How Meditation May Help People with Problems

We cannot escape from suffering because it has its roots in our own mind. Suffering develops from the grasping attitude we have due to the belief in illusion. We usually take things seriously and believe in the solidity and permanence of things. This creates many negative emotions. Only working with our own mind can really give us freedom from suffering. We have to deal with the emotions, things and situations that we face in our lives. We have to try to change the things that we can and deal with the ones we cannot.

Many problems that we have arise from the tightness of our mind. We take things seriously and thus create negative emotions and other problems. Through meditation, we can learn to open our mind and relax in different kinds of situations. Meditation develops flexibility and openness of the mind that will help us in dealing with problems. When you meditate, you get to know your mind and heart more. Opening your mind reveals the natural kindness of your heart and relaxing means less grasping. Knowing yourself and developing loving kindness and compassion usually means that you will have more self-confidence and better self-esteem. You become more aware of your needs and that way decisions are easier to make. The result of this is usually that you are not so bothered about other people's talk and your mind is not constantly changing according to others' opinions. Meditation helps to calm your mind and it becomes more stable.

We want and desire many things. It is good to differentiate between wanting and needing. Sometimes we really need something and then we need to get it. Usually, however, we want things even though we actually do not need them. After getting that something, for a moment the desire goes away but soon it will return again. By running after our desires all the time, we create a restless and unsatisfied mind. Of course we cannot give up on everything but we need balance.

Let us be happy and satisfied with what we already have. When our mind relaxes, we shall find more pleasure and happiness from this present moment.

As we look at our life now, it seems that happiness comes only momentarily and dissatisfaction and suffering prevail most of time. By practising with our mind, this begins to turn the other way round. We develop a deeper understanding of our mind and thus this present moment begins to seem very precious. Meditation helps us to find a balance in our mind. A balanced mind is more relaxed and does not have so many problems.

Chapter Summary

This chapter has explored the nature of meditation and how this may be used in dealing with people's problems. It has focused on one approach to meditation, based on Buddhism, but there are many other approaches. The Further Resources below offer some suggestions about where to find these.

REVIEW QUESTIONS

1 What is a negative emotion?

2 How can we use the words 'here and now', 'our heart' and 'our head' to explain what meditation is?

3 In Buddhism, what are samsara and moksha?

CHAPTER LINKS

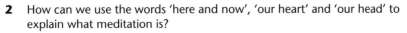

For further discussion of aspects of Buddhism, see Chapter 20.

FURTHER RESOURCES

Bhikkhu, T. (1994) *The Buddhist Monastic Code*, Valley Center, CA, Metta Forest Monastery. Basic introduction to Buddhist beliefs and practice.

Leshan, L. (1999) *How to Meditate: A Guide to Self-discovery*, New York, Little, Brown. Practical guide to types and methods of meditation, dealing with many practical questions, including which techniques to develop and whether it is necessary to have a teacher.

Queen, C. (2000) *Engaged Buddhism in the West*, Boston, Wisdom. Good study of the applications of Buddhism.

Part VI

Resource file

Mind-body Approaches

This resource file gives supplementary information on mind-body approaches, over and above the individual areas of practice referred to in the preceding chapter, and offers suggestions for further reading.

This category of approaches has somewhat imprecise boundaries since some can be categorized here and elsewhere. It includes a variety of approaches that bring together the mind and the body in an integrative way, so as to heal or enhance wellbeing. This category includes some therapeutic approaches such as hypnosis and hypnotherapy, as well as those involving touch, such as therapeutic touch and the Trager approach, which uses movement and touch to benefit the mind and body.

- *Gestalt therapy* is holistic in the sense that it emphasizes the integration of the person through the authenticity of experience in the present. Gestalt refers to a 'whole', which cannot be taken apart without destroying it and which means more than, and is different from, the sum of its parts. Fritz Perls and others developed Gestalt therapy. Another theorist, Kurt Goldstein, who apparently did not see himself as a Gestalt psychologist (Votsmeier, 1996), linked Gestalt psychology with field theory, associated with systems theory and the systemic notion of working with the person as a whole, in relation to their wider environment.

Further Resources

Perls, F., Hefferline, R. and Goodman, P. (1951) *Gestalt Therapy: Excitement and Growth in the Human Personality*, London, Souvenir Press.

Zinker, J. (1989) *Creative Process in Gestalt Therapy*, London, Vintage Books.

- *Guided imagery* is an ancient form of helping that involves the helper suggesting to the person the use of the senses in creating images in order to enhance understanding, whether of problems or an aspect of knowledge.

Further Resources

Naparstek, B. (1995) *Staying Well with Guided Imagery*, New York, Warner Books.

Rossman, M. (2000) *Guided Imagery for Self-healing*, 2nd edn, H.J. Kramer, New World Library.

- *Clinical biofeedback* lies within conventional as well as complementary and alternative approaches. Biofeedback is a cognitive behavioural therapy based on aspects of behavioural psychology, which, ideally, enables a person to gain control of a particular behaviour and consequently control or extinguish a specific personal problem (Bandler and Grindler, 1982).

Further Resource

Danskin, D. and Crow, M. (1981) *Biofeedback: An Introduction and Guide*, Palo Alto, CA, Mayfield.

- *Hypnosis* is a form of treatment in which the therapist uses relaxation and other techniques such as suggestion to enable the person to focus on a particular issue or problem and, perhaps, bring about changes in behaviour. Hypnotherapy uses a combined approach based on hypnosis and therapy to bring about change while the patient is deeply relaxed.

Further Resources

Alman, B. and Lambrou, P. (1993) *Self-hypnosis: The Complete Guide to Better Health and Self-change*, London, Souvenir Press.

Mackenzie, R. (2005) *Self-change Hypnosis*, Milton Keynes, Trafford Publishing.

- *Kinesiology*, sometimes known as applied kinesiology, refers to the holistic use of body movement and energy patterns as an aid to diagnosis and treatment in healthcare. It may be used in association with different systems of medicine, such as TCM.

Further Resource

Diamond, J. (1979) *Behavioural Kinesiology*, New York, Harper Row.

■ **Kriotherapy** (or cryotherapy) involves activating temperature receptors in the skin to stimulate the circulation of the blood and increase the release of 'feel-good' hormones.

Further Resource

Light, K. (1995) *Cryotherapy in Sport Injury Management*, Champaign, IL, Human Kinetics Publishers.

■ **Light therapy** is used to combat such conditions as seasonal affective disorder (SAD), based on the theory that it can improve people's mental, as well as their bodily, health.

Further Resource

Lam, R. (ed.) (1998) *Seasonal Affective Disorder and Beyond: Light Treatment for SAD and non-SAD Conditions*, Washington, DC, American Psychiatric Press.

■ **Neurolinguistic programming** could be viewed either as a conventional or as an alternative strategy, in mental health work. In this connection, I am grateful to the therapist Nancy Blake for her ideas and writing, particularly for her personal communication to me in which she suggests that neurolinguistic programming offers an alternative empowering strategy for the relatively powerless person for whom becoming mentally ill may have been an unconscious attempt to exercise power and gain control.

Further Resources

Bandler, R. and Grinder, J. (1982) *Neuro-linguistic Programming and the Transformation of Meaning*, Moab, UT, Real People Press.

Blake, N. (2002) Psychoneuroimmunology and NLP, *Positive Health*, 78: 14–20.

■ **Psychosynthesis** is not a school of thought, but an approach to psychology based on existential ideas (the notion that what happens in the present is paramount), developed by Dr Roberto Assagioli, and used by him to work with people holistically, that is, bodily, emotionally and spiritually.

Further Resource

Assagioli, R. (2000) *Psychosynthesis: A Collection of Basic Writings*, Amhurst, MA, Synthesis Centre.

■ **Prayer** is an approach used variously in different faiths, one of which may combine it with healing, through focusing on the mind, body and spirit. A healer may use prayer individually or in a group, to mobilize the healing energy of the person who is sick.

Further Resources

Dossey, L. (1989) *Recovering the Soul: A Scientific and Spiritual Search*, New York, Bantam Books.

Lonegren, S. (2007) *Spiritual Dowsing*, Glastonbury, Gothic Image.

■ **Psychotherapy** is the generic term used to refer to a variety of approaches used to tackle mental health problems and to promote mental well-being. It is not generally regarded as a complementary therapy or an alternative medical approach, although in structural terms it shares several features with many of these, including the lack of state regulation and statutory registration of practitioners in many countries and in the UK its location partly outside the NHS framework.

Further Resource

Clarkson, P. and Pokorny, M. (eds) (1994) *Handbook of Psychotherapy*, London, Routledge.

■ **Qigong**, which in Chinese means cultivating the life energy, uses exercises, postures and meditation to enhance the qi of the body (see Chapter 20). It is sometimes called Taiji Qigong.

Further Resource

Jarmey, C. (2003) *The Theory and Practice of Taiji Qigong*, Chichester, Lotus Publishing.

- *Thought field therapy* (Chapter 30) was developed by Roger Callahan during the late twentieth century. It involves using a tapping technique with the fingers at meridian points on the body and hands to bring about mental and physical changes.

Further Resource

Callaghan, R. and Trubo, R. (2002) *Tapping the Healer Within: Using Thought Field Therapy to Conquer your Fears, Anxieties and Emotional Distress*, New York, McGraw-Hill.

- *Trager therapy* was developed by Milton Trager in the 1920s and relies on gentle movements to bring about relaxation and improved mental focus and physical mobility. It uses mentastics, a related series of gentle exercises.

Further Resource

Trager, M. and Hammond, C. (1995) *Movement as a Way to Agelessness: A Guide to Trager Mentastics*, Barrytown, NY, Station Hill Press.

- *Transcendental meditation* is an approach to meditation that sets out to achieve a deep state of relaxation, in the process aiming to achieve contentment, recharged energy and creativity. Transcendental meditation uses techniques such as a repeated sequence of words, known as a mantra, as a means of achieving a focused and concentrated state of mind.

Further Resources

Chopra, D. (1990) *Perfect Health*, New York, Harmony Books.

Goldsmith, J.S. (1990) *The Art of Meditation*, 2nd edn, New York, HarperCollins.

Kabat-Zinn, J. (1991) *Full Catastrophe Living: Using the Wisdom of Your Body and Mind to Face Stress, Pain and Illness*, New York, Delta.

Keown, D. (2003) *Buddhist Ethics: A Very Short Introduction*, Oxford, Oxford University Press.

Kulananda (1996) *Principles of Buddhism*, London, Thorsons.

Singh, R. (1996) *Inner and Outer Peace through Meditation*, Rockport, MA, Element Books.

Herbal Medicine 23

ANDREW STABLEFORD

What is Herbal Medicine?

In its simplest form, herbal medicine is the use of plants in the treatment of illness, but in reality this covers a wide range of approaches. It is true to say that plants have always had an important role to play in the human condition. There are examples of the use of herbs as medicine in all ancient cultures and herbal medicine remains the primary medical system for many indigenous societies.

The fact of the action of plants on human physiology is not surprising. We rely on plants for food and our biochemistry is interrelated with the chemicals found in plants, both food substances and those which are called secondary metabolic compounds. These compounds serve many purposes within plants, for example to repel or kill pathogens, for communication, to affect the animals who eat them, and many of their effects on humans are well demonstrated.

Traditional uses include the pragmatic treatment of everyday conditions, for example the treatment of infectious conditions, the treatment of wounds and contusions. Some traditional remedies have been developed as mainstream medicines. A typical example is aspirin, originally derived from willow bark, and used as a **herbal decoction** (the extraction of substances by boiling plants) for the pain and inflammation of arthritic joints and for temperature control in the treatment of fevers, in exactly the same way that aspirin is used today.

Herbal Medicine and Holism

Orthodox or allopathic medicine largely follows the **reductionist** (simplified) biomedical **approach** to health that espouses evidence-based practice. The foundations of this therapeutic approach are in orthodox pathophysiology, which in turn is derived principally from studies in pathology. Pathology is informed by **dissection** (cutting up and separating parts, for example in the study of anatomy) and gives a structural understanding of the body in terms of the anatomy of the tissues and organs and a functional understanding in terms of underlying **biochemical** (involving chemical activity) **processes**. This approach lends itself to the understanding and intervention in medical matters concerned with structure and health management and can be effective in these areas, particularly in surgical techniques and the management of acute illnesses and symptoms. However, this therapeutic approach does not allow for the understanding of the process by which people become ill and allows little conceptual understanding of people in terms of their functional modalities, which we know as mind and spirit. This has led to the development of a medical system that does not recognize the emotional nature of people or the importance of the processes of feeling, thinking, intuition and belief. The same can, of course, be said for the practice of herbal medicine from a biomedical perspective. Illness is conceptualized as an unfortunate circumstance.

In many traditional systems of medicine, however, illness is seen as a consequence of the breakdown of the integration of the individual both internally and in relationship to the world. A holistic view of wellbeing conceives wellbeing as engendered by living in accordance with the laws of nature so that the health of the body, mind and spirit is supported by a fundamental balance and integrity. The person is not sick because of a disease, they are diseased because they are sick. The goal of the physician is to assist the patient in treating illness and to educate them in the ways in which they are hindering themselves. There is a danger that incorrect treatment of disease conditions can hinder the understanding of the real nature of the causative factors. Wellbeing of the spirit is associated with desirelessness and unconcern, which allow for the uninterrupted, spontaneous and harmonious expression of life. Overconcern, overwork, striving, negative emotional states and negative experiences all corrupt this expression, creating disharmony and leading to disease. In modern society, people are ill in complex ways and a complex therapeutic understanding and therapeutic foundation are required to intercede effectively.

This holistic perspective has much in common with the ideas of Taoism and other Eastern approaches and is generally understood as originating from the Eastern tradition, but an understanding of a dynamic and integrative approach to health is also part of the Western tradition. With their concept of the 'wyrd', Anglo-Saxons had much in common with the traditions of the East. Wyrd in this sense means unfathomable or mysterious and refers to the idea that the individual lives in a web of creation of their own making and that disease patterns are the consequence of disturbances created by the individual's intent and actions. It may be the case that there is a common root to both East and West traditions through the Indo-European stem of language and culture. The Anglo-Saxon tradition and other early traditions are poorly recorded, having been predominantly an **oral tradition** (handed down by word of mouth rather than through printed words). Present-day holistic medical systems mark a re-emergence of a different way of looking at the individual and the way he relates to the world.

Contemporary Herbal Medicine Practice

There are many contemporary approaches to the use of herbs in medicine, including those that use the biomedical, evidence-based approach. The majority of Western medical herbalists, however, adopt an approach that has its roots in a system of therapeutics developed in North America in the late nineteenth century called **physiomedicalism**. Physiomedicalism developed from the same root as naturopathy and osteopathy and involved the integration of holistic ideas of natural therapeutic healing, modern medical understanding and the botanic healing system then in current use by the indigenous native Americans. Physiomedicalism was introduced into the UK by herbalists from the USA who were being harried by the orthodox medical profession and the system was adopted in the UK as the primary form of herbal medicine practice. Herbal medicine was used primarily at this time for the treatment of endemic infectious diseases, for which orthodox medicine had little to offer. Herbal medicine has adapted over the years to meet the changing needs of society and the developments of orthodox medicine. Now orthodox medicine is efficient at dealing with endemic diseases and acute illness, the role of herbal medicine is the adoption of the holistic counterpart, looking at the origins of disease in a complex society where people are subject to the imbalances of mind and spirit on the body. In alignment with this transition, the actions of herbs need to be developed from those of purely physiological engagement to those which work upon the integration of all aspects of the body.

The physiological processes are controlled and regulated homeostatically by complex factors, some of which are topical to the tissues and organs and some of which are concerned with the regulation of the physiology in relationship to the external environment. This neurobiological homeostatic control is regulated principally by the autonomic nervous system (ANS) in conjunction with the central nervous system (CNS). The ANS is largely, from a structural classification, operated by the older centres of the brain, in particular the limbic system, and forms a large part of what we regard as the subconscious part of the mind. The limbic system is largely concerned with maintaining homeostasis in the body, that is, control over the physiological processes of the body such as temperature, appetite, memory and predictability, emotional experience and expression and the coordination of involuntary behaviour and emotional response.

The sense of self is, however, more concerned with the conscious mind. We are used to making decisions and having a sense of autonomy and free will, which are functions connected with processes connected structurally with the higher brain centres and the cerebral cortex in particular.

There is a tendency for modern people to experience a disassociation between the conscious and the unconscious and to regard physiology as being unconnected with brain function. It is imperative to recognize that physiological function is inseparable from the energy associated with it and the feeling that either created it or accompanies it. To change physiological function is to change the energy and the feeling associated with it and demonstrates holistic resolution. In fact, the physiological pattern can inform the practitioner of the subconscious experience of the patient.

The physiomedicalists classified herbs into categories based on their main physiological actions on the tissues and organs, for example stimulants, relaxants, astringents, sedatives, demulcents (relieve irritation and have soothing properties) and nerviness. The same herbs can be seen in a different way and their actions interpreted, labelled and applied differently to demonstrate how they may bring about a deeper integrating action within the body, between the physiological processes and the unconscious and conscious processes. This process can lead to a change in personal concept and feeling and consequently a change in one's appreciation of the ability to interrelate in one's life process.

Herbal Medicine Actions

Table 23.1 gives details of examples of herbal actions that integrate psychological and physiological functions to bring about associated changes in personal feeling. Actions may require several herbs combined together to attain the required effect and herbs may fit several categories.

Table 23.1 Different herbal actions

Contemporary action	Physiomedical action	Intervention	Examples of herbs
Diffusive Creates an outward and upward movement of blood and energy	Diaphoretic (produces perspiration). Relaxant and stimulant action on blood vessels. Encourages peripheral circulation in fever management, cardiovascular disease	Engenders a sense of freedom and liberation. Maintains a sense of boundaries, integration and control. Leads to the release of conditions featuring fear, overregulation and control	*Achillea millefolium* (yarrow) *Angelica archangelica* (angelica)
Harmonizing An action that unites functions together and integrates action throughout the nervous system. Action is centred in the head	Relates to herbs that regulate and balance the ANS and CNS and promote normal function of the neuroendocrine system. Stimulating and relaxing	Creates a sense of balance and integrity. Promotes the feeling of being in control	*Rosmarinus officinalis* (rosemary) *Hyssopus officinalis* (hyssop) *Hypericum perforatum* (St John's wort)
Stabilizing An action that creates tone (balance between stimulation and contraction) in the visceral organs. Action is centred in the body	Relates to herbs that have a regulating action on the central metabolism; includes astringents and many herbs that work on the liver, pancreas and digestive tract	Creates a grounding action. Promotes the feeling of having personal authority	*Agrimonia eupatorium* (agrimony) *Carbenia benedictus* (blessed thistle)
Resolving Removes negative impression by a process of transformation. Involves a change in the emotional valency attached to important life events	Depurative or cleansing herbs concerned with the removal of toxicity and combined with herbs with an aromatic quality. An extension of physical cleansing action to that of energetic cleansing action, that is, the 'impression' associated with toxicity	Removes complexes or internalized and unresolved emotional issues, giving a sense of resolution and peace	*Paeonia laterifolia* (paeony root) *Schizandra chinensis* (schizandra) *Citrus aurantium flores* (orange blossom)
Restoring An action that is positive and uplifting. Counteracts the often self-punitive feelings people have about themselves	Relates to herbs with a reputation as tonics or having nutritive benefit to the vital organs and tissues. The physically nutritional benefit relates to a sense of being nurtured	Engenders a sense of being nourished, loved, supported and respected	*Hydrocotyle asiatica* (gotu cola) *Panax ginseng* (ginseng)

Taking a Case History: Case Example

The consultation starts with taking a comprehensive and detailed case history that explores the presenting complaint and related symptoms, checks the body systems for other disturbances, investigates the personal and family previous medical history and endeavours to construct a context in terms of the patient's life circumstances in order to understand a possible connection with the complaint. This is followed by a physical examination. The blood pressure, pulse and tongue are routinely checked by a herbal practitioner but other physical examination is carried out as determined by the particular case.

This case involves a 25-year-old woman who had seen the herbalist four years previously. The presenting complaint on this occasion was that she has been suffering from frequent and increasingly worse migraines for some months and these are now occurring at a rate of three or four attacks per week. The symptoms start with blurring of the vision and reddening of the left eye and progress to a severe headache, which forces her to retire to bed. The following day she feels drained of energy and has a dull headache. A review of systems reveals that she also has persistent nasal catarrh and sinus problems. Her energy is poor. Her sleep is disrupted and of poor quality, she finds it difficult to settle to sleep and she wakes in the early hours of the morning. Her menstrual cycle is regular and of normal flow and duration.

She is of attractive, slim, healthy and well-groomed appearance. She is sociable and communicates well.

Upon questioning, it was discovered that she is living in a unhappy relationship in which she suffers mental abuse but from which she cannot find the strength to leave. She works for the family firm of her partner and her best friend is the brother of her partner.

Clinical examination reveals the following findings. Her blood pressure is 110/70 mmHg (very weak) (the previous day it had been 110/80). Her radial pulse is 76 beats per minute and very weak, the right pulse being stronger than the left. Her tongue shows a swollen and pale body that has a slippery surface and red papillae in the anterior third of the surface (Figure 23.1).

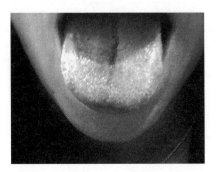

Figure 23.1 Photograph of the patient's tongue

Analysis

The clinical signs are expressions of the balance of the ANS. The ANS determines the balance of how the body's physiological processes are oriented.

The significance of the blood pressure readings is as an indicator of physiological functioning rather than that of the reading per se. Two days previously her blood pressure as measured by her GP was 110/80 and her blood pressure four years previously following a course of herbal treatment had been 110/60. The day before the consultation she had had a migraine. The differences in diastolic blood pressure are significant. The diastolic blood pressure is the pressure in the artery when the heart is not contracting and is primarily determined by the degree of constriction of the smooth muscle of the artery. There are a number of determinants of smooth constriction, but the major factor, particularly in young people, is emotional tension. Emotional tension results in constriction of smooth muscle as a reflex 'guarding' or defensive action by the unconscious. The significance of the migraine is that in migraine there is a spastic vasoconstriction within the circulation that acts as a mechanism to resolve tension. Her blood pressure measurements clearly reflect a build-up of tension that is dissipated by the migraine, leading to a reduction in diastolic blood pressure. Persistently elevated diastolic blood pressure leads to chronic constriction within the organ systems and throughout the body as whole, and over a long period of time results in a reduction of the energy potential of the visceral organs. A pale and swollen tongue indicates that the perfusion of blood to the tongue is diminished and demonstrates that this has taken place. The slippery surface of the tongue is the result of excessive release of saliva and demonstrates that the visceral processes of the digestive tract are overworking. The red papillae in the tongue are the result of the irritation of immune complexes or 'toxic heat' circulating in the bloodstream and demonstrate disturbance within the immune system. This is related to the internalization of energy and emotion.

In summary, the clinical signs suggest that there is a pattern of deficient functioning within the ANS, which involves a pattern of poor blood and energy perfusion to the exterior and the congestion of blood in the internal organs, the liver in particular. The internalization and congestion of blood and energy are related to the direction of the immune function, which also becomes internalized and corrupted, leading to the production of immunological complexes or 'heat'. The internalization of the blood and energy and the actions of the immune system relate directly to the internalization of emotional expression. Her emotional experience is one of being subject to external controlling actions and being deprived of her own authority and independent decision making, with the internalization of unexpressed anger, fear and resentment.

The Prescription

The prescription is a combination of different herbal tinctures formulated together into a complex medicine. Tinctures are alcoholic extracts of plants, which have excellent extraction qualities so that the plant is closely represented in liquid form, a long shelf life, they can easily be mixed together and, most importantly, they represent, in a small dose, the qualities of the plant in an energized form. By combining different herbs together, complex actions can be achieved that can work on multiple sites in the body simultaneously.

The herbs prescribed for the patient are: *Angelica archangelica radix, Hydrocotyle asiatica, Schizandra chinensis, Agrimonia, Paeonia laterifolia, Carbenia benedictus, Rosmarinus officinalis* (see Figure 23.2), *Hypericum perfoliatum* and *Citrus aurantium flores*. Table 23.1 describes the herbal actions. The patient takes a 5ml dose of the medicine twice daily.

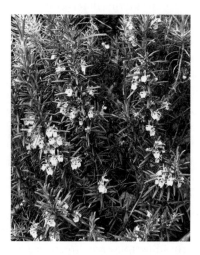

Figure 23.2 Rosemary (*Rosmarinus officinalis*)

This particular formula is designed to create appropriate movement and adjustment within the ANS to create balance and to move the underlying psychological processes towards resolution. Essentially, by changing the physiology, the underlying energy and emotion associated with the physiology pattern will also be changed, leading to a change in the experience of the patient and a different perception of herself with regard to the situation she is in.

Treatment Assessment

The patient experienced no further migraines after commencing the treatment and over a period of several weeks gained in energy. Two months after the start of treatment, she changed her job and after four months, she found the strength to break from her relationship and moved out to her own house. The decision to leave the relationship was of her own making. If the circumstances had been different, the changes she has experienced in herself might have enabled her to act differently so as to retrieve the relationship.

Risk Assessment

The medicine is of a low dose, nontoxic nature and its subtle psycho-physiological repatterning actions do not carry the potential risks and side effects that materially acting symptomatic medicines may have.

Professional Qualification and Regulation

Herbal practitioners have always and continue to practise outside statutory regulations, essentially being subject only to common law. Many herbal practitioners belong to the National Institute of Medical Herbalists (NIMH), which was founded in 1864 and provides professional voluntary regulation with a strict professional code of ethics, accreditation of training and a register of members. The profession has recognized that lack of statutory recognition is a situation that will have to change, given the growth in complementary medicine and the movement towards EU centralization and harmonization of qualification and regulation in the professions. The origin of the recent movement towards statutory regulation of herbal practitioners was the House of Lords (2000) Select Committee on Science and Technology's report on complementary and alternative medicine and the government's response. The committee identified that herbal medicine was a part of complementary medicine that met the criteria for regulation, these being the potential risk to the public through poor practice, an existing voluntary system of self-regulation and the foundations of an evidence base for the discipline. Regulation would ensure that suitably qualified practitioners, capable of recognizing the limitations of practice and when to refer, could be identified by a statutory title and placed on a register of practitioners. After much delay and consultation with the profession, the process led to the White Paper (DH, 2007) *Trust, Assurance and Safety: The Regulation of Health Professionals in the 21st Century*, in which the government proposed that herbal medicine should be regulated by the Health Professions Council (HPC). Ongoing and constructive debate between the HPC and the Steering Group representing herbal medicine continues.

In addition to professional regulation, there is a parallel process of regulation concerning herbal medicine products. The Medicines and Healthcare Products Association (MHRA) is an agency of the Department of Health concerned with ensuring that medicines, including herbal medicines, are safe for public use. The MHRA registers products under the EU's Traditional Herbal Medicinal Products Directive. This makes provision for practitioners who supply their own herbal medicines to be exempt from licensing.

Chapter Summary

This chapter has dealt with the nature of herbal medicine and what distinguishes it from conventional medicine. It has examined what the principle of holism means in herbal medical practice. It has discussed how herbs work and how the process of practice, from history taking through to prescription and treatment, takes place.

REVIEW QUESTIONS

1. What is allopathic medicine?
2. What is the main body in the UK responsible for the professional and legal regulation of treatment with herbal medicine?
3. What is a diaphoretic?

CHAPTER LINKS

For further discussion of other aspects of traditional herbal medicine, see Chapter 21.

FURTHER RESOURCES

Bartram, T. (1998) *Bartram's Encyclopedia of Herbal Medicine*, London, Robinson. A comprehensive compendium and information source book for herbal medicine remedies and treatments.

Buhner, S.H. (2002) *The Lost Language of Plants*, White River Junction, VT, Chelsea Green Publishing. Argues for the ecological contribution of plant-based medicinal practice.

Hoffmann, D. (2003) *Medical Herbalism: The Science and Practice of Herbal Medicine*, Rochester, VT, Healing Arts Press. Deals with the principles and practice of herbalism.

Mills, S. and Bone, K. (2000). *Principals and Practice of Phytotherapy*, London, Churchill Livingstone. Textbook of mainstream herbal medicine therapeutics.

Oschman, J.L. (2000) *Energy Medicine: The Scientific Basis*, London, Churchill Livingstone. Readable and general introduction to energy medicine.

Wood, M. (2004) *The Practice of Traditional Western Herbalism*, Berkeley, CA, North Atlantic Books. Deals with traditional energetics and the nature and uses of different categories of medicinal plants.

Web Links

www.herbmed.org – HerbMed is an interactive, electronic herbal database that provides hyperlinked access to the scientific data underlying the use of herbs for health.

www.herbs.org – The Herb Research Foundation is a nonprofit organization dedicated to responsible, informed self-care with medicinal plants.

www.nimh.org.uk – The National Institute of Medical Herbalists is the main professional association for Western herbal medicine. It accredits professional training associations, provides a register of practitioners and information and advice for the profession and the public.

www.ehpa.eu – The European Herbal Traditional Practitioners Association (EHTPA) was set up in 1994 as an umbrella body for professional associations across Europe wanting to benefit from joint working and strengthening the role of the herbal profession. It currently represents practitioners from Ayurveda, Western, Chinese and Tibetan herbal medicine, and TCM.

www.bhma.info – The British Herbal Medicine Association (BHMA) includes companies involved in the manufacture or supply of herbal medicines, herbal practitioners, academics, pharmacists, students of phytotherapy and others. The BHMA supports its members with advice and comments on legislation and labelling.

The following are more general web links of relevance not only to herbal practitioners but to other complementary practitioners as well:

www.emea.eu.int – The European Medicines Agency (EMEA) is a decentralized body of the EU set up in 1995 and is responsible for the protection and promotion of public and animal health through the evaluation and supervision of medicines for human and veterinary use. Relevant committees include the Committee for Medicinal Products for Human Use and the Committee on Herbal Medicinal Products, which provides scientific opinions on traditional herbal medicines.

www.hpc-uk.org – The Health Professions Council is a healthcare regulator of 13 professions including professions allied to medicine.

www.wmin.ac.uk/sih/page-1005 – Integrating Complementary and Alternative Medicine (iCAM) is a new centre based in the School of Integrated Health providing information and intelligence on CAM integration and professional development.

www.mhra.gov.uk – The Medicines and Healthcare Products Regulatory Agency (MHRA) is an executive agency of the Department of Health responsible for ensuring that medicines, including herbal medicines, and medical devices work and are acceptably safe. Relevant committees include the Herbal Medicines Advisory Committee and the Committee on Safety of Medicines. The MHRA registers products under the Traditional Herbal Medicinal Products Directive.

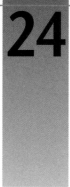

Aromatherapy

KAREN TINKER

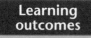

Learning outcomes

By the end of this chapter, you should be able to:

■ demonstrate an understanding of the origins of aromatherapy and its concepts

■ outline what aromatherapy practice entails

■ summarize the main treatment methods and options used by qualified aromatherapists

■ discuss the effectiveness of aromatherapy/essential oils using the evidence base

What is Aromatherapy?

Aromatherapy means simply treatment or therapy by scent or smell, or 'healing through the senses'. Aromatherapy is a complementary and holistic healthcare practice using essential oils to prevent and/or bring relief for physical, mental and emotional conditions in the client after a full medical case history has been taken.

As the name 'aromatherapy' suggests, the scent is important, so in practice, it is essential to ensure that the client actually likes the aroma of the oil(s) being used, although the application is often physical, 'pushing' the oils into the skin for absorption, by gentle massage. However, treatment can be applied via bathing/showering, body lotions, vaporization, compresses and, in some case, neat application.

In France, aromatherapists first have to be qualified as doctors and can prescribe essential oils for ingestion. In the UK, qualified aromatherapists are not registered by the state. They would not prescribe for ingestion owing to the strength of the oils and the fact that some can be toxic. As aromatherapy is a holistic therapy, the practitioner is able to give advice on diet, lifestyle and relaxation techniques. Aromatherapists do not diagnose or give any kind of medical advice, unless also qualified in this respect, nor will they give advice on over the counter/prescribed medication.

It is not the aim of the practitioner to advise for or against a doctor's opinion, but to work with the condition(s) presented in a complementary manner. It is necessary to have some idea of how over the counter (OTC) and prescribed medications affect a person, in order to ensure that the oils do not contraindicate/adversely affect the medication and vice versa. The qualified aromatherapist can treat people of all ages, including babies from birth, if need be, with very low dilution of essential oils.

The History and Philosophy of Aromatherapy

The origins of aromatherapy can be found as far back as ancient Egypt, where essential oils were found in Tutankhamun's tomb, and papyrus documentation exists from 2,800 to 2,000 BC describing the use of plant extracts and essences in healing, cosmetics, ritual and perfumery; from the Vedic scripts of ancient India, the *Rig Veda* describes the use of 700 plant extracts/essences in healing; to China, dating back to the *Yellow Emperor's Classic of Internal Medicine*, which documents the use of plant extracts and essences in healing and ritual. The Bible mentions the bringing of gifts of frankincense, myrrh (and gold), showing the use of plant essences pre-Christianity. The Phoenicians transported oils, gums and other plant essences for sale during their merchant 'reign' throughout the East, bringing the plants as well as their essences, as far west as the Mediterranean area.

At the time of the Great Plague in London (1665–66), doctors would attend their patients with a stick containing a bag of lavender hanging from their hats. This would prevent disease, lavender being antibacterial, antiviral and antifungal and would also prevent disgust in the doctor from the stench of the 'unwashed'.

In more modern times, plants were used more in cosmetic and perfume preparations until Gattefosse, a French perfumer, discovered the healing properties of lavender. During a perfumery process, he burnt his hand badly and plunged it into a vat of lavender oil, with the result that the burn stopped stinging and healed very quickly, compared with usual burns of that degree. There was no scarring on the burned hand. After this, Gattefosse studied the healing properties of plant oils and coined the term 'aromatherapy', the title of one of his books published in 1928. He discovered that the essential oils were more effective in their totality than their synthetically produced counterparts and their isolated active ingredients.

Following Gattefosse, Valnet, a French doctor, used plant extracts to treat physical and psychiatric disorders in his patients, publishing his results as *Aromatherapie* in 1964.

Madame Marguerite Maury (1895–1968) was a pioneering researcher and practitioner of aromatherapy, who followed Valnet, having studied his works. Her book was first published in French in 1961 and has been published in English translations since then (Maury, 2004). She took into account the patients' temperaments and health background and devised cosmetic preparations for them, taking the science of aromatherapy further than anyone else had previously. In her practice, she created a prescription that took account of the person's unique health problems and provided a medicinal combination of perfumed essences that transcended merely aesthetic goals.

Part VI

Many modern medicines are based on the chemical compounds of plants and follow on from the use of herbs and plant essences in healing.

The term 'aromatherapy' can be misleading, as it suggests that the healing effects simply occur through the sense of smell, although the scent is the primary application in any treatment, as the oils are smelled by the client and affect the brain and physiological system via the limbic system before any use of massage/bathing and so on. However, each oil has its own unique blend of components that interact with the body chemistry directly in different ways, affecting the organs or the system as a whole. Via the skin, in massage or bathing, the essential oils are readily absorbed and transported through the body via blood and lymph. The classic test for this is to rub a clove of garlic on the sole of the foot – the skin absorbs the volatile oils from the garlic and the smell can be detected on the breath approximately 10 minutes later, or more, depending on the efficiency of the person's system. Different oils will be absorbed at different rates. For example, eucalyptus and thyme will be absorbed in 20–40 minutes, lavender and geranium in 60–80 minutes.

The main ways in which essential oils can affect the body are:

- *Pharmacological:* chemical changes take place when the oil enters the bloodstream and affects hormones and enzymes
- *Physiological:* systemic changes take place, stimulation/sedation and so on
- *Psychological:* inhalation creates a response to the aroma, which can, in turn, cause a physiological response
- *Spiritual:* many practitioners believe that some oils have a spiritual healing effect, easing soul pain and disharmony, bringing one closer to one's 'god'.

With the first two methods, aromatherapy has much in common with traditional herbal medicine; here it is not only the scent, or aroma, that is important, but the physiological and chemical changes that can take place when the oil(s) enters the body and interacts with the organs or the complete system.

The actual philosophy or aim is to bring the client into balance of mind, body and spirit, the state of homeostasis. Aromatherapy is not a primary healthcare discipline, which means that its practitioners are not regulated by the state in the way medical nurses and doctors are, but nevertheless, practising aromatherapists should be qualified and insured/indemnified, and, when asked, willing to show evidence of both.

What Practice Entails

Although people do not need to be referred by a doctor to a practitioner, this can happen with open-minded doctors/healthcare providers. Other complementary therapy practitioners may also refer clients for this treatment. The client may decide that aromatherapy is the appropriate way to be treated and approach the relevant professional.

Taking a full consultation, to include lifestyle, skin type (in case of sensitivity or contraindication to some oils), dietary and medical conditions, the aromatherapist will be able to determine whether the client is suitable for aromatherapy or should be redirected to another, more appropriate practitioner. It is usual for an aromatherapist to have an understanding of other complementary therapies, a knowledge of anatomy and physiology that 'allows' a decision to refer the client to a medical doctor or to pursue a doctor's permission for aromatherapy treatments to go ahead.

Practice example

M was a 47-year-old Bosnian, who had suffered in the war between Bosnia and Herzegovina in 1992–5. Ten years later, he presented with severe mood swings, flashbacks, headaches/migraines, nightmares, irritability, depression, insomnia and lethargy/apathy. His body language was 'closed' and his attitude somewhat truculent. He often felt suicidal.

M had been treated with Prozac (an antidepressant), but that had been stopped prior to his attending for aromatherapy treatments, as he and his doctor agreed that it was not improving his condition. At the time of attending for his first treatments, he was not taking any doctor-prescribed or OTC medication apart from occasional painkillers for the headaches/migraines. A full medical history was taken, including as many details of M's war history as he was able to discuss, but mostly the memories were too traumatic. In Bosnia, it is difficult to gain a diagnosis of post-traumatic stress disorder as doctors are constrained by so many conditions/regulations, and aromatherapists cannot diagnose unless they are also doctors, but it would appear from the symptoms that it could be what M suffered from. Details were also taken of any shrapnel/bullet injuries, shrapnel/bullets still in the body, metal plates/pins from repair operations and other similar features.

In taking the medical history, care is taken to check for conditions that can:

1. contraindicate the use of massage/skin application of oils, for example severe and spreading skin infections, illnesses such as colds/flu, recent injuries/operations, osteoporosis/brittle bone disease and so on
2. contraindicate the use of certain oils, for example eucalyptus should not be used on pregnant women, epileptic people or diabetics, and nut allergies would preclude the use of almond oil.

The family medical history is also taken to give the practitioner an awareness of any disease/illnesses that may be familial such as cancer, epilepsy or diabetes.

Some practitioners may use a patch test, to ensure that the oils proposed are non-irritating to the client; however, this is not usually the case, as the treatment generally follows straight on from the consultation, provided the client is not contraindicated. There are always substitutes for oils that may sensitize or irritate.

Before beginning the treatment, the aromatherapist should explain which oils they propose to use and why, allow the client to smell them to ensure beneficial psychological effects/responses and explain how the client can use the oils at home between treatments, if appropriate.

The practitioner will also advise on dietary/lifestyle matters, such as exercise and eating healthily, and aftercare, such as drinking plenty of plain water and avoiding alcohol/tea/coffee/cigarettes immediately after a treatment.

If a client has issues that contraindicate them to the aromatherapy massage or aromatherapy as a whole, they can be advised where to find appropriate help.

After being informed as to the proposed treatment, the client should sign their consent and the therapist should also sign the form; notes should be kept for every treatment the client has, documenting the oils used, their effects and the client's feedback, and these should be signed by the relevant practitioner, in the case of a business/practice where more than one therapist treats the client.

Methods of Treatment/Application

The following are the main methods used in aromatherapy:

- *Massage:* a blend of essential oils in a carrier oil (preferably of vegetable/plant origin, not mineral oil, see lotions below) will be massaged into the skin, covering the whole body (except 'private' areas) using a series of formal movements, usually designed to relax the client. If the client needs a stimulating/ energizing massage, appropriate oils to enhance/match the process can be used. There will be a limit to how many drops of essential oils can be used and there will be a synergistic blend of oils appropriate for the client.
- *Bath:* a blend of essential oils, sometimes mixed with a little honey or milk to aid dispersal in water, can be added to the bath; this is useful where massage is contraindicated. Again there will be a finite number of drops advised by the practitioner.
- *Footbath:* the soles of the feet are some of the most absorbent areas of the body and if the client cannot have massage or a full bath, this is a good method of treatment.
- *Vaporization/inhalation:* by steam, use of burners/lamp rings, oils on tissues; the aroma is extremely important, as previously mentioned – the oil molecules are carried to the brain, via the nose and the limbic system, creating an instantaneous response in the client; many practitioners will smear some of the blend just under the client's nose before beginning massage.
- *Hot and cold compresses:* dilute 4–5 drops of essential oil in hot or ice-cold water – depending on condition(s) to be treated – and soak a cotton cloth in the water, wring out and apply to the relevant area.
- *Skin lotions/oils/shower gels/shampoos:* skin lotions will be more effective as they will not be rinsed off and they are unlikely to break down the oils as detergent mediums would. Again, a determined blend and number of drops per amount of medium will be applied. It is advisable to use lotions that do not contain

mineral oil derivatives as the molecules are too large to allow absorption into the skin, thus limiting the effect of the essential oils to the aroma only.

■ *Flower waters:* particularly useful in skin complaints and can be made by the client, much as children do with rose petals. The resulting liquid is not as strong as an essential oil, but will contain the plant's properties and aroma, so can be effective to a degree. If the client is to make their own flower water, the aromatherapist should advise which plants to use for best therapeutic effect.

■ *Douche:* can be used to combat genitourinary infections.

■ *Neat application:* several oils can be used neat. Lemon oil can be used externally only on warts, lavender oil on burns and tea tree oil on insect bites, stings and infections. It is possible to use other oils neat, although they may irritate sensitive skin.

■ *Internal use:* as previously stated, this is not practised in the UK. The International Federation of Aromatherapists recommends external use by the above methods.

Practice example (cont)

In M's treatments, a strong blend of anti-stress, antidepressant/anti-grief and calming oils was used – sandalwood, lavender, frankincense and others, totalling 24 drops in 30 ml of grapeseed carrier oil. The treatment was massage of the whole body, back, back of legs, front of legs, chest/abdomen and head and face. The first treatment was shorter, owing to time being taken for the consultation – and was just massage of the back and back/front of legs.

M was informed of the oils to be used, how to use them at home and provided with enough to use as massage oil after bathing/showering until his next appointment. As M had a fairly balanced lifestyle and healthy dietary habits, he did not need any advice with this. He was a smoker, so was advised to avoid cigarettes immediately after the treatment; he did not feel ready to quit smoking, although his family kept 'nagging' him about this.

From the first treatment, he relaxed totally, falling asleep. He reported feeling like he never had before, so relaxed, cheerful and happy. M had come to the treatment session believing that nothing and no one could help him. He left feeling 'on top of the world, like I can fly'.

When he arrived for his second treatment – an hour early, he was so eager – he reported that his family, friends and colleagues were asking him to bottle what he had had, commenting that he was even better tempered than before the war. He felt so, too. M had been a basketball player before the war and said that even the 'feel-good' factor of the exercise did not compare with the feeling from massage and the oils. When he used the oils at home, they reminded him of how much he had relaxed during the massage and that memory helped as much as the actual oils did.

In terms of M's symptoms, his feedback from the first treatment was that:

■ the flashbacks had reduced drastically, by about 75–80%

■ there was no insomnia and his sleeping patterns were normal

- his headaches and migraines had disappeared completely
- his nightmares had reduced by 80%
- his irritability had disappeared
- his stress levels had reduced to zero
- his suicidal thoughts and feelings had gone
- his mood swings were drastically minimized, by approximately 90%
- his depression was gone. He felt that life was now worth living
- his lethargy and apathy had disappeared. He was full of energy and motivation, to the point where he asked to learn aromatherapy in order to help others who had suffered as he had
- as a 'side effect', M cut down on smoking, because his stress levels had dropped and he did not feel the need to smoke as much.

The improvements continued throughout his four initial treatments, one per week; by the end of the second treatment, he reported feeling 20 years younger, physically, emotionally, mentally and spiritually. He certainly looked younger – the stress lines and expression were gone from his face, the body language was open. M was now laughing out loud in sheer joy.

Research into Essential Oils and Aromatherapy

There are many books on the market to discuss/explain the effects of essential oils and their benefits. In order to know these effects and benefits, an increasing number of trials and research studies have been undertaken.

Kowalski (2002) notes the effectiveness of aromatherapy in work with hospice patients to reduce pain, anxiety and depression and increase wellbeing.

Han et al. (2006) conducted a randomized clinical trial on the effectiveness of aromatherapy on dysmenorrhea symptoms (menstrual pains) and found that aromatherapy involving abdominal massage with two drops of lavender (*Lavandula officinalis*), one drop of clary sage (*Salvia sclarea*) and one drop of rose (*Rosa centifolia*) in 5 cc of almond oil significantly decreased the severity of menstrual cramps.

Chapter Summary

This chapter has discussed the origins and nature of aromatherapy. It has explored what practice entails, with reference to some of the main benefits, as well as the need for caution in usage and the avoidance of aromatherapy in some cases. This chapter has used an example from practice to indicate how it may be used and has referred briefly to the effectiveness of aromatherapy in reducing pain and enhancing wellbeing.

REVIEW QUESTIONS

1   Is aromatherapy a modern or an ancient form of practice?

2   What are the four particular ways in which aromatherapy affects a person?

3   Can you name at least 10 different forms of aromatherapy treatment?

CHAPTER LINKS

For further discussion of the regulation of aromatherapy, see Chapter 5.

FURTHER RESOURCES

Buckle, J. (ed.) (2003) *Clinical Aromatherapy: Essential Oils in Practice*, 2nd edn, Edinburgh, Churchill Livingstone. A text on the uses of aromatherapy by healthcare professionals.

Lawless, J. (1995) *An Illustrated Encyclopaedia of Essential Oils*, Shaftesbury, Element Books. Useful guide for the practitioner, covering the use of 160 essential oils in aromatherapy.

Schnaubelt, K. (ed.) (1998) *Advanced Aromatherapy: The Science of Essential Oil Therapy*, Rochester, VT, Healing Arts Press. Exposition of the research into how essential oils affect the body.

Schnaubelt, K. (1999) *Medical Aromatherapy: Healing with Essential Oils*, Berkeley, CA, Frog Books. An evidence-based guide to the uses of essential oils.

Tisserand, R. and Balacs T. (1995) *Essential Oil Safety: A Guide for Healthcare Professionals*, Edinburgh, Churchill Livingstone. Helpful guide to the safe use of essential oils.

Web Links

www.rccm.org.uk – Research Council for Complementary Medicine. Useful source of information about a wide range of complementary approaches, including aromatherapy.

www.acponline.org/journals/ecp/julaug00/aromatherapy.htm – An archive of effective clinical practice.

www.cancer.org/docroot/ETO/content/ETO_5_3X_Aromatherapy.asp – The American Cancer Society provides information about the uses of aromatherapy, not to prevent or treat cancer, but to enhance the quality of life of people with cancer.

www.library.nhs.uk/cam/SearchResults.aspx?searchText=aromatherapy – A useful source of relevant research.

Resource file

Biologically based Therapies

This resource file gives supplementary information on biologically based approaches, over and above the individual areas of practice referred to in the preceding two chapters, and offers suggestions for further reading.

A great many approaches are rooted in part or in whole in biologically based theories and perspectives, such as dietary therapy and supplements, macrobiotics and a wide variety of herbal approaches. Some techniques, such as herbal medicine, are also used in complete medical systems such as TCM. Others, such as nutritional medicine, form part of conventional medicine, although there is much overlap between this and complementary and alternative approaches. While preparing this book, I was engaged in an extended debate with a group of medically based nutritionalists – academics and researchers – who stated that they had worked hard to attain their present position of recognition in conventional medicine and so preferred not to contribute directly to this book.

A growing group of therapies have their origins in advances in scientific and medical research, as well as in the motivation to seek alternative therapies where conventional approaches appear ineffective, as in cancer treatment. Approaches in these categories include chelation therapy, enzyme therapy, orthomolecular therapy, light therapy, neural therapy and biological cancer therapies. Herbal and dietary approaches have expanded greatly since the early twentieth century and include herbal therapy, anti-cancer diets, macrobiotic diets, fasting and juice therapy.

■ *Apitherapy* involves using multiple stings by bees as a treatment for such conditions as multiple sclerosis and to reduce the inflammation from arthritis.

Further Resource

Kismatullina, N. (2005) *Apitherapy: Guidelines for More Effective Use*, Cambridge, International Bee Research Association.

■ *Bach flower remedies* based on the tree and flower extracts and essences were developed by Dr Edward Bach in the 1930s. They are the best known of a cluster of flower remedies used as remedies and in traditional medicine in many parts of the world by nonindustrial societies. Their uses include the treatment of the emotions as well as bodily conditions.

Further Resources

Bach, E. and Wheeler, F.J. (1997) *The Bach Flower Remedies*, New Canaan, CT, Keats Publishing.

Barnard, J. (ed.) (1987) *The Collected Writings of Edward Bach*, Hereford, Flower Remedy Program.

Chancellor, P.M. (1971) *Handbook of the Bach Flower Remedies*, New Canaan, CT, Keats Publishing.

Howard, J. and Ramsell, J. (eds) (1990) *The Original Writings of Edward Bach*, Saffron Walden, C.W. Daniel.

Wildwood, C. (1995) *Flower Remedies: Natural Healing with Flower Essences*, Rockport, MA, Element Books.

■ *Ear candling* (also Hopi ear candling, ear coning or thermal auricular therapy) is a popular therapy based on burning a hollow candle with its lower end inserted into the ear. It has been found ineffective at improving health and wellbeing (Rafferty and Tsikovdas, 2007) and also hazardous in terms of the risk of causing ear injuries and, less relevant to evidence-based practice but extremely important, leading to house fires (McCarter et al., 2007). Despite its name, Hopi ear candling does not correspond with any traditional healing practice of the Hopi native American people.

Further Resources

McCarter, D.F., Courtney, A.U. and Pollart, S.M. (2007) Cerumen impaction, *American Family Physician*, 75: 1523–8.

Rafferty, J. and Tsikovdas, A. (2007) Ear candling: should general practitioners recommend it?, *Canadian Family Physician*, 12: 2121–2.

■ *Iridiology* is the use of the study of the eye to help with the diagnosis and treatment of diseases and conditions.

Further Resources

Colton, J. and Colton, S. (1991) *Introductory Guide to Iridology*, 2nd edn, London, Thorsons.

Jensen, B. and Bodeen, D. (2002) *Understanding Iridology*, New Dehli, B. Jain Publishers.

Shelby-Riley, J. (1999) *Iridology Simplified*, Hastings, Society of Metaphysicians.

■ *Nutritional therapy* is the use of food, nutrition and dietary supplements to treat illnesses and promote health.

Further Resources

Lazarides, L. (1996) *Principles of Nutritional Therapy*, London, Thorsons.

Sharon, M. (1989) *Complete Nutrition*, Garden City Park, NY, Avery Publishing.

■ *Urine therapy*, urotherapy, urinotherapy or uropathy are terms used to refer to the use of urine for therapeutic purposes.

Further Resource

Kroon, C., Moritz, V., Dranow, M. and Saraswati, S. (1996) *The Golden Fountain: The Complete Guide to Urine Therapy*, Mesa, AZ, Wishland.

Chiropractic

JACQUELINE RICHARDS AND HUGH GEMMELL

By the end of this chapter, you should be able to:

■ outline what chiropractic practice entails

■ summarize the main treatment options used by chiropractors

■ demonstrate an understanding of the origin of chiropractic and early chiropractic concepts

■ discuss the effectiveness of chiropractic using the evidence base

■ discuss the issue of the possibility of a significant serious event in chiropractic

What is Chiropractic?

The word chiropractic comes from a combination of the Greek words *cheir* and *praxis*, and means 'done by hand'. Chiropractic is a primary contact healthcare discipline that specializes in the examination, diagnosis, management and prevention of mechanical disorders of the musculoskeletal system and the effects of these disorders on the function of the nervous system and general health.

In practice, there is an emphasis on manual treatments including spinal manipulation, which chiropractors may refer to as an 'adjustment'. Treatment consists of a wide range of manipulative techniques designed to improve the function of the joints as well as relieve pain and muscle spasm. Chiropractors are qualified to treat all joints of the body including extremities such as shoulders, elbows and hands, hips, knees and feet.

Chiropractic treatment is not limited to manipulation of joints. Chiropractic management may encompass soft tissue therapy such as myofascial trigger point therapy, massage, heat, cold, electrical stimulation, dry needle therapy (acupuncture), ultrasound, traction and postural support, as well as advice on exercise, diet, lifestyle and over the counter (OTC) medications. Chiropractors often provide support for pain management, sports injuries and functional rehabilitation. The goal of care is to relieve pain and improve function of the neuromusculoskeletal system.

Chiropractors take an integrated and holistic approach to the health needs of their patients. A holistic outlook means that the practitioner focuses on the whole person, rather than the sum of their parts. This is known as the **biopsychosocial** model of healthcare. Chiropractors are concerned with not only the biological aspect of a patient's care, but also the psychological and social impact of their condition. They take into consideration a patient's home and work environments, sporting activities, hobbies and anything else that could have an effect on their physical and mental health. A chiropractor can treat patients of all ages, ranging from infants of one week to geriatrics, as well as pregnant women.

Chiropractic History and Philosophy

Chiropractic began as a heterodox health system claiming to be a complete alternative to orthodox medicine. Heterodox is defined as being something new and original, not derived from something else. This is no longer the case; chiropractic has evolved into one of the neuromusculoskeletal specialities complementary to general medical care.

Manipulation has been used in many cultures across the world, probably for many thousands of years. A form of manipulation was practised in China as early as 2,700 BC. Hippocrates, the father of medicine, clearly defined techniques of spinal manipulation in his book *On Joints*. Many early inhabitants of North, South and Central America practised some form of spinal manipulation, and the custom of having children walk on troubled backs has been reported from both America and Polynesia. However, bone-setting might be viewed as a precursor to chiropractic. Bone-setters were men and women, usually not formally qualified, who set broken or dislocated bones and treated joint problems.

The founder of chiropractic was Daniel David Palmer. The origin of chiropractic can be traced back to 18 September 1895 when Harvey Lillard, a janitor, was treated by D.D. Palmer. Harvey Lillard had been deaf for 17 years. An examination showed a vertebra 'out of place' from its normal position. D.D. Palmer manipulated the vertebra back into position by using the spinous process as a lever and as soon as the manipulation was done, the man could hear as before. D.D. Palmer claimed to be the first to use the spinous and transverse processes of the vertebra as levers to replace 'displaced' vertebra.

D.D. Palmer later began to teach chiropractic to others. Bartlett Joshua Palmer, Daniel David's son, received his diploma from his father in 1902. From D.D. Palmer's initial school, chiropractic education spread rapidly across the USA. By the mid-1920s, there were more than 50 chiropractic schools in North America.

D.D. Palmer espoused the following early chiropractic concepts:

1. *Vitalism:* Characterized by the belief in a universal intelligence and innate intelligence. Universal intelligence is the life force of creation. Innate intelligence is a part of universal intelligence. It is the vital force that maintains health and controls the reparative processes within each body. Innate intelligence is able to transmit impulses via the nervous system.
2. *Subluxation:* Palmer believed that the flow of impulses through the nervous system could be interrupted by a vertebral displacement or subluxation.
3. *Tone:* Describes an equilibrium in nerve tension. Palmer considered life to be an expression of balance or tone.
4. *Adjustment:* Describes the specific chiropractic spinal manipulation of a subluxation.

D.D. Palmer was described as the 'discoverer' of chiropractic, and his son Bartlett Joshua described himself as the 'developer'. B.J. Palmer took over the school that his father had set up. He worked hard at marketing and took a young profession and made it an established, better known profession. B.J. Palmer developed new spinal assessment strategies as well as new chiropractic techniques and ideas.

Chiropractic has had an interesting past filled with external and internal disagreements. However, in chiropractic today, most of the conflict has been resolved. D.D. Palmer's initial chiropractic theories have evolved and through research, chiropractic has become more scientifically grounded. There is currently extensive research being done into the profession and, according to the General Chiropractic Council (GCC), the profession is required to be evidence based. There can be little doubt that chiropractic is now generally more accepted by the general public, governments and other healthcare workers than it was 50 years ago. The standard of chiropractic education has improved, the standard of regulation of chiropractic practice has improved and the healthcare system has evolved and doctors are now encouraged to work with a number of other specialized professions, including chiropractic. Today, chiropractic is a fast-growing independent healthcare profession in the UK, regulated by the GCC. Since 14 June 2001, the title of 'chiropractor' has been protected by law and it is a criminal offence for anyone to describe themselves as any sort of chiropractor without being registered with the GCC.

What Practice Entails

As a primary contact discipline, patients do not need to be referred to a chiropractor. Thus chiropractors are qualified to examine effectively to determine whether a condition is within their therapeutic scope of practice or not. If a condition is deemed to be not within their therapeutic scope of practice, the patient will be referred to the appropriate professional.

Practice example

Mr Smith, a 50-year-old construction worker, presents to the chiropractor complaining of right-sided lower back pain and occasional right leg pain. Mr Smith's pain is a constant ache with occasional shooting pain down his right leg. The pain is worse on walking and activities such as bending and lifting, and relieved by rest and OTC pain medication.

History Taking and Examination

During the first visit, a detailed medical history will be taken. This includes details of the current complaint or reason for attending the appointment, past medical history, psychosocial history, family history and a systems review.

The history is followed by an examination. The examination will include vital signs and, if indicated, further physical examination, for example an abdominal examination and cardiovascular system review can be done to rule out other causes of Mr Smith's condition. The physical examination is followed by a focused neurological examination, which includes cranial nerves, superficial and deep tendon reflexes as well as pathological reflexes, myotome testing for muscle strength grading and sensory testing. An orthopaedic examination is done on the area of complaint. This includes observation, palpation and special provocative testing to gain an insight into the condition. Special testing includes range of motion, joint play and muscle length and strength testing to assess musculoskeletal impairments. If indicated, further investigations will be done.

Before treatment starts, the chiropractor will explain to Mr Smith what the diagnosis is, what treatment methods will be used, alternatives to care, the management plan, including approximate number of treatments per week and number of weeks of care, and, finally, the risks of care. While the risk of serious adverse effects is rare in chiropractic, the risks are discussed with Mr Smith in detail, with the opportunity for him to ask questions. Informed consent will be obtained from Mr Smith before treatment commences.

Further Investigations

Chiropractors are able to identify when further investigations are needed and act on this need in the patient's best interests with the patient's consent. Chiropractors are qualified to take and read X-rays. The typical circumstances where an X-ray may be necessary are recent injuries, older patients whose bone structure may have altered over time, unusual examination findings, or a history of serious disease. An X-ray aids the chiropractor in making a more accurate diagnosis of the patient's condition. An X-ray is not required for all patients presenting to a chiropractor, only about 20% of patients require X-rays to rule out serious complications. Chiropractors may also order blood tests, MRI and CT scans as well as ultrasound imaging to help in diagnosis.

Approaches and Techniques

The type of treatment a patient will receive is dependent on the patient's complaint, their physical condition and patient preference. Treatment of dysfunctional joints may involve spinal manipulation or adjustment, mobilization, instrument-assisted manipulation or soft tissue therapy such as muscle relaxation techniques and myofascial trigger point therapy:

- *Manipulation* involves a high velocity, low amplitude gentle thrust specifically to the involved joint using a short lever technique, which takes the joint slightly beyond the passive range of joint motion. This can result in a cracking sound. The 'crack' is the result of overcoming negative intra-articular pressure. When joint surfaces are forced apart, the intra-articular pressure drops to a point where it reaches the partial pressure of carbon dioxide. Carbon dioxide and other gases are suddenly released from the synovial fluid to form a gas bubble within the joint space. A flow of fluid into this low pressure region collapses the gas bubble, which is perceived as an audible crack.
- *Mobilization* is defined as the application of manual force to the spinal joints within the passive range of joint motion. Mobilization does not involve a thrust.
- *Instrument-assisted manipulation* uses an activator adjusting instrument to produce a short lever mechanical thrust to a specific joint segment.
- *Post-isometric relaxation* is a muscle relaxation technique. A muscle group is passively stretched by the chiropractor until a gentle stretch is felt by the patient. The patient is asked to contract isometrically, using 10% of the patient's power, against resistance while in the stretched position. The patient is then asked to relax completely and the muscle group is then further stretched passively through the resulting increased range of motion. The process is repeated up to three times.
- *Trigger point therapy* is a soft tissue therapy technique used to release myofascial trigger points in muscle. A myofascial trigger point is a hyper-irritated spot in skeletal muscle that is associated with a hypersensitive palpable nodule in a taut band. The spot is painful on compression and can give rise to characteristic referred pain, referred tenderness, motor dysfunction and autonomic phenomena. Trigger points are treated using trigger point pressure release, muscle stretching, and dry needle therapy (an optional postgraduate course).

A chiropractor may use massage, heat, cold, electrical stimulation, ultrasound, traction and postural support, as well as advice on exercise, diet, lifestyle and OTC drugs as part of their management plan. Functional rehabilitation is becoming more prominent in chiropractic practice and it is not uncommon for a patient to be given active rehabilitation exercises.

Contraindications

A contraindication to manipulation is defined as a problem identified during the medical history or examination that would make the application of manipulation inadvisable, due to the potential to cause harm or worsen an associated condition. There are two types of contraindications to manipulation, absolute and relative. An absolute contraindication means that under no circumstances should the patient be manipulated. A relative contraindication means that the chiropractor may use their judgement and determine if manipulation is safe on the patient. It is judged on the patient's individual needs.

Activity

List as many conditions/diseases that would affect the integrity of a joint. Think in terms of conditions that would affect the bone, ligaments, nerves and blood vessels.

There are many conditions/diseases in which a chiropractor needs to consider whether manipulation is the best treatment option. If we look at bone, the following conditions may affect the integrity of bone: tumour, bone infection, arthritides (plural of arthritis), metabolic disorders and trauma. However, the decision is not black and white. Some arthritides can be treated when not in an acute inflammatory stage. Trauma, once X-rayed and cleared for fractures and dislocations, may be treatable.

Activity

A 55-year-old male patient presents to the chiropractor with lower back pain (LBP). The condition is generally worsening; the pain is constant and wakes him from sleep. The patient is a smoker; he is also losing weight without a change in his eating habits.

1. Is there any further information you would like from this patient to make his condition clearer?
2. Would you do any further investigations for this patient? If so, what?
3. Would you consider chiropractic treatment to be appropriate for this patient?

When considering contraindications, it is important to obtain a thorough history from the patient, for example: What makes the condition better or worse? Has the patient had this condition previously and how was it treated then? Are there any associated symptoms? Diseases such as cancer can be familial, therefore a family history should be taken as well. Symptoms such as night pain, weight loss without a change in eating patterns and the patient's smoking habit are termed 'red flags' and may indicate a serious condition. In terms of further investigations, the guidelines need to be followed. In this patient's case, an X-ray is justifiable. If the X-ray reveals a lesion, MRI can be considered, as well as blood tests. Considering the patient's history and the possible lesion, both of which are suggestive of cancer, the patient is not a candidate for spinal manipulation.

What Research Tells us about Chiropractic Effectiveness

In August 1993, a study on the effectiveness and cost-effectiveness of chiropractic management of LBP was published, otherwise known as the Manga Report. The study was funded by the Ontario Ministry of Health. One of the findings stated that 'spinal manipulation applied by chiropractors is shown to be more effective than alternative treatment for lower back pain' (Manga et al., 1993: 221).

A significant amount of research on the topic has been done since the Manga Report was released. In 2004, a systematic review and best evidence synthesis was done on the efficacy of spinal manipulation and mobilization for LBP and neck pain (Bronfort et al. 2004). For acute LBP, there is moderate evidence that spinal manipulative therapy (SMT) provides more short-term pain relief than mobilization, and limited evidence of faster recovery than physical therapy. For chronic LBP, there is moderate evidence that SMT and prescription non-steroidal anti-inflammatory drugs (NSAIDs) have similar effects. In the short term, SMT and mobilization are effective when compared with GP care and placebo, and in the long term, SMT and mobilization are effective when compared with physical therapy. For a mix of acute and chronic LBP, SMT and mobilization provide a better outcome in the short and long term when compared with placebo and other treatments. For chronic neck pain, there is evidence to suggest that SMT and rehabilitation exercises are superior to SMT alone. SMT and mobilization are superior to GP management for short-term pain reduction. Thus recommendations of SMT for LBP and neck pain can be made with some confidence.

In 2004, the UK BEAM Trial Team (2004) published the results of a randomized trial, which had studied the effectiveness of physical treatments for back pain in primary care. It concluded that relative to 'best care' in general practice, manipulation followed by exercise achieved a moderate benefit at three months and a small benefit at twelve months. Manipulation alone achieved a small to moderate benefit at three months and a small benefit at twelve months.

The North American Spine Society sponsored a special focus issue of *The Spine Journal* entitled 'Evidence-informed management of chronic low back pain without surgery'. Articles were contributed by leading spine practitioners and researchers. Among them, Bronfort et al. (2008) studied 'Evidence-informed management of chronic low back pain with spinal manipulation and mobilisation'. They concluded that SMT and mobilization are viable options for treatment and are, at the very least, as effective as other interventions. Table 25.1 presents a summary of these research findings.

In conclusion, the evidence of efficacy for spinal manipulative therapy has been established. However, perhaps there are other factors to consider when looking at the evidence for efficacy. There is evidence to suggest that treatment outcomes may be influenced by predictors. These predictors may include duration of symptoms, demographics and psychosocial circumstances. There is also evidence to suggest that chiropractic treatment may include a placebo effect. The term 'placebo effect' is taken to mean not only the narrow effect of an imitation intervention, but also the spectrum of nonspecific effects present in any patient–practitioner relationship. For example, patients of chiropractors are more satisfied with their care in terms of time spent with the patient, communication with the patient and rapport building. This may lead to a certain placebo effect being present during treatment.

Table 25.1 Messages from research

Author	Summary
Manga et al. (1993) *The Effectiveness and Cost-effectiveness of Chiropractic Management of Low Back Pain*	The Manga Report found chiropractic to be more effective than alternative treatments for LBP. It recommended that chiropractic services be integrated into the healthcare system and reasonable steps should be taken to encourage cooperation between healthcare providers
UK BEAM Trial Team (2004) United Kingdom back pain exercise and manipulation (UK BEAM) randomised trial: effectiveness of physical treatments for back pain in primary care, *British Medical Journal*	When compared with 'best care', SMT achieved benefit at 3 and 12 months
Bronfort, G. et al. (2004) Efficacy of spinal manipulation and mobilization for low back pain and neck pain: a systematic review and best evidence synthesis, *The Spine Journal*	There is evidence to suggest that SMT provides similar or better outcomes when compared with placebo and other treatments such as McKenzie therapy, medical care, management by physical therapists, soft tissue therapy or back school
Bronfort, G. et al. (2008) Evidence-informed management of chronic low back pain with spinal manipulation and mobilization, *The Spine Journal*	The review indicated that there was a lot of evidence for the efficacy of chiropractic and estimated a very low risk of adverse effects. This supports SMT and mobilization as viable treatment for LBP
Van der Velde et al. (2008) Identifying the best treatment among common nonsurgical neck pain treatments, *Spine*	Five treatments were evaluated, including NSAIDs, selective cox-2 inhibiting NSAIDs, exercise, mobilization and manipulation. The study concluded that when the object is to maximize life expectancy and treatment-related harms and benefits are considered, no treatment is clearly superior. However, the study assumed a risk of stroke with neck manipulation, yet the evidence suggests no risk

Practice Issues

The most important issue to consider is the possibility of a significant serious event and 'stroke'. As with all manual therapies, the hand on skin contact with a patient may cause a reaction to treatment. An adverse reaction to manipulation is described as 'a transient subjective discomfort of the patient, not influencing his or her working ability'. It appears within six to twelve hours and resolves spontaneously within hours to two days. Reactions include local soreness at area of manipulation, headache, light-headedness and increased tiredness. Reactions such as this are relatively common (Peterson and Bergmann, 2002).

In terms of serious adverse events, chiropractic has come under a lot of unfounded criticism concerning the issue of spinal manipulation and stroke. The evidence suggests that the risk of a serious adverse event, immediately or up to seven days after treatment, is low to very low. Thiel et al. (2007) investigated the safety of chiropractic manipulation of the cervical spine. Data were obtained from 28,807 treatment consultations and 50,276 cervical spine manipulations. There were no reports of significant serious adverse events. This translates to an estimated risk of a serious adverse event of, at worse, ≈ 1 per 10,000 treatment consultations immediately after cervical spine manipulation, ≈ 2 per 10,000 treatment consultations up to seven days after treatment and ≈ 6 per 10,000 cervical spine manipulations ($\approx$ is approximately equal to). According to Thiel et al. (2007: 2376), a significant serious adverse event was defined as:

> referred to hospital A&E and/or severe onset/worsening of symptoms immediately after treatment and/or resulted in persistent or significant disability/incapacity.

The Bone and Joint Decade 2000–2010 is a global initiative to promote research to combat musculoskeletal disorders, recognized as a chronic care challenge of the new century. The initiative is endorsed by the United Nations, the World Health Organization, the Vatican, 44 governments and 750 organizations. The studies thus far have been published in a *Spine* journal supplement in February 2008. In one of the studies reported by the Neck Pain Task Force, Cassidy et al. (2008) investigated the risk of vertebrobasilar artery (VBA) stroke and chiropractic care. They found that VBA stroke is a rare event in the population. There is an association between VBA stroke and chiropractic visits in those under 45 years of age; however, there is a similar association between VBA stroke and GP visits in all age groups. This is probably explained by patients with vertebrobasilar dissection-related neck pain and headache consulting both chiropractors and GPs before their VBA stroke. Patients with head and neck pain due to vertebral artery dissection seek care for these symptoms, which precede more than 80% of VBA strokes. No evidence was found of excess risk of VBA stroke associated with chiropractic care.

In conclusion, a mild reaction to chiropractic treatment is an accepted risk. These reactions are relatively common and the majority of cases resolve spontaneously. Serious significant adverse events are rare and during the data collection period for the study done by Thiel et al. (2007), no serious adverse events were reported. Cassidy et al. (2008) reasoned that the association between VBA stroke, chiropractic and GPs may be explained by patients visiting these healthcare providers with pre-existing VBA conditions. No excess risk of VBA was found in association with chiropractic.

Chapter Summary

Chiropractic is concerned with the diagnosis, treatment and prevention of mechanical disorders of the musculoskeletal system and the effects of these disorders on the function of the nervous system and general health. There is an emphasis on manual treatments including spinal manipulation or adjustment (World Federation of Chiropractic, www.wfc.org).

The evidence for the efficacy of spinal manipulation in patients with nonspecific LBP is reasonably well established. The evidence of efficacy of spinal manipulation is not as well established for the cervical spine. It is suggested that SMT as well as rehabilitation are more effective than other treatments; however, there is the issue of serious adverse effects to consider. The risk of a serious adverse effect is a rare occurrence.

REVIEW QUESTIONS

1   What is the definition of chiropractic?

2   Who is the founder of chiropractic and what were his early chiropractic concepts?

3   What are the five main types of chiropractic treatment? Give a brief description of each.

4   Chiropractors are qualified to take and read X-rays. What are the typical circumstances where an X-ray may be necessary?

CHAPTER LINKS

For further discussion of the anatomical and physiological basis for practice, see Chapter 14.

FURTHER RESOURCES

Haldeman, S. (ed.) (2005) *Principles and Practice of Chiropractic*, 3rd edn, New York, McGraw-Hill. Comprehensive book designed to be a core text for students and a reference book for professionals focusing on chiropractic principles, diagnosis and treatment. Covers theory, philosophy and practice principles.

Peterson, D.H. and Bergmann, T.F. (2002) *Chiropractic Technique: Principles and Procedures,* 2nd edn, St Louis, Mosby. Describes the rationale and application of spinal manipulative therapy. Includes the basic anatomical, biomechanical and pathophysiological principles necessary for applying spinal manipulative therapy.

Wilson, F.H. (2007) *Chiropractic in Europe: An Illustrated History*, Leicester, Matador. Documents the history of chiropractic from its origin in the USA to the present day, focusing on a European perspective.

Web Links

www.gcc-uk.org – The General Chiropractic Council was established by the Chiropractors Act 1994 to regulate and develop the chiropractic profession. Chiropractors must be registered with the GCC.

Part VI

www.chiropractic-uk.co.uk – The British Chiropractic Association is the largest and longest established association for chiropractors in the UK.

www.chiropractic-ecu.org – The European Chiropractors' Union was established to promote the development of chiropractic in Europe and to pursue the interests of chiropractic as a science and a profession by research, teaching, publications and legal activities.

www.aecc.ac.uk – The Anglo-European College of Chiropractic, Bournemouth and http://hesas.glam.ac.uk/subjects/chiropractic/ – the Welsh Institute of Chiropractic, University of Glamorgan are internationally accredited and GCC-recognized chiropractic schools in the UK.

Osteopathy **26**

ANDREW MADDICK

Learning outcomes

By the end of this chapter, you should be able to:

- define osteopathy and understand the legal basis for osteopathic treatment
- explain the history of osteopathy
- discuss the theoretical aspects of osteopathy
- understand the principles, practice and techniques of osteopathy
- clarify how osteopathy differs from other treatments such as chiropractic

This chapter is concerned with osteopathy, which is also known as osteopathic medicine and osteopathic manipulative treatment, and includes cranial osteopathy.

What is Osteopathy?

Osteopathy is a system of medicine developed to treat infectious diseases, and is capable of treating any illness, based on the scientific understanding that the body is capable of making its own remedies against disease. Osteopaths use their hands to detect and correct problems and to assist the natural mechanics of the body to work better. Osteopathic treatment aims to improve the way the body works by improving the way it moves.

The musculoskeletal focus of much of today's osteopathy represents a speciality within the broad concept of osteopathy. Osteopaths are extremely good at treating backs, necks and other minor musculoskeletal problems, and these problems account for the majority of osteopathic consultations. However, osteopathy is a total system of medicine, and osteopaths treat patients with a remarkable range of conditions, from relatively simple pain and discomfort to asthma, epilepsy, cerebral palsy and contagious diseases.

The Osteopaths Act 1993 defines osteopathy as 'what an osteopath does'. Rather than a definition, the General Osteopathic Council (GOsC) includes a 'description of osteopathy' in the statutory register of osteopaths, and states:

> Osteopathy is an established, recognised system of diagnosis and treatment that lays its main emphasis on the structural and functional integrity of the body. It is distinctive by the fact that it recognises that much of the pain and disability we suffer stem from abnormalities in the function of body structure ... Its main strength, however, lies in the unique way in which the patient is assessed from a mechanical, functional and postural standpoint and manual methods of treatment applied that suit the needs of the individual patient rather than the specific treatment for a specific problem. (GOsC, 2008: 835)

History of Osteopathy

Osteopathy was invented by Andrew Taylor Still (1828–1917), who had originally trained as an engineer before studying medicine. He graduated from Kansas City School of Physicians and Surgeons in 1855 and worked as a military surgeon in the American Civil War, and then as a frontier doctor (Still, 1908).

After the death of three of his children from meningitis, Still became disillusioned with the medical practices of the time. He spent many years studying anatomy, researching disease and experimenting with new forms of treatment (Still, 1899). He was influenced by his early training as an engineer and eventually devised a theory of new medical philosophy based on mechanical principles and the innate healing capacity of the body. He used his new approach to treat many patients and claimed great success. In 1874, he first used the term 'osteopathy' and in 1892, he opened the first School of Osteopathic Medicine in Kirksville, Missouri.

Osteopathy was established to reform the practice of medicine and surgery, which in the late nineteenth century was relatively primitive. Osteopathy was used to treat every type of condition, and although it relied primarily on manual manipulation, it also encompassed surgery. Unfashionably for the period, Still and early osteopaths placed a great deal of emphasis on evidence and research, understanding the aetiology of diseases and osteopathic treatment.

Osteopathy was introduced into the UK by Martin Littlejohn (1828–1917), who founded the British School of Osteopathy in 1917. In 1936, the voluntary General Council and Register of Osteopaths was formed.

Theory of Osteopathy

Osteopathic diagnosis is complicated, and each diagnosis is individual to each patient. Osteopathy treats the person, not the illness. This is not a politically correct platitude, but an essential tenet of osteopathic theory. Pathology, aetiology and response to disease are specific to each patient, and therefore osteopathic treatment is specific to the person. The self-healing capacity is also a vital part of osteopathic theory and most osteopathic treatment has the objective of restoring this self-healing capacity rather than simply fixing the presenting problem. For example, a child with pneumonia presents with typical signs and symptoms. The diagnosis and basic medical aetiology are both obvious, but where allopathic medicine seeks to remove the bacterial agent and gives antibiotics, osteopathic medicine looks to the body's ability to combat the pneumonia, and asks: 'Why was this child not able to fight the pathogen successfully? A healthy body can overcome the disease, why not this one?'

In osteopathy, the aetiology of the disease is an important part of how it is to be treated. Similar symptoms may have widely varying aetiology in each patient. The patient succumbed to the pneumonic pathogen for a reason, perhaps because of the poor shape of the ribcage, the poor mechanics of breathing, because lymphatic drainage from the lungs is compromised, or the nerve supply to the area may have been deficient. It may, however, be nothing to do with the chest; it may be the overall function of the immune system, or a problem affecting the function of the whole body such as generalized dehydration. It may be something highly specific like a mild posterior displacement of the left fibular head. Whatever the cause, it is specific to each patient.

Principles of Osteopathy

The basic principles of osteopathy have not changed since Still's time. Osteopathy's original principles of aetiology and treatment remain as relevant to osteopaths today as they were to osteopaths 100 years ago. It is sometimes argued that Still's original vision of osteopathy as a reforming movement in medicine is outdated and that developments in medical science have improved orthodox medicine and rendered osteopathy obsolete (Hamonet, 2003). But osteopathy has maintained a coherent and comprehensive philosophy for the cause and treatment of disease and remains a popular system of 'alternative' medicine (Vickers and Zollman, 1999). The basic principles of osteopathy are theoretically the same for any patient with any condition. Osteopathic diagnosis is often more detailed and accurate than normal medical diagnosis and may not necessarily be limited by condition. Buxton (2002: 23) suggested restating osteopathic principles. His principles include professional and educational issues in addition to traditional osteopathic tenets such as:

> self-healing powers; unity of the individual; movement is the essence of health; the importance of the axial skeleton; and the relationship of structure and function.

The application of these principles governs the osteopathic approach to diagnosis and treatment, rather than providing a protocol for each condition, with a set of predefined diagnoses and techniques.

Practice of Osteopathy

Osteopathy is a small profession, with currently around 4,000 osteopaths registered in the UK. Most osteopaths work in private osteopathic clinics as individuals or with other osteopaths, or in multidisciplinary clinics with other healthcare practitioners. There is no official grading of osteopaths, such as consultant, registrar or senior house officer. All osteopaths are simply osteopaths and while many osteopaths claim specialist interest or expertise in particular areas, at present there is no official certification or qualification of practice other than the undergraduate osteopathic degree. The owner or senior osteopath in a clinic is usually referred to as the 'principal' and the other osteopaths as 'associates'. These terms imply a degree of clinical seniority, and in some clinics, this reflects the reality of one experienced practitioner who takes responsibility for the education and development of his osteopaths. However, in many clinics, the principal is simply the owner of the business and the assistants may have equivalent experience and clinical seniority.

Almost all osteopathic clinics see patients without referral – most patients seek osteopathy before visiting their GP and book appointments themselves. An increasing number are referred by their GP, although most fund the treatment themselves (or use health insurance), while some GP practices have osteopaths funded by local PCTs.

The vast majority of osteopathic diagnoses are made clinically, that is, without the use of X-rays, MRI scans, blood tests or other investigations. Osteopaths have an excellent grounding in clinical examination and pathology and are always aware of potentially dangerous signs and symptoms, and referrals to the GP and immediate referrals to A&E are not uncommon. The past rivalry between GPs and osteopaths has all but disappeared and most osteopaths have an extremely good relationship with their local GPs.

Osteopathic consultations involve a detailed case history, with questions about the presenting problem, as well as past medical history. This is followed by an examination, where the patient undresses to their underwear, posture is observed and some movements are performed. The osteopath will then palpate (feel or touch) the patient's body to assess motion and may perform some more movements. After examination, the osteopath will formulate a diagnosis and plan of treatment, telling the patient the cause of the problem, and what can be done, as well as the risks of osteopathic treatment and the likely course of the problem without treatment. Most initial consultations will include treatment.

First consultations usually last longer than subsequent treatment sessions, and are therefore usually more expensive. The cost of osteopathic treatment varies around the country; smart osteopathic practices in the West End of London may well charge in excess of £100 per session, and small town practices, often operating from a room in the osteopath's house, may charge as little as £30, while PCT-funded osteopathic treatment will be free to the user. The cost of treatment usually reflects the price of rent and hours of availability, and while good, popular osteopaths are able to command high fees, the cost of treatment is not always a reliable indication of quality of care. The osteopathic schools are an excellent place to get effective osteopathic treatment at low cost, and at many, pensioners and children may be seen free of charge.

Osteopathic Techniques

Palpation and Manipulation

Osteopaths use case history, observation and clinical examination to reach a broad diagnosis, and rely mainly on **palpation**, that is, a sense of touch, for an accurate osteopathic diagnosis. The osteopath uses palpation (as well as observation) to assess biomechanics and to detect abnormal structure or abnormal motion that has the potential to lead to disease.

Osteopathic diagnosis is extremely complicated and sophisticated. Rather than labelling the problem, a diagnosis will incorporate the structural aetiology.

Once a problematic area (or 'lesion', or 'dysfunction') has been identified, it can be treated. Osteopathic treatment relies on manipulation, but it is important not to confuse the broad term 'manipulation' with the cracking or clicking of 'spinal manipulation':

> Most people think of the thrusting [cracking or clicking] type of techniques when they hear the word 'manipulation', however, osteopathic manipulative medicine includes many forms of manipulation in which there is no thrusting force and many treat the soft tissues of the body. (DiGiovana, 2001: 62)

Manipulation includes all types of osteopathic treatment, put simply, it is the 'therapeutic application of manual force' (Glover, 2002).

Spinal Manipulation

'Spinal manipulation' usually refers to the high velocity thrust (HVT) technique (also known as high velocity low amplitude thrust) that is commonly used in osteopathy. The purpose of an HVT may be to increase the movement between vertebrae, to alter muscle tone around an area of the spine, or to change the nerve activity around a spinal segment. The technique usually involves placing the patient in a contorted position with a twisting or squashing of the back or neck, with a quick jerking movement. The contorted position restricts motion to one or two vertebrae, while the quick jerking motion increases the motion between the isolated joints. This is often accompanied by a popping or cracking noise, called 'cavitation', which may sound rather dramatic, but is quite safe. Cavitation is not a reliable indicator of a successful technique, although many patients place great importance on the popping of a joint. There has been much publicity about the efficacy of spinal manipulation, mainly due to poor quality reviews of small disparate research papers. Despite the uncomfortable position and the dramatic noise, there is an extremely low risk of serious adverse effects from spinal manipulation. The most catastrophic adverse reaction is a cerebrovascular accident, which has a very low risk, but because of the small numbers of these reactions, the exact risk is unknown. A study published in 1996 identified 185 reports of injuries as a result of spinal manipulation from 1925 to 1993, which translates as a risk significantly smaller than one in a million (Vick et al., 1996). When used by an osteopath who is trained to recognize risk factors and taught to execute safe, efficient HVT, the risk is negligible.

Cranial Osteopathy

Cranial osteopathy is a popular form of osteopathic treatment. It is not a type of osteopathy, as the name implies, but a group of techniques – osteopathic cranial techniques. These use small amounts of movement, with the osteopath palpating small movements of the body and applying small amounts of force. Cranial osteopathic techniques are difficult to learn and require a fair degree of technical skill, although often these techniques are impalpable to the patient and it may appear as if the osteopath is just laying hands on the patient without doing anything.

These techniques can be used on the head, but are widely used on all parts of the body. Cranial osteopathy was first developed by William Garner Sutherland (1873–1954), one of Still's students. Sutherland emphasized that the principles of cranial work are an extension of Still's original osteopathic principles rather than a new theory (Lee, 2001). He also applied his theory to the whole body, but because it was first discovered and described in the cranium, the term 'cranial osteopathy' has stuck.

Because the term 'cranial osteopathy' is technically inaccurate, it also has a number of different names – 'osteopathy in the cranial field', 'the involuntary mechanism' and 'craniosacral osteopathy'. Anyone doing cranial osteopathy is an osteopath, but cranial osteopathy is not to be confused with 'craniosacral therapy', which is an unregulated derivative of the cranial technique usually taught to non-clinicians and non-osteopaths.

Traditionally, osteopaths have used a rather anachronistic explanation to explain how cranial techniques work. In the 1930s, Sutherland proposed 'five phenomena' – movements that helped him to understand the motion of the body. These include the movement of:

- the cranial bones
- the cerebrospinal fluid
- the central nervous system, that is, the brain and spinal cord
- the reciprocal tension membrane
- the sacrum.

There has always been debate about this theory, but the clinical results, the usage among osteopaths and the popularity with patients indicate the clinical effectiveness, despite the absence of a clearly understood theory.

Classical Osteopathy

'Classical osteopathy' is a term coined by the osteopath John Wernham (1907–2007). Classical osteopathy concentrates far more on osteopathy's original aims of treating disease and sickness, rather than purely musculoskeletal pain. It also strongly advocates osteopathic diagnosis and treatment (the 'total body adjustment'), acknowledging that most pain and disease are the result of mechanical dysfunction in the body as a whole, not necessarily at the location of the pain or illness. The techniques may appear similar to most osteopathic techniques, but 'long lever' techniques (using a limb to add leverage) are common. Routine treatment of important areas such as the pelvis, upper thoracic spine, thoracolumbar junction and mid-lumbar spine are frequently used.

In 1949, Wernham established one of the oldest osteopathic schools in the country, now known as the John Wernham College of Classical Osteopathy, which trained osteopathic students. At the beginning of the twenty-first century, osteopathic education changed radically, with osteopathic courses needing degree status, standardized delivery and academic, rather than vocational, tutoring. Rather than dilute the osteopathy taught at the college, Wernham changed the course between 1996 and 1998, so as to teach osteopathic graduates. This left the college free to teach osteopathic concepts, philosophy, theory and technique, without having to cover basic biochemistry, study skills and generic healthcare.

Paediatric Osteopathy

Paediatric osteopathy is the osteopathic treatment of children. Like cranial osteopathy and classical osteopathy, paediatric osteopathy tends to see patients with a wide variety of complaints. Because of the breadth and depth of paediatrics, it is taught at only a very introductory level at undergraduate level, if at all. As a result, most osteopaths working with children will study paediatrics as graduates. Both cranial and classical osteopathy place great emphasis on the treatment of children and include paediatric modules in their teaching. The Foundation for Paediatric Osteopathy runs the world-renowned Osteopathic Centre for Children, with clinics in London and Manchester, and specializes in paediatric osteopathy and provides the clinical training for the Masters degree in Paediatric Osteopathy. The foundation delivers osteopathy for every child, on a donation basis, and treats children of all ages with all conditions, providing osteopathic care in two London hospitals for premature babies, children with colic, gastro-oesophageal reflux, cerebral palsy, autism, dyslexia, growing pains and any other condition a child may present with.

Osteopathy requires the body to be assessed as a whole, so osteopaths do not specialize in complaints the way that doctors do. Osteopaths cannot specialize in shoulder problems, knees, cardiology, immunology and so on. However, osteopaths can and do specialize in children. Good reports from parents have led to an increasing number of doctors and other health professionals seeking the help of osteopaths in treating children (Sullivan, 1997; Hayden, 1999).

Animal Osteopathy

Osteopathy is used increasingly in the treatment of animals. Horses and dogs are especially popular, but in theory any animal can be treated. Of course, the osteopath must be familiar with the anatomy, physiology, common conditions and normal function of the different animals, and new techniques must be learned or developed to deal with the movement of large horses or small dogs, but the osteopathic theory and principles remain the same.

Professional Training and Education

In the UK, osteopathy is independent from medicine. Osteopathy is generally taught in small independent colleges in association with overseeing universities. In the UK, there are currently eight osteopathic degree courses. The common degrees are of equivalent status, but have disconcertingly different titles. Osteopaths who trained before graduate status was introduced or those who trained abroad often hold a Diploma in Osteopathy (DO). More recent graduates have a Bachelor of Science in Osteopathic Medicine (BSc OstMed), or a Bachelor of Osteopathy (BOst). From 2010, all degree courses will be standardized as a Masters degree in Osteopathy (MOst).

In the UK, training is of an excellent standard, with programmes lasting four to five years. Three good A levels are usually required and must include biology and one other science. Bridging courses or different entry programmes may be available to graduates or mature students with a professional background.

The basic teaching provides a good medical grounding and includes anatomy, biochemistry, physiology, pharmacology, pathology, pharmacology, clinical methods, osteopathic theory, osteopathic techniques and osteopathic clinic. At qualification, all osteopaths will have completed hundreds of hours in a supervised clinic, observing and examining patients, and eventually diagnosing and treating patients

Osteopaths must complete continuing professional development annually. For most osteopaths this comprises short courses, conferences, and in-house practice education meetings. Some osteopaths teach, undertake Masters degrees or further structured education.

Osteopathy is different around the world. In the USA, osteopathy was integrated into the orthodox medical system and American osteopaths are fully trained medical practitioners. Relatively few practice as osteopaths and most go on to work as GPs, specialists, surgeons or in other fields of medicine. In Germany, osteopaths are usually doctors or physiotherapists who study osteopathy at graduate level. Until recently, osteopathy was illegal in France. However, it is now practised legally but rather unsatisfactorily; the osteopath needing a doctor's permission to perform some techniques. The British GOsC has helped to provide support and a framework for regulation across Europe and other parts of the world. In many countries where no regulation is present, the GOsC is still used by British trained osteopaths as a regulator.

The Regulation of Osteopathy

In 1993, the Osteopaths Act was passed and the GOsC was formed to regulate osteopathy. The title 'osteopath' is protected and all new osteopaths in the UK must now be graduates of accredited colleges, or foreign trained with GOsC conversion. The GOsC is primarily a body to protect patients, and is responsible for investigating patient complaints, removing osteopaths from the register for professional reasons, and approving education and continuing professional development.

The British Osteopathic Association is a sort of trade union for osteopaths, which is responsible for the promotion of the profession, and provides support for osteopaths, legal and business advice, professional indemnity insurance and independent representation to the GOsC, the Department of Health and so on.

Research Evidence for Practice

There is relatively little modern research in osteopathy. The main reason for the lack of research today is the lack of funding. As osteopathy is external to the NHS, the NHS provides no funding. Pharmacological companies have no interest in osteopathy, and without a large sponsor, there is no access to funding, which is essential for good research.

The *International Journal for Osteopathic Medicine* and the *British Osteopathic Journal* are good osteopathic research publications that almost exclusively contain osteopathic studies. The *Journal of the American Osteopathic Association* is very good and frequently publishes some historical papers, has free online access to a large proportion of its content, but is primarily a 'family medicine' or general practice journal, with little osteopathic research and much pharmacology.

The National Council for Osteopathic Research is a relatively new organization that aims to provide a strategic plan for osteopathic research. It has recently commissioned research into adverse effects in osteopathy and will soon produce a database of osteopathic research.

Practice example

Glue ear

Sue brought her five-year-old son Arnold to the clinic. Sue complained that Arnold had started saying 'what?' a lot, turned the TV up loudly, and had been misbehaving in school. This had started after a cold, and had been going on for six weeks. Arnold's ears were examined and the ear drum looked red and dull. He could not follow basic instructions and was clearly deaf. There was a degree of muscular tension around his neck and thorax, and his head was held forward. A diagnosis of otitis media with effusion was made. This was a result of poor drainage from the head and neck, and partly poor mechanics of the anterior fascia and nasopharynx, which stopped full opening of the Eustachian tube on swallowing. Arnold was treated three times to improve the mechanics of the head, neck and thorax; the treatment included muscle stretching and articulation of the neck and thorax and some gentle 'cranial' techniques. There was a small but significant improvement after each treatment. After the third treatment, Arnold's hearing had returned to normal, his behaviour had improved, and he no longer needed to turn the sound up on the TV.

Practice example

Colic

Lizzie was a six-week-old baby who had developed colicky symptoms of regular prolonged bouts of crying that worsened towards evening. Lizzie was the first child and her mother had experienced a quiet pregnancy. The labour started spontaneously two days before her due date and started well, but after several hours of pushing, the mother started to tire and there were some concerns about Lizzie's heart rate, so a vacuum extraction (ventouse) was performed. Lizzie was born pink and healthy, she breast-fed well and slept a lot in her first week. She had been unsettled since the second week and seemed to be getting worse. On examination, the osteopath discovered a feeling of axial compression through the whole body, particularly around the area of the diaphragm. The osteopath gently stretched and balanced Lizzie's body over two treatments to reduce the feeling of compression. After these two treatments, there was an improvement in symptoms, Lizzie was calm through the day and only cried for up to an hour in the evenings.

Practice example

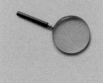

Headaches

Ellie was a 30-year-old primary school teacher who visited the clinic complaining of headaches. These had started two weeks ago for no apparent reason, and were described as dull throbbing headaches that appeared in the late afternoon. On examination, the osteopath found a slouched posture with hunched shoulders and the head held forward. This posture was a result of leaning over to talk to small children, and sitting in children's seats. The osteopath found tight musculature in the back of the neck and the front of the thorax, the tension in the neck was in the top of the neck and spreading forward over the head. Two treatment sessions concentrated on releasing the spinal restriction in the thorax and stretching the neck. Ellie was given exercises to do twice a day to help the stretching. Her headache was worse on the evening of the first treatment, then disappeared completely. The headaches only recurred six months later, during an Ofsted inspection of her school, and resolved after one visit to the osteopath.

Practice example

Back pain

Donald was a 43-year-old insurance broker working in London. He visited his osteopath with low back pain. The pain had first started four months ago and had been gradually getting worse until a game of squash last week, when he had twisted awkwardly and the pain had worsened significantly. The osteopath found that the deep muscles in the lowest part of the back had been badly strained and other muscles were in spasm to protect them. The rest of the low back was painless, but movement was restricted. The poor movement in the back had been compensated for by increased motion in the lowest part of the back, the extra stretch on these muscles had been causing the pain over the last four months and playing squash had been the last straw for the low back. The osteopath performed an HVT to the painless part of the back to increase movement and take the strain off the lowest part of the back, allowing it to heal. The low back improved significantly after treatment and required two further sessions to normalize the movement of the whole spine. Donald was given some exercises to maintain movement of his back and advice on how to sit at work.

The Differences between Osteopathy, Chiropractic and Physiotherapy

For basic musculoskeletal problems, there is little difference in the way that osteopaths, chiropractors and physiotherapists work. Many of the techniques are similar and we have more in common than we have in difference. Physiotherapists tend to be NHS based so they are accessed through hospitals or GPs, and they tend to be free at access, but there is often a waiting list. Physiotherapists tend to focus on rehabilitation post surgery or injury, or on particular conditions, for example cerebral palsy, cystic fibrosis and strokes. In contrast, osteopaths and chiropractors tend to work privately, so appointments are charged to the patient, but there is rarely a waiting list. Both osteopaths and chiropractors tend to see a wider variety of problems, particularly painful problems. Osteopaths tend to see more sickness and disease and chiropractors traditionally have a more spinal focus. Chiropractors use X-rays regularly and often use the title 'Dr'. However, there is a great range of difference within each profession. Some chiropractors work in a similar way to osteopaths, and two osteopaths may work completely differently. Because of the personal nature of touch and manual therapy, finding the right practitioner is a personal thing – it is often the practitioner, rather than the discipline, who is more important. If a patient is unsure about who to see, or whether a problem is amenable to treatment, most physiotherapy, chiropractic and osteopathic clinics will be happy to talk to prospective patients and give advice about suitability.

Chapter Summary

Osteopathy is a system of medicine based on the premise that the healing capacity of the body works best when the mechanics of the body are sound; sound mechanical function can prevent illness and restore health. Osteopaths improve the mechanics of the body by osteopathic manipulation, ranging from gentle cranial-type techniques to joint articulation and high velocity thrusts.

Part VI

REVIEW
QUESTIONS

1   Who regulates all osteopaths in the UK?

2   When was osteopathy first invented?

3   What is the difference between osteopathic manipulation and a high velocity thrust (HVT)?

4   How many osteopaths currently practice in the UK?

CHAPTER
LINKS

For further discussion of the anatomical and physiological basis for practice, see Chapter 14.

FURTHER
RESOURCES

Collins, M. (2005) *Osteopathy in Britain: The First Hundred Years*, Charleston, SC, BookSurge. Fascinating history, tracing osteopathy in Britain from bone-setting through the introduction of osteopathy, the early failed attempts to regulate osteopathy, Stephen Ward and the Profumo affair, to the Osteopaths Act and the profession in the 1990s.

Kuchera, M.L. and Kuchera, W.A. (1994) *Osteopathic Considerations in Systemic Dysfunction*, Columbus, OH, Greyden Press. Technical book that explains osteopathic considerations in pathology from the common cold to cardiovascular disease and irritable bowel syndrome.

Still, A.T. (1908) *Autobiography of AT Still*, rev. edn, Kirksville, MO, A.T. Still, available at www.interlinea.org. The story of Still's life in America in the nineteenth century, from childhood to his development of osteopathy. The language is a little old-fashioned, but the book gives a general view on how osteopathy came about, is easy to read, with not too much osteopathic theory.

Triance, E. (1986) *Osteopathy: A Patients Guide*, London, Thorsons; Chaitow, L. (1982) *Osteopathy: A Complete Healthcare System*, London, Thorsons. These two short volumes are written with patients in mind, and are good accessible introductions to osteopathy, covering some of the basic theory and principles.

Ward, R.C. (ed.) (2002) *Foundations for Osteopathic Medicine,* 2nd edn, Philadelphia, Lippincott, Williams and Wilkins. Technical manual of osteopathic principles, techniques, applications and approaches. It is thorough, with some excellent introductions, but some of it is rather technical for general readers.

Web Links

www.osteopathy.org.uk – General Osteopathic Council

www.osteopathy.org – British Osteopathic Association

www.bcom.ac.uk – British College of Osteopathic Medicine

www.bso.ac.uk – British School of Osteopathy

www.fpo.org.uk – Foundation for Paediatric Osteopathy/Osteopathic Centre for Children

www.jwcco.org.uk – John Wernham College of Classical Osteopathy

www.brighton.ac.uk/ncor – National Council for Osteopathic Research

www.jaoa.org – *Journal of the American Osteopathic Association*

www.interlinea.org – Inter Linea (osteopathic website)

Reflexology 27

NICOLA HALL

What is Reflexology?

Reflexology is a form of complementary medicine that involves treatment to specific areas (reflex areas) found in the feet and hands using a precise form of massage given mainly by the thumbs and sometimes the fingers. There are reflex areas in the feet and hands that correspond to all the parts of the body, so it is possible to treat a wide variety of conditions using this method. Conditions that might be helped include migraines, sinus congestion, back and neck problems, IBS and other digestive problems, menstrual and menopausal problems and many stress-related conditions. Most commonly, reflexology will involve treatment to the feet rather than the hands, which will usually only be used if the feet are not accessible, or for self-treatment when the hands are more easily reached. Although treatment is given to the feet, the method is not really one to treat actual foot problems, which will be best dealt with by a podiatrist.

A holistic approach to treatment is followed and within a treatment session, all the reflex areas in both feet will be treated, which will, in turn, treat the whole body. Depending on the symptoms that are present, extra attention will be given to the reflex areas that will be most helpful in clearing or easing these symptoms. Although most practitioners will be following an approach to treat the physical side of a person, treatment may also benefit people emotionally or spiritually. Treatment can be used to help people in different stages of illness from acute conditions to chronic conditions. In general, treatment is given once a week for a course of between three to six treatments each at weekly intervals, although with acute conditions, treatment may be given twice weekly. In addition, it is not necessary to be unwell to receive treatment and reflexology can be an excellent way to maintain good health by having regular maintenance treatments at intervals of four to six weeks, which may help to prevent subsequent illness. One of the great benefits of reflexology treatment experienced by nearly all who receive treatment is one of relaxation, and this relaxation effect is most important especially since so many conditions can be considered to be stress related.

The method is suitable for all age groups from the very young through to the elderly. With babies, treatment may help with problems such as colic and eczema. For babies and young children, the treatment session will be shorter due to the smaller foot size and also to prevent restlessness during treatment. With the elderly, treatment can help to clear or alleviate symptoms that may be present, while other benefits can include the physical touch of the practitioner to the feet of the patient and the chance to have someone to talk to for an hour. The majority of patients who visit a reflexologist are probably within the 35–65 age group and it appears that more women seek reflexology treatment than men, although treatment can be equally effective in both sexes.

Reflexology History and Philosophy

The exact origins of reflexology are not fully understood but it is thought that the method has evolved from types of pressure therapy used within TCM thousands of years ago. The first pictorial evidence of a method of treatment using pressure to parts of the feet and hands comes from a drawing found in the so-called physician's tomb of Ankhmahor at Saqqara in Egypt dated 2500 BC, which shows one man holding onto another man's foot and applying pressure with the fingers and one man holding onto another man's hand and applying pressure with the fingers. Other early evidence of therapies involving the application of pressure to the feet has also been traced back to India, Tibet and Japan, where drawings showing mapping of the body on the feet have been found. It is thought that the Incas used foot treatment, which is still being used in North American Indian tribes, in particular the Cherokees, who practise a form of reflexology.

Modern day reflexology is based on a method called 'zone therapy', which was rediscovered in the early 1900s by Dr William Fitzgerald (1872–1942) an American ear, nose and throat specialist. Fitzgerald described how the body could be divided into 10 longitudinal zones, with each zone extending from the toes up the body to the brain and down to the fingers. Each zone was of equal width at any point in the body, and the zones were numbered according to which toe or finger they were in line with. Therefore, zone 1 was in line with the big toe and thumb and zone 5 in line with little toe and little finger. The method of zone therapy involved applying pressure to a part of the body to influence the functioning of another part of the body situated in the same longitudinal zone but distant from the part of the body to where pressure was applied. By applying pressure to a zone, it was considered that any disturbance or energy block within that zone could be cleared, and with the correct flow of energy, the body parts in that zone would function correctly. Fitzgerald would use various gadgets (rubber bands, clothes pegs, metal combs and clips) to apply pressure and the method was mostly used to relieve pain and also to act as an anaesthetic.

The work of Fitzgerald was not widely recognized but Dr Jo Shelby Riley, one of his medical colleagues, used reflexology in his practice and introduced the method to Eunice Ingham who worked with him. Eunice Ingham (1889–1974) was the first person to separate work on the reflexes of the feet from zone therapy in general, and in the early 1930s, she described reflexology as it is widely known today. She compiled a foot chart to show the positions of reflex areas in the feet relating to all of the parts of the body and established that these areas were arranged to form a map of the body in the feet. Whichever zone or zones of the body an area was situated in, there was a reflex area in the same zone or zones of the feet, with the right foot corresponding to the right side of the body and the left foot corresponding to the left side of the body. She termed her method of working on the feet 'The Eunice Ingham method of compression massage'. The work of Eunice Ingham was introduced to Great Britain and parts of Europe in the 1960s by Doreen Bayly (1899–1979), who was trained by Eunice Ingham. Over the years, a number of variations in the way reflexology is practised have developed but the method first introduced by Eunice Ingham and then Doreen Bayly is still the method on which nearly all these variations are based.

Another contribution to identifying the position of the reflex areas in the feet was from the German practitioner, Hanne Marquardt. In addition to the longitudinal zones of the feet, she described how there were important transverse zones at the level of the shoulder girdle, waist and pelvic floor. These areas could be identified in the feet in relation to the bones of the feet and offered a more accurate way to locate the position of the reflex areas. All areas above the shoulder girdle in the body would be represented above shoulder girdle level of the foot (between phalanges and metatarsals), all areas between shoulder girdle and waist level in the body would be represented between shoulder girdle and waist level (between metatarsals and tarsals) in the foot, and all areas below waist level and above the pelvic floor in the body would be represented between waist level and the level of the pelvic floor (across tarsal bones between the malleoli) in the foot. A further transverse zone to the diaphragm level was later introduced and in the foot, this is found just below the arch of the foot extending below the ball of the foot. These transverse zones together with the longitudinal zones give a grid-like pattern on the feet to help the practitioner identify the position of the reflex areas, which can be most useful since no two pairs of feet are identical.

There are some who now discount the theory of zones to explain how reflexology works and feel that by treating the feet and hands this is connecting to the meridians as used by acupuncturists. The acupuncture meridians all start or end in the feet and hands and although these may be stimulated by reflexology, most practitioners feel that zone theory is a more appropriate explanation of how their treatment is working as opposed to the meridian theory. The overall result, however, is the same, as the practitioner is trying to balance the flow of energy within the reflexology zones in a similar manner to the acupuncturist balancing the flow of energy or chi within the meridians.

With the growing interest in receiving complementary therapies, the need for regulation in the UK was put forward by a House of Lords Select Committee report published in 2000. Following the report, National Occupational Standards for reflexology were developed (Healthwork UK, 2002) and a core curriculum for reflexology courses in the UK was published in 2006 by the Reflexology Forum. The Stone Report (2005) recommended a federal approach to regulation of complementary therapies that were not statutory regulated, and a regulatory process involving 12 therapies, including reflexology, was set up by the Foundation for Integrated Health in 2006. The Federal Working Group report on how a regulatory body might look resulted in the setting up of the Complementary and Natural Healthcare Council (CNHC) in April 2008 to act as a voluntary regulatory body to regulate those complementary healthcare professions not seeking statutory regulation. To date, the CNHC has not set up its register and other groups have also become established to offer regulation, so the current situation regarding regulation is confusing but will hopefully become more clear in the not too distant future. The main purpose of regulation is to offer one central place to which the general public can refer when wanting to find a qualified practitioner of the different therapies so they can be assured that the person will be qualified and working to set standards and that procedures are in place should a complaint need to be made.

What Reflexology Practice Entails

It is not necessary for a person to receive permission from their general practitioner before going for reflexology treatment, although it is recommended that patients inform their doctor that they are having treatment. The decision to try reflexology treatment is usually based on knowing someone who has benefited from having treatment and the client base for practitioners is usually by personal recommendation.

Practice example

Mrs L, a 45-year-old primary school head teacher, presents for treatment complaining of frequent migraines. She thinks these are possibly stress related and has always suffered from migraines about three times a year but now they occurring more frequently – about once a month. She has to resort to OTC painkillers when they occur, and on one occasion had to go to bed when the migraine occurred. She is concerned that this might happen again and prevent her from getting to work.

At the first treatment session before treatment commences, the practitioner will take details of the patient's present and past medical history. This will include asking about any medication the person may be taking and any other treatments currently being received.

Once these details have been recorded, the practitioner will ask the patient to remove their footwear and then seat them in a reclining position. A recliner chair is the ideal arrangement for treatment – the patient is sitting comfortably with their legs raised to a convenient height for the practitioner to be able to treat them when sitting on a low stool.

First, the feet will be examined to identify any areas that might need to be avoided, such as an ingrowing toenail, a verruca, a corn or athlete's foot. It is sometimes the case that problems in an area of the feet can reflect a problem in the corresponding part of the body. A small amount of talc will then be placed on the feet and the feet massaged generally for a few moments to enable the person to get used to the touch of the practitioner and to warm the feet up if necessary. Some practitioners prefer not to use talc and may instead work with cornstarch or may use neither. The concern about the use of talc is because there is asbestos in talc that might be absorbed by the practitioner or patient, although there is no evidence to support this and the levels of asbestos in talc are very low. The use of cream or oil on the feet for reflexology treatment is not normally advised, since it makes the foot too slippery for the precise form of massage that is to be applied to the reflex areas.

The practitioner will then explain to the patient how treatment will be given and what the patient might feel as treatment is given. As pressure is applied to the reflex areas, the patient will be aware of pressure but this may vary from one point to another. In some areas, it may feel as if more pressure is being applied (which will not be the case) and sometimes there might be a degree of sharpness felt (as if the fingernail was being applied to the foot). If there is tenderness in an area of the foot when pressure is applied, it means that the corresponding part of the body is out of balance. It might be expected that at the first treatment, there would be the most tender areas, and then at subsequent treatments, as the person felt better, the tender areas would reduce in number. In practice, this is not always the case, as sometimes a patient's feet become more sensitive to reflexology and they feel more tender areas in the feet even though they are feeling in better health. Sometimes the practitioner may feel 'gritty' areas in the feet, which suggest 'grittiness' in the corresponding part of the body. These 'gritty' areas have been described as crystals in the feet, although the exact nature of the crystals has not been analysed. These areas are particularly common in, for example, reflex areas relating to the neck and shoulders, and if massage was given directly to these areas in the body, the 'grittiness' would probably be felt. By massaging the 'gritty' areas in the feet, the 'crystals' can be dispersed. The patient will be asked to inform the practitioner if areas of the feet are tender and this will be noted by the practitioner. With experience, the practitioner may feel differences in the feet and would then question the patient about problems in the corresponding areas, but the main interpretation of treatment will be based on what the patient feels in the feet.

A treatment session will last about one hour and during this time the patient may either lie back and relax or may prefer to talk with the practitioner. The practitioner will need to assess whether the patient wants to relax or talk. The fact that the patient is being seen on a one-to-one basis by the practitioner for one hour is an important one, as the patient will feel more comfortable in an unrushed situation to talk about their problems, which can in itself often be beneficial.

At the first treatment, the practitioner will probably not rework reflex areas, preferring to wait to see how the patient responds to treatment. Provided there is no strong reaction to treatment, then at subsequent treatments, important areas will be reworked. In the example of Mrs L's migraine, areas to the head, neck and spine will be important, with other possible important reflexes to include the solar plexus (for relaxation), adrenal glands (for stress), liver (for toxins), large intestine (for healthy elimination) – depending on the cause of the problem. By talking to the patient and establishing which reflex areas in the feet are found to be tender, this will help the practitioner to decide which reflex areas are going to be the most important.

At the end of the treatment, the practitioner will discuss the need for further treatments. For most conditions, a course of treatment is recommended, with a patient being advised to try three treatments at weekly intervals. Any possible reactions to treatment will also be mentioned in case the patient should experience them. It is quite possible that a person who suffers from headaches and migraines may experience a headache following treatment. Also the person might feel tired after treatment and would be advised to rest. Some patients may feel thirsty after treatment so would be advised to drink plenty of water.

Approaches and Techniques

There are now a number of different approaches to reflexology treatment, but in the true sense, reflexology will involve treatment to the feet or hands. There are practitioners who practise methods called 'ear reflexology' and 'facial reflexology', but these methods are more similar to types of acupressure rather than reflexology.

The basic technique used to apply pressure to the feet and hands can also vary from one practitioner to another, but most are based on two slightly differing techniques. The Ingham method involves using a 'caterpillar' movement to work the reflex areas, with the thumb continually bending and straightening to move quite quickly from one point to the next. The Bayly method involves working with the thumb held bent to apply pressure without bending and straightening in between working the reflex points. This approach is slower and more precise.

The pressure applied to the reflex points will be firm but not heavy, although there are approaches to treatment that use the extremes of pressure – a much firmer pressure or a much lighter pressure. Certainly the pressure used will be adjusted to suit the person being treated so that treatment is not uncomfortable. For those with ticklish feet, it is unlikely that reflexology treatment will appear ticklish, since with confident handling of the foot, the practitioner will apply a definite pressure to the various points, and once the patient knows what to expect, they do not usually find it ticklish.

Most practitioners will follow a set order of treatment to work the two feet. Some may work all the points in one foot and then all the points in the other foot;

some practitioners may work the right foot first and others the left foot first; some may treat 'systems of the body' by working a few points in one foot and then the same points in the other foot that relate to a particular system, for example the digestive system. The individual practitioner will follow the approach they think is preferable and will normally always follow the same approach to treatment.

Activity

In the light of what you have read so far, consider whether you feel reflexology is appropriate for everybody.

With the method of reflexology, there are very few occasions when it is not appropriate to give treatment. However, there are a number of conditions when the practitioner may need to exercise particular care. These would include cases where a person is on medication for their condition, such as thyroid problems, high blood pressure, diabetes, or where there is a heart condition. Most people who come for reflexology will have already received a medical diagnosis of their condition and it is not within the scope of reflexology treatment to make a medical diagnosis. Should a patient come for treatment without a medical diagnosis and not show any improvement in their condition as a result of reflexology treatment, they should be advised to see their doctor.

One of the times it would not be appropriate to treat a person would be if they were suffering from a deep vein thrombosis or phlebitis. In these cases, there is always a risk that the blood clot might move in the body and cause a more serious problem. Although there is no evidence to suggest that reflexology would cause a blood clot to move, it is best not to treat in these conditions.

Another particular area of debate is the treatment of a woman who is pregnant. There are some who feel it is not appropriate to treat a pregnant woman but there is no evidence to suggest that reflexology is contraindicated at this time. Many pregnant women benefit from treatment to help with nausea and sickness, backache, sciatica and tiredness during their pregnancy and to help at the end of pregnancy if they are overdue. As a general rule, treatment would be given with particular care to a pregnant woman who had never had reflexology treatment before and who had never been pregnant before or had a history of miscarriage.

Research

There is little scientific research into the effectiveness of reflexology since it is difficult to carry out studies of the method using double-blind trials. Some projects have been carried out when general foot massage is given (as a placebo) as opposed to a group receiving reflexology treatment, but this cannot really be considered as a suitable placebo effect, since benefits will be achieved from foot massage and, to a small degree, some reflex areas may be worked on at the same time.

However, the British Reflexology Association (BRA) has carried out a number of surveys involving its members and after an initial structure and symptom audit to establish which conditions were most commonly treated, further surveys concentrated on the most common conditions that practitioners saw patients for, namely stress, IBS and insomnia (www.britreflex.co.uk/_Research.html). All these surveys of conditions showed positive outcomes, although the numbers participating were quite small (see Table 27.1).

A number of research projects have been carried out in China but often these do not involve traditional reflexology. Interesting results have been found from more recent studies by researchers at the University of Hong Kong (www.reflexology-research.com/fmri.html) using functional magnetic resonance imaging (fMRI) (Table 27.1). They carried out three separate studies to explore what happens in the brain when pressure is applied to specific areas in the foot – the adrenal gland reflex, the eye reflex and a part of the big toe. In one of studies, there was a comparison of foot reflexology and electro-acupuncture.

Table 27.1 Reflexology research findings

Author/study	Summary
BRA (1998) Structure and symptom audit	Showed which conditions were most commonly treated by reflexology
BRA (2000) To test the effects of reflexology on clients who report unabating symptoms of stress affecting their qualify of life	Results showed that reflexology treatments reduced perceived levels of client stress and their ability to cope with stress had increased
BRA (2002) To test the effects of reflexology on clients who report a diagnosis of IBS or are complaining of the symptoms of IBS affecting their qualify of life	Reflexology was found to have had only a small effect on mild symptoms, but its effect on severe symptoms was highly significant. It seemed to be most effective in reducing severe cases of abdominal pain, hardness of stools (constipation), stomach distension, and least effective for reducing severe symptoms of feelings of anxiety and frequent feelings of fatigue
BRA (2004) The effects of reflexology on insomnia	Showed a significant improvement for half the group treated, but for the other half, where the causes of insomnia prevailed, the improvement was less significant
Tang, M., Li G., Chan, C., Wong, K., Li, R. and Yang, E. (2005) Brain activation at temporal lobe induced by foot reflexology: an fMRI study, 11th Annual NeuroImage Meeting	Results showed the activation of brain areas including the temporal lobe, cerebellum, right claustrum and right anterior central gyrus when working the left big toe
Tang, M., Li G., Chan, C., Wong, K., Li R. and Yang, E. (2005) Vision related reflex zone at the feet: an fMRI study, 11th Annual NeuroImage Meeting	Results showed the activation of brain areas including the cerebellum and left frontal lobe and left insula, but not the cerebral cortex (which matched results for acupoints), when working the eye reflex in the left foot

Practice Issues

As a result of treatment, there should be no serious reactions provided that treatment has been given correctly without overworking – either by working with too heavy a pressure or by working for too long a period of time. General 'healing' reactions to treatment can result as the elimination systems of the body become activated to clear unwanted toxins from the system. These reactions may include the need to visit the toilet more frequently, developing symptoms of a cold, developing a headache. If they are to be experienced, all these reactions will occur within about 24–48 hours following treatment and should last for a similar period of time. Other common reactions to treatment include tiredness, deep sleep and a general feeling of wellbeing.

Chapter Summary

Reflexology is a simple form of treating the body and often its simplicity detracts from the powerful effects that the treatment can achieve. As with many complementary therapies, there will be examples of treatment being helpful to people with a wide range of disorders, so it is certainly worth people trying treatment. There are very few people who will not benefit from a course of treatment even if just benefiting from the relaxation effect.

To achieve wider recognition, it is often stated that more scientific evidence is required to show how the treatment works; however, this is unlikely to happen. Hopefully, people will continue to try treatment based on personal recommendation, regardless of the lack of scientific evidence. The treatment is a safe one and unlikely to cause harm if given correctly.

REVIEW QUESTIONS

1 On which parts of the body do reflexologists focus during treatment?

2 What is zone therapy?

3 What are the main differences between the Ingham and Bayly methods of applying pressure to the feet and hands?

CHAPTER LINKS

For discussion of issues regarding the evidence base for practice, see Chapter 12.

FURTHER RESOURCES

Bayly, D.E. (1998) *Reflexology Today*, Rochester, VT, Healing Arts Press. One of the first books written on reflexology to explain the subject (originally published in 1978). Offers a basic introduction to the subject.

Part VI

Hall, N. (1994) *Reflexology for Women,* London, Thorsons. This easy-to-follow illustrated book focuses in particular on specific concerns that affect women and how they can be helped by reflexology, although many of the conditions referred to will also affect men. Suitable text for students of reflexology as well as the layperson.

Hall, N. (2000) *Reflexology: A Way to Better Health,* Dublin, Gill & Macmillan. Straightforward guide to the background and application of reflexology, written for the student and layperson.

Web Links

www.britreflex.co.uk – The British Reflexology Association

www.reflexologyforum.org – The Reflexology Forum

www.cnhc.org.uk – Complementary and Natural Healthcare Council

www.fih.org.uk – Foundation for Integrated Health

www.reflexology-research.com – Reflexology Research Project

www.britreflex.co.uk/training – The Bayly School of Reflexology (official teaching body of the British Reflexology Association)

The Alexander Technique **28**

LENA SCHIBEL-MASON

Nature of the Alexander Technique

The Alexander technique (AT) is based on the discovery that how we use ourselves affects our functioning. We can get into bad habits, which in turn can become the cause of many discomforts and illnesses from high blood pressure to back pain, from digestive disorders to breathing problem, stress and depression.

By addressing that which has taken us 'out of true', out of our centredness, we can regain balance and ease and gracefulness, which will also have a beneficial effect on our aches and pains. We can address our harmful habits with the AT, be they physical, emotional or mental. F.M. Alexander, the founder of this technique, was very clear about the importance of applying it to our entire life, not just to our physical discomforts.

It is a technique that teaches us to learn from our mistakes/bad habits by giving them our compassionate attention. Mostly we are not even aware of having acquired these habits. In this way, we start learning from them and become able to let go of them rather than perpetuating bad use through not wanting to know or through judging ourselves. It is a technique that helps us free ourselves from overuse and underperforming.

My own first step towards AT was curiosity and I knew nothing about it other than that it had been recommended as a bodywork with a 'spiritual' approach (in

Part VI

the widest sense of the word). I took that to mean that it encompassed much more than my physical wellbeing. My first lesson gave me a profound experience of space and peace and wholeness and 'hooked' me for life. I soon trained and then taught the technique for more than 20 years to a wide spectrum of students (musicians, actors, riders, dancers, as well as those coming with pain or wishing to improve any daily activity). I was also involved in training students to become AT teachers for 12 years before opening my own school in York in 2003. I am still exploring the technique and I am deeply attracted by the range and depth of its application.

History of the AT

Frederick Matthias Alexander (1869–1955) was born in Tasmania and had an inquisitive mind from early childhood, for example he asked his teachers how they knew the truth of what they taught him. As a young man, he became a successful Shakespearian actor and orator. Not long after he started his career, he suffered acute laryngitis, which led to hoarseness on stage but not in normal speech. At first, he followed his doctor's advice and took the recommended remedies, but when he did not get any better, he had a unique/ingenious insight that he himself might be contributing to his loss of voice when performing.

His excellent observational skills – equalling scientific research – and his patience led him to discover the root of the soreness of his throat. By using mirrors and reciting in front of them, he found out that when projecting his voice, more than with normal speaking, he shortened his neck and pulled his head back, thus restricting his larynx. He realized that in order to speak freely, he needed to release his neck, so that his head would not be pulled back and down, into coming 'forward and up' – basically allowing it to rest freely/potentially movable on top of the spine. He also observed that any shortening of the neck shortened and narrowed the whole stature.

So the releasing of the neck became the starting point for the unravelling of an habitual pattern that being startled or straining can put us in – the 'startle pattern' (see Figure 28.3 below).

Alexander called the balanced relationship between neck, head and back the 'primary control', later 'primary direction'. By preventing himself from going into a version of 'startle pattern', he succeeded in not straining his voice. The steps between finding this pattern in himself as a reaction to the stimulus to speak and actually being able to prevent it from happening took years of continued observation.

He found that his habit was stronger than his reasoning (recognizing the force of habit). He went on stage wanting not to pull his head back, but could not prevent himself from doing it. His next discovery was 'inhibition' and 'non-doing'. He realized that he could prevent his habitual preparatory response to a planned action by giving himself a choice:

1. I could speak
2. I could lift a hand
3. I could do nothing at all.

He kept the options open for as long as possible and when he finally acted, hardly any preparatory habit had kicked in.

What Happens in a Course of Lessons

There is a wide variety of reasons for someone to start lessons in AT. The spectrum ranges from curiosity to severe pain, from the wish to enhance the quality of life to addressing emotional and thinking habits as well as physical ones that have led to discomfort. Some of the aches and pains in the shoulder, neck, back and head can be traced back to certain activities or they can come about without particular awareness of what causes them. Stress and its wide-ranging impacts are also an important field of application.

An AT teacher does not give a diagnosis and does not treat. Yet through observation and questions, the teacher can soon identify patterns/habits that lead to or contribute to the 'dis-ease' experienced by the student. Someone coming for a lesson will become aware of how they themselves can address their discomfort through the guidance and gentle feedback of the teacher with words and hands. The student can make new experiences and unlearn the strain they are putting themselves under.

Body mapping was originally developed by Alexander teachers Barbara and William Conable, who have had a particular focus in working with musicians. Body mapping is a way of coming in contact with the hazy/inaccurate sense of self that many of us have, and allows more wholeness to evolve.

In the course of the first lessons, the five principles that make the AT different from other approaches are introduced. They are:

1. Faulty sensory awareness
2. Recognition of the force of habit
3. Giving directions
4. Non-doing and inhibition
5. Primary control.

Use affects functioning and only when I look at the whole person will I be able to become aware of how that person is misusing themselves. Faulty/unreliable sensory awareness can jeopardize the new findings to become part of ourselves. For example, I can realize that I have no clear sense of my hip joints or sitting bones (ischial tuberosities) and so overuse my lower back and thighs. The means to get out of this habitual overuse into a more balanced and coordinated use are not doing the new 'posture' or movement, but allowing it to happen, first through stopping/inhibition of the immediate response to a request/stimulus, like getting up from a chair, and second through giving directions. So, after exploring the hip joints with pictures, a skeleton and on the pupil himself, I ask the pupil to allow the hip joints to be spacious and free (this is giving directions) and to stop before changing mode (from sitting to standing) and reiterate to himself the directions before getting up. Giving directions is mentally allowing something new to happen, which also creates physical space for it to happen, especially with the feedback, the guiding hands and words of an AT teacher. Primary directions are directions aiming at the neck, head and back, the area most sensitive to overwork when we get out of balance. Alexander found that this area needed to be included in our mental realigning of our activities through thinking. 'Allowing my neck to be free' is a primary direction that may be given in conjunction with a direction to my hip joints for example. 'Ends and means' describes the overall attitude towards achieving. If primarily focused on the goal of building up muscles in our stomach or legs, for example, we may become end focused, not realizing how much we overuse other parts of our body like the neck or hold our breath.

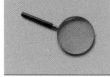

Practice example

Mr M comes because of feeling unduly tired and listless, thinking of maybe needing to change his job as it means long hours of sitting at the computer.

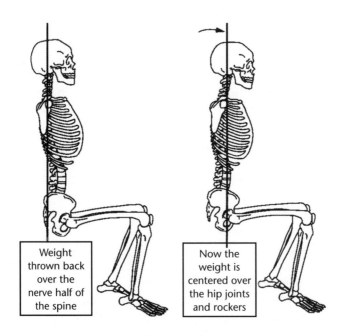

| Weight thrown back over the nerve half of the spine | Now the weight is centered over the hip joints and rockers |

Figure 28.1 Finding balance on the sitting bones

Source: © Conable and Conable, 2000. Distributed by GIA Publications, Inc. All rights reserved. Used by permission

Faulty Sensory Awareness

We discover together that the way Mr M is sitting doesn't allow him to breath enough and he experiences, through guidance with words and hands, how sitting on his sitting bones gives him a base from which he can grow tall without pulling himself straight. This stops him sinking into his middle, squashing his diaphragm (this caused him originally to breathe too little) and rounding his back (which originally caused a strain on his back, neck and head). The new experience of sitting and breathing, although it feels easier and lighter, doesn't 'feel right', the sitting balance has changed. This shows us that a more balanced use of ourselves is not instantly acceptable to our whole being, because it feels strange – our habits are upset.

Activity

To experience the power of habit, you could explore the following. Interlock your hands/fingers as if you were praying. Look at which thumb is on top, and then unfold and refold your fingers by first changing the folding of the thumbs and then the rest of the fingers. This new, unfamiliar handhold might feel odd/uncomfortable, 'not you'. The same sense of unfamiliarity might occur when you fold your arms – notice which one is on top and then fold them the other way round.

Despite Alexander's insight that a free neck allows free alignment of the head with the neck, and the torso with the head and the neck (primary control), he could not instantly apply this principle. Through force of habit, he ended up with his head pulled back even when he thought he was not pulling his head back. This led him to realize that he could not trust his sensory appreciation. His body, all his senses, especially his kinaesthetic sense (which tells us where we are located in space) didn't give him appropriate feedback as to where in space he was moving and being. He had faulty sensory appreciation/awareness.

Recognition of the Force of Habit

Learning the new is not 'feeling for what is right', but is less specific and more indirect. Mr M might try to recreate the same feeling when he sits at his computer that he had in the lesson. But his habit will make him feel that the old, which he knows, is right – and not his experience from the lesson. He cannot approach learning by directly going for what he perceives as favourable. The new experience feels wrong, the usual/habitual way of sitting feels right.

One effective indirect way of unlearning habits and linking to new experiences is the **balanced resting state**: a way of generally unwinding by lying on one's back, knees up and head on a comfortable amount of books, just high enough for the head to be a continuation of the direction of the back, without it being pulled back or pushed into the throat. (This procedure is described in the introductory books listed at the end of the chapter.)

To guide the client through this resting state could be the next step in the lesson. Different from relaxation techniques, this lying down time aims at a restful awareness through inviting appropriate muscle tone and lively eyes. It is not about switching off or listening to something else – music/TV – or asking yourself to relax in certain areas of your body.

Giving Directions

You 'walk' consciously through yourself, inviting certain areas to do less and allow them to be supported/carried (back, head, feet), other areas (joints, neck) to be free/not holding extra tension, and you foster awareness of the whole self from head to toe, rather than homing in on specific, less comfortable areas. This inviting of ease and release in joints and muscles of head, neck, back, arms and legs, which also invites ease and release from troubling thoughts or feelings, is called 'giving directions'.

Better than any wish 'to do the right thing', these 10–20 minutes on our back prepare us for doing less, investing less unnecessary effort into the activities of daily life.

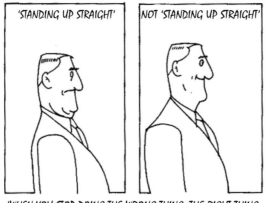

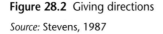

Figure 28.2 Giving directions

Source: Stevens, 1987

When Mr M gets back up from the floor to standing, he might feel more at ease or more grounded/in touch with the floor, more lively, having shed extra effort, or more tired initially, having come in touch with how much effort he normally invests in keeping things going and how hard he pushes himself.

The end of the lesson could be an exploration of sitting at a desk/computer with awareness of the sitting bones and how that allows more breathing and support from the floor and chair.

The practice between lessons will ideally consist of at least one lying down session in the balanced resting state a day and a wish for growing awareness of his breathing (as it is, not 'bettering' it) and his sitting bones. Each lesson (at least one a week to begin with), Mr M will come back with a growing awareness of his breathing pattern and the accumulative freedom gained from regular lying on his back.

The hardest part of the AT seems to be that we can learn by not doing, non-doing and by inhibiting the impulse to (re-)act in the old habitual way.

You can experience this phenomenon with another person. One of you is the observer, the other the active one (then switch round). The active one stands with eyes closed and takes her arms straight out to each side so they are shoulder high. The observer looks at the arms and if one of them is not level with the shoulder gently lifts or lowers it. The active person, now with eyes open, probably reports that this levelling feels wrong.

If you were too well balanced with this activity, the next one might give you this odd sense. Walk and, without looking down, come to standing (feet not together, slightly apart, which will probably happen anyway) and, still not looking down, place your feet parallel. Then have a look and if they are slightly off, correct them into being parallel and then look up again. You might feel wrong, pigeon toed.

Non-doing and Inhibition

Let's stay with the example of breathing and sitting in Mr M. If he comes out of the lesson with the idea 'I need to breathe more' and deliberately starts to breathe more deeply, he will soon become strained and uncomfortable. Breathing is a reflex in us and can well look after itself, provided we don't override the reflex. So the indirect way to freer breathing is to perceive how he is breathing (awareness/non-doing) to inhibit any preparations for 'better' breathing and to allow his breathing to expand his ribcage (giving directions) without designing how that should come about.

Similar could be his dealing with the awareness that he is 'not on his sitting bones'. Instead of instantly pulling himself up and into the perceived 'right' place, he inhibits this first reaction, allows his neck to be free and his sitting bones to support his sitting (giving directions) and then follows these directions with a movement that aligns him into more ease, which now comes from a much more integrated space in him. Inhibiting and directing are the lifeblood of the AT.

After the first joy of more freedom and ease, his learning curve may plummet and there might be a question: am I getting anywhere? This may occur when faulty sensory awareness, or the need to 'do the right thing', needs detecting: the student thinks he is doing the right thing but actually he is putting more pressure on himself to succeed in something and through that stands in his own way. He might say for example: 'I am bending now with a straight back and when the object is on the floor, I bend and go on my knees before taking the object.' Both examples aim at more economy of movement as is the intention when learning the AT, but they are too prescriptive. A much more general approach needs to be strengthened: of stopping what he is about to prepare for and giving directions to allow the neck to release so that the head can rest freely on top of the spine and the back can lengthen and widen.

Reading this, you could experiment with this yourself. The activity could be getting in and out of a chair.

1. Get in and out of a chair as you would normally do.
2. The second time, instead of instantly responding, give yourself a choice:
   – you could get up
   – you could start speaking
   – you could stay seated doing nothing.

When tuning in to this choice has allowed you to 'unprepare' for any of those options, get up and sit down. The quality of effort might be slightly less or different, depending how much you actually came back to 'neutral' and believed in your choice.

The 'non-doing' aspect of the principle of inhibition is about not aiming to do the 'right' thing once you get into action, but to stay in the open space that gradually develops when we stop our habits. In this open space, we act much more as a whole – with ease.

We realize how strong habits are when we consider how long it takes us to develop them. The unlearning, like the learning, needs patience and perseverance. This aspect of the AT has most fascinated me over the years. I do not need to do something new, better – which is what we mostly associate with learning: to do something. I just need to *not do* what I habitually do. This 'not doing something habitual' sets free my potential of more efficiency and economy, and I can access a wider range of my capacity to do things like walking, standing, talking, playing the piano and so on.

Primary Control

Primary control is the relation between neck, head and back, which is vital for any wellbeing and economy of movement. This relation between neck, head and back is most easily upset with anything fast, loud, unexpected coming our way and the reaction to, for example, a slammed door starts with the neck shortening, which in turn pulls the head back and down, which in turn shortens the whole stature. F.M. Alexander found out when observing himself in mirrors that even his wish to project his voice to an audience elicited this pattern in him. It is called the startle pattern (Figure 28.3).

This more general, indirect approach to relearning daily activities (by stopping and giving directions to neck/head and back and other areas) will keep the fire of change kindled and stop Mr M running into cul-de-sacs.

Parallel to this development went an exploration of his way of playing his instrument and teaching it. Mr M brought his guitar now and then to lessons and worked on how to let go of overrelying on specific areas (like arms, shoulders, eyes, 'listening in', or looking at fingers) and worked on connectedness to the world around, which again fed into freer breathing and greater flow through his whole being.

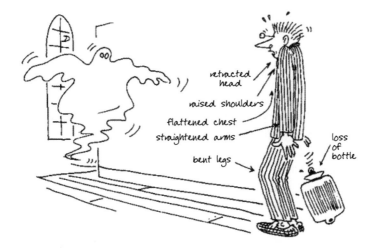

Figure 28.3 Startle pattern
Source: Stevens, 1987

A next step towards more space, freedom in breathing and connectedness in himself through a stronger back led him to want to realize his potential by becoming self-employed, which is where he is now, successful and breathing. He is a good example of how, although the way into working with these principles is the physical body, the whole being is affected and changed. He is happier and more confident, besides having fewer aches and pains and, if they crop up, he generally knows how to deal with them.

In his book *The Alexander Technique as I See It* (1989), Patrick Macdonald, a first generation teacher, lists the above five ingredients as being specific to the AT and as a way of discerning between other methods of bodywork and this technique. These five principles make the AT unique among bodywork as this technique acknowledges the force of habit and our false ideas and perceptions of ourselves and of the remedies. It is like an underlying principle to all activities of life, be they exercise or meditation, bricklaying or juggling.

Recognition of F.M. Alexander and the Technique Today

Alexander came to London in 1906 and soon became acknowledged in many quarters. He gave lessons to George Bernard Shaw and Aldous Huxley (who wrote about the technique in two of his books), and to actors, scientists and physicians (the latter soon sending pupils to him). Nicolas Tinbergen, professor of animal behaviour at Oxford, gave his Nobel Prize speech about the AT in 1973, and the educationalist John Dewey wrote introductions to three of Alexander's books praising the technique as the most profound and far-reaching discovery in education.

Part VI

Research has confirmed the freeing of breathing capacity in asthma sufferers and the re-establishing of antigravity reflexes, thus lightening the impact of movement on force plates under the feet of those examined (Jones, 1997). Recent research has confirmed its effectiveness in helping with back pain (UK BEAM Trial Team, 2004). The conclusions of the research were that 'one to one lessons in the Alexander technique from registered teachers have long term benefits for patients with chronic back pain. Six lessons followed by exercise were nearly as effective as 24 lessons.' Research is also in progress at the psychology department of Hull University to assess the effect of the AT on emotional wellbeing.

The Society of Teachers of the Alexander Technique was founded in 1958 by teachers who were trained personally by F.M. Alexander and is, with its affiliated societies throughout the world, the biggest professional body of AT teachers today (about 4,000 worldwide). Go to the website (www.stat.org.uk) to read about how to find a teacher and about the three-year full-time training courses and weekend taster courses.

Any amount of lessons can be beneficial. Bear in mind that learning the technique is comparable to learning an instrument (you are the instrument) or a language. You can get along quite well with some basics or you can become an expert in a constantly widening and deepening field of application. An article in the *British Medical Journal* on research into the Alexander technique confirmed that just six lessons can make a significant difference to lower back pain sufferers (Little et al., 2008).

Chapter Summary

The Alexander technique is an invaluable skill for all walks of life and for all kinds of ailments. It teaches the individual how to unlearn those unwanted patterns that interfere with an innate poise, balance and coordination.

REVIEW QUESTIONS

1   What are the five principles that comprise the AT and make it different from other bodywork?

2   What is meant by 'giving directions' and 'primary control'?

3   How does the Alexander teacher assess and help their client?

CHAPTER LINKS

For further discussion of different ways of categorizing complementary approaches, see Chapter 5.

FURTHER RESOURCES

Gelb, M. (2004) *Body Learning: An Introduction to the Alexander Technique*, London, Aurum Press. Gelb started out as an professional juggler and, as an AT teacher, inspires clients such as IBM, General Motors, Microsoft and the US Army. Wonderfully clear and lively, with many pictures.

De Alcantara, P. (2007) *The Alexander Technique: A Skill for Life*, Marlborough, Crowwood Press. A professional cellist, his book is very clear and has inspiring case studies.

UK BEAM Trial Team (2004) United Kingdom back pain exercise and manipulation (UK BEAM) randomised trial: effectiveness of physical treatments for back pain in primary care, *British Medical Journal*, www.bmj.com/cgi/content/abstract/329/7479/1377. Over 500 patients with chronic or recurrent back pain from 64 GP practices in England were involved in this research. Normal care, exercise, massage and AT were compared in their effects. Exercise and AT lessons but not massage remained effective at one year.

Web Link

www.stat.org.uk – The Society of Teachers of the Alexander Technique (STAT) is the oldest and largest professional society of teachers of the Alexander technique.

Part VI

Resource file

Manipulative and Body-based Approaches

This resource file gives supplementary information on manipulative and body-based approaches, over and above the individual areas of practice referred to in the four preceding chapters, and offers suggestions for further reading.

Manipulative and body-based approaches form a reasonably coherent category, in that they share the distinctive characteristic of concentrating on reducing pain and dysfunction of the skeleton, muscles and associated tissues and improving health and well-being. The term 'bodywork' is sometimes used in this connection.

■ *Bowen therapy* focuses on the musculoskeletal system and is used to encourage self-healing by the body, to alleviate problems with joints and soft tissues.

Further Resource

Baker, J. (2002) *The Bowen Technique*, Lydney, Corpus Publishing.

■ *Craniosacral therapy* originated in osteopathy and focuses on manipulating the bones and tissues of the head and neck, with a view to affecting the membrane around the brain and the spinal chord. It is often associated with osteopathy.

Further Resource

Cohen, D. (1995) *An Introduction to Craniosacral Therapy: Anatomy, Function and Treatment*, Berkeley, CA, North Atlantic Books.

■ *The Feldenkrais method* is a system of exercises originated by Moshe Feldenkrais in the 1940s, akin to the Alexander technique, enabling people to improve their bodily efficiency.

Further Resource

Sharfarman, S. (1997) *The Feldenkrais Method for Dynamic Health*, Cambridge, MA, Da Capo Press.

■ *Hydrotherapy* involves using water as a treatment for a variety of skeletal and muscular complaints, using, for example, hot and cold baths and underwater massage.

Distinct from hydrotherapy, water therapy involves consuming a quantity of water in order to cleanse the bowels.

Further Resource

Ruoti, R.G., Morris, D.M. and Cole, A.J. (1996) *Aquatic Rehabilitation*, New York, Lippincott Raven.

■ *Lymphatic pumping* may be used – perhaps where conventional medicine has little to offer, apart from surgical tights, as in a case of the often hereditary condition lymphodema – as a gentle form of massage (often referred to as lymphatic massage), aiming to engage the lymphatic system in removing waste substances from the body.

Further Resource

French, R. (2003) *Milady's Guide to Lymph Drainage Massage*, New York, Milady Publishing.

■ *Massage* covers a vast range of approaches, the common focus being on touching the body, with softer or firmer movements, to relieve stress, stimulate blood flow or treat particular muscular inflammations or injuries. Physiotherapists use sports massage in sports injuries clinics and hospitals, and complementary therapists may use a wide range of approaches, such as Thai, Indian head massage, shiatsu or Swedish massage. Baby massage or hand, foot and leg massage are also used. Therapeutic massage may be used alone or in conjunction with other complementary approaches such as aromatherapy (Vickers, 1996). Hot stone massage originated with Mary Hannigan in 1993 and entails heat treatment using a combination of massage, thermotherapy (heat therapy) and hydrotherapy (aquatherapy or water therapy) to relax and heal. Flat stones such as basalt (a very ancient, dense and therefore heavy rock) are often preferred, placed on the body or used for deep tissue massage. Indian head massage is a method of massage given with the client fully clothed and in the seated position. It is often used to relieve stress and tension. Seated acupressure massage is a Japanese method that uses more than 100 acupressure points on the body. It is used to relax and relieve muscular tension.

Further Resources

Beck, M.F. (1994) *Milady's Theory and Practice of Therapeutic Massage*, 2nd edn, Albany, NY, Milady Publishing.

Cassar, M. (1994) *Massage Made Easy*, Allentown, PA, People's Medical Society.

Mitchell, S. (1997) *The Complete Illustrated Guide to Massage: A Step by Step Approach to the Healing Art of Touch*, Shaftesbury, Element Books.

Myotherapy (from 'myo' – muscle – and 'therapy' – treatment) is a form of massage that uses pressure on trigger points throughout the body to relieve musculoskeletal pain. Trigger point therapy is a similar approach, involving the application of pressure to trigger points on the body, to relieve pain.

Further Resource

Prudden, B. and Tivy, D. (1985) *Myotherapy: Bonny Prudden's Complete Guide to Pain-free Living*, New York, Ballantine Books.

Rolfing is a form of manipulation of the deep tissues, which aims to release physical and emotional stress, and improve muscle tone.

Further Resources

Anson, B. (1992) *Rolfing: Stories of Personal Empowerment*, Kansas City, Heartland Personal Growth Press.

Bond, M. (1996) *Balancing Your Body: A Self-help Approach to Rolfing Movement*, Rochester, VT, Inner Traditions International.

Ultrasound involves directing high frequency sound waves at the body so as to treat damaged muscles or tissues with the heat generated.

Further Resource

Rumack, C., Wilson, S. and Charbonneau, J. C.V. (1998) *Diagnostic Ultrasound*, St Louis, MO, Mosby.

29 Reiki

ROSEMARY PHARO AND DOREEN SAWYER

By the end of this chapter, you should be able to:

- have a basic understanding of what reiki is
- appreciate the history and philosophy of reiki
- state the importance of lineage for UK practitioners
- describe what practice entails
- discuss relevant research on reiki
- explore relevant practice issues

What is Reiki?

Reiki is a term used to describe an ancient energy, which in modern times is used as a hands-on healing technique. Although it is a personal spiritual practice, it is more generally understood as a complementary therapy. Reiki is pronounced 'ray key' and is usually translated as 'universal life energy'. There are various definitions and explanations of reiki, which is the result of reiki being taught orally and the history being passed on by word of mouth over the decades.

The rediscovery of reiki is attributed to a Japanese man called Mikao Usui. The term 'reiki' describes what the energy is and what we are doing when using it; it is not actually the name of the system, although it is commonly called reiki in the West.

Reiki is practised professionally for the benefit of people and, increasingly, animals. For example, equine reiki now forms part of one degree course in the UK (www.reaseheath.ac.uk/courses/equine/foundation_degree_natural_horsemanship.html).

History and Philosophy

Mikao Usui was born in Taniai, a small village in Japan (now called Miyama) on 15 August 1865. He was born into a Tendai Buddhist family. Tendai is one of the many schools or sects of Buddhism. In his early life, Usui contracted cholera and had a near-death experience, which included a vision of the Buddha Dainichi Nyorai – he felt that this experience and vision saved his life. He later made contact with a Buddhist bonze (priest) and asked about the vision. It was at this point that he converted from the Tendai school to the Shingon school of Buddhism. As a result, his family disowned him; even in her will, his daughter said that his name was never to be used in her household.

Usui's original teachings were a spiritual practice based on Tendai Buddhism, and took many, many years of teaching. They were for personal development and were not about healing others, that is, they were not what we call reiki. This was Usui's original system, which was a 'method to achieve personal perfection'. This is different to the 'hands-on'-type healing that we have been taught in the West, which we call reiki. Usui studied for many years, had a long journey and out of that journey and the spiritual teachings came reiki.

Although until recently the reiki story has been full of mysteries and blind alleys, in a strange way, it nowadays gets us closer to what is going on. Usui did not run formal classes or workshops (they are a Western idea), instead he worked informally at a clinic from his home, healing and teaching. It would appear that Usui modified what he taught depending on the understanding and ability of the individual. People went to him for healing, but in healing them, he would also give a blessing. He would teach the basic principle of how people could heal themselves, give them some guidelines, which we know now as the 'precepts' or 'principles', and a simple meditation. He would do all this with the proviso that they kept notes and wrote down any questions and queries the next time they met. If they were dedicated and interested, he would teach them more. In those early days (1900s), communication and travel were not easy, so he would only see them perhaps every three to six months, or even longer.

When teaching those with Buddhist backgrounds, he taught by a process of meditations, which helped the individuals to use and to become the energy. Usui taught many naval officers from various backgrounds and beliefs; several of them were Christian, several of them were dualistic in belief, that is, part Shinto, part Buddhist, or part Christian, part Buddhist and so on. Many found it difficult to connect to the energy through meditation, either because of their beliefs, which may not have acknowledged the energy, or their military training. So Usui modified the system to help them experience the energy, and introduced the use of tools that enabled the naval officers, and those less spiritually aware, to practise their healing. These tools were in the form of symbols at what we would call the second level.

Some sources say that over 2,000 people were taught reiki by Usui, 21 of whom were trained to teacher level. One of his students was Dr Hayashi, a former naval officer and surgeon, who spent 10 months learning with him in 1925–26. Usui travelled throughout Japan and eventually the sheer workload proved to be detrimental to his health, and on 9 March 1926 he died of a stroke. Usui was cremated and his ashes placed on an altar in Saihoji Temple in Japan. Before his death, Usui gave his notes to a man referred to as the 'Soke Dai', with the instruction that they be kept safely for use in the world in the future.

Hayashi went on to open a clinic in Tokyo where he then trained others in reiki. Using what he had learned from Usui, he changed some of the format of the teachings using symbols and mantras and broke down the training into degrees or levels. Hayashi was a doctor and observed what happened when hands were put in different positions. From his medical experience and observations, he formulated a number of hand positions, which we now learn in the West as the basic 12 hand positions for giving reiki. Hayashi used to offer training in exchange for the students working unpaid in his clinic; level 1 students worked for three months, level 2 students for nine months and those at teacher level for two years. One of Hayashi's most well-known pupils was Hawayo Takata, who was a Japanese woman from Hawaii who had come back to Japan for a short period. It was Hawayo Takata who took reiki to America, from where it spread across the world when she began teaching openly in the 1970s.

The teachings of Usui equated to seven levels, each divided into three parts; the three parts of the first level are generally now known as a first degree, second degree and Master and that is what is generally included in Western teachings.

Importance of Lineage and Training for Practitioners

The reiki student will come across various descriptions and styles of reiki. When referring to Western reiki, this may be generally understood as having a lineage (a family tree or flow chart) tracing the teachings back teacher by teacher to Usui via Hayashi. In some instances, these may be described as Japanese lineages, where the teachers are predominantly Japanese. There are also lineages that go back to Usui through other teachers, but not through Hayashi and these may be described as Eastern lineages, but may also be described as Japanese lineages. From the learner's point of view, it does not really matter whether it is described as Western, Eastern or Japanese, provided the lineage can be traced back to Usui as the 'originator' of the system. There are other 'channelled' systems described as reiki but these may include other techniques that were not part of those used by Usui and/ or Hayashi. It is important for those wishing to train as professional reiki practitioners that they are able to provide a clear lineage for their reiki or 'hands-on healing', back to Usui via Hayashi or other direct students of Usui; this is a recommendation of the Reiki Council in the UK for those wishing to be included on any national register for reiki practitioners. It is a requirement of the current National Occupational Standards for Reiki practitioners in the UK.

Reiki is something that people often initially choose to study for their own benefit and not with the intention of practising as a professional therapist. Its first focus is on self-treatment, personal wellbeing and spiritual development, although people can give effective treatments from the very start.

It has traditionally been taught by independent reiki teachers, with the techniques being passed on by word of mouth. Reiki is also taught through educational establishments, such as colleges or private schools. Whichever route is selected, if people now wish to work professionally as reiki practitioners in the UK, it is important that the training encompasses additional information such as dealing with clients, local and national legislation, business awareness and so on.

In 2006, the first National Occupational Standards for Reiki were produced. To our knowledge, there are currently no recognized qualifications that have been mapped to those standards. The revised 2009 standards are now available on the Skills for Health website (www.skillsforhealth.org.uk). The standards indicate the minimum level of training that would be expected from a professional reiki practitioner, but do not differentiate between levels such as level 1 and level 2. A practitioner is deemed to be competent, provided they meet the minimum standards specified.

In addition to the National Occupational Standards, the Reiki Council has produced a core curriculum, which teachers should refer to when planning their courses. The core curriculum is a framework on which courses can be developed, and is there to help teachers to plan their courses. It is not prescriptive regarding the order of training, so teachers may decide the order in which they teach various topics, and it can be expanded and developed to include additional topics that may be required as part of that particular reiki style. The current recommendations in the core curriculum are that the training period for a reiki practitioner working professionally should be at least nine months, it should be a minimum of 140 hours' training, which will include at least 50 hours face to face with a tutor. Part of the requirements is that a number of treatments are completed and recorded and some of these would need to be supervised by an occupationally competent reiki practitioner.

During the course of training, a student will learn techniques for using reiki and other topics under the title of practitioner skills and practice management. The beginner will receive what is called an 'attunement' or 'initiation' to the first level of reiki. The attunement or initiation is what gives practitioners access to the reiki energy, and without it, reiki cannot be practised. Students would then be given a reiki history, depending on the style of reiki they are being taught. There would be a description of reiki, and how it can be used. Students would learn about the reiki principles or precepts, which are used as a focus when working with reiki. Practical uses of reiki would include guidelines for self-treatment, plus opportunities to practise and use reiki on other people, both seated and lying down. The most important part of reiki is using it on oneself in order to be able to understand and experience the reiki energy, prior to using this energy on other people. Reiki should be used by the practitioner for self-treatments on a daily basis.

Under the National Occupational Standards, it is not a requirement that what we know as level 2 is necessarily taught. However, most teachers would probably wish to give an attunement or initiation to level 2, together with what is recognized as level 2 training. At this level, individuals are taught the use of the reiki symbols, their origins and their meanings. These symbols may be used during normal reiki treatments, and to send reiki distantly.

In addition, meditations may be taught that will help the individual to focus on and develop the reiki energy. Different meditations may be used depending on the style of reiki being taught. Students should be aware that there are many different styles of reiki, with many different names. The most familiar ones are Usui shiki ryoho (the Usui method for natural healing) and Usui reiki ryoho (the Usui method for universal life energy healing).

As well as reiki-specific training, individuals would be made aware of the standards expected of them as practitioners, and may be referred to the code of ethics produced by the Reiki Council or by a professional reiki organization. Individuals may be asked to keep a reiki diary, which records their journey from when they start using the reiki and is ongoing. Students should also ensure that their communication skills are sufficient so as to provide a professional impression to their prospective clients.

It may be that the teacher of the reiki aspects is different from the teacher of the business and practitioner aspects, and if being assessed against National Occupational Standards, it may be that the assessor is a different person, who is a qualified assessor.

The National Occupational Standards and core curriculum also require the student to have received an initiation or attunement from their teacher in person. This would put those who choose to receive their initiation or attunement through a website at a disadvantage if they wished to meet the National Occupational Standards. Some insurers may also not grant cover to therapies that have been learned at a distance.

When looking for a course for professional training in reiki, the student should ideally satisfy themselves that the teacher, or training establishment, is fully aware of the requirements of the National Occupational Standards and the core curriculum for reiki. In addition, these students may wish to ask the teacher whether they are currently practitioners of reiki as well as teaching. Reiki teachers should be qualified practitioners with at least two years' practical experience as a practitioner and they should also hold a Master or Master teacher's certificate in reiki. Questions that students may ask include information about the student's time with the tutor, additional study time required, the length of the course, supporting materials provided, which may include manuals or textbooks, and what support there is after the training is complete. They may also ask about certification and whether this is through independent certification by a teacher, or is a fully accredited course through a college or other training establishment. At the time of writing, either is acceptable, as there is no formal procedure for individual teachers to have their personal courses accredited. Prices for training can vary greatly, and a higher price does not indicate a superior level of training. Students should satisfy themselves that they have obtained as much information as possible about the cost and length of training and exactly what they will get as part of the training package; it is vitally important that information should also include clear details on what will be required by the teacher prior to issuing the final certificates to the student.

What Practice Entails

Reiki is a wonderful tool for anyone to have, whether working as a professional practitioner, or just wishing to use it for themselves. The point has already been made that the most important recipients of reiki are practitioners themselves: both through their daily practice and through regularly receiving reiki from others.

One of the tremendous advantages of reiki is that it can be used alongside other complementary therapies, as well as orthodox medicine. However, if a practitioner wishes to include reiki while using other therapies, they should always ensure that they have the specific consent of their client before giving reiki.

There are two forms of practice:

- *Self-practice:* A reiki practitioner's daily self-practice could generally include, for example, saying the reiki principles or precepts and giving themselves a reiki treatment.
- *Professional practice:* While reiki is available in some hospitals and hospices, most clients will self-refer to a practitioner, either as a result of personal research or word-of-mouth recommendation by friends and acquaintances. The practice may be either in person or at a distance.

Approaches and Techniques

What approach to a reiki treatment is chosen depends very much on the style of reiki the practitioner has learned or they choose to use for a particular treatment.

Practice example

Mr B presents with recurring headaches, stress and depression. As a minimum, the practitioner will begin by taking personal details for a record card. Some practitioners will, however, take a full medical history and details of medication. The decision is style dependent.

Mr B will usually be asked to remove just his shoes as treatments are given fully clothed. He could receive his treatment sitting in a chair or lying on a couch, either is acceptable. The practitioner may begin by scanning Mr B to find areas of imbalance or proceed directly to placing their hands in a standard sequence of places around the body and allowing the reiki to flow. The hands may be placed directly on the body (except in sexually sensitive areas) or close to the body but not touching. Where touch is used, it is good practice to gain permission for this from the client. The hands may be kept still, or they may move, depending on the specific reiki techniques used.

The reiki may be felt very strongly or not at all by the client. Mr B could experience subjective sensations such as heat, cold, tingling or pulsing as the energy moves through his body. He may go into a deeply relaxed state to aid his body in its healing, which may also produce personal insights into changes that could improve his quality of life in general.

Depending on the style of reiki, the practitioner may also combine work with affirmations with the healing treatment in which the client can participate.

At the end of the treatment, the practitioner will gently bring Mr B back into an everyday waking state and will offer him the opportunity to feed back and evaluate his experience of the treatment where appropriate. Mr B will also be given appropriate aftercare information.

Over the next few days, Mr B may experience what is termed a 'healing reaction' as his body moves into a state of greater balance. These may include a 'flu-like' feeling, a lessening or initial worsening of headaches, tiredness. They are all positive signs of change within his body-mind system.

Generally, Mr B will benefit most from a series of treatments as the effect tends to be cumulative. Sometimes just one treatment is enough to produce helpful results. Sometimes, as with any orthodox or complementary therapy, no direct initial benefit is felt but changes are seen over a longer period. The effects of reiki can be very subtle or very obvious.

As well as being able to give a treatment without touching, which may be helpful where people have severe injuries that would contraindicate touch or where the client has a preference for not being touched, treatments can also be given at a distance. This can mean in the same room but not near the person or at considerable physical distance from the client. This feature of reiki gives tremendous flexibility to the practitioner and offers an opportunity to reach people therapeutically who may not physically be able to come to a clinic, are in hospital or are far away.

It may also make it easier to treat hyperactive or autistic children who may not be comfortable initially sitting or lying still. The autistic child would be able to be in the room, find their own 'safe' space, possibly playing with toys. The practitioner can carry out a treatment initially from a distance and gradually, over a number of sessions, as the child becomes more comfortable, may be able, if appropriate, to treat the child on a chair or couch. Reiki offers tremendous flexibility for treating children. The authors' experience is that reiki brings welcome feelings of calm and peace very quickly to children.

Reiki may also be given to animals. However, under the Veterinary Surgeons Act 1966, the practitioner needs the owner to confirm that their animal has seen a vet for any condition that needs treating as this is a legal requirement. An example might be a dog who has had a road accident and is under veterinary treatment. The owner is concerned to speed the recovery of the dog and to help the dog feel more comfortable. The practitioner will treat the dog according to their style of reiki, using either hands on or hands off, as appropriate to the needs and temperament of the dog.

There are no proven contraindications to reiki when given on its own. It is an extremely safe and low-risk treatment to give. There are, however, some different schools of thought on the subject, although these are not based on any research facts. However, if reiki was being given in conjunction with other modalities, the contraindications for those modalities would then come into play. It is important to advise clients who are taking medication to check if the dosage they are taking may need to be changed as a result of any improvements in their condition.

Notwithstanding reiki being a low-risk therapy, there are certain circumstances in which it would not be appropriate to give reiki. For each of the listed circumstances, can you give a reason why?

1. The reiki practitioner is feeling shocked, upset, low or vulnerable.
2. The reiki client presents as violent or abusive.
3. The reiki practitioner is presented with a sick child whose parents have not first visited a medical professional.
4. The reiki practitioner believes the client has food poisoning.

1. Practitioners need to be in good emotional health to handle clients and give treatments.
2. Practitioners have the right to refuse treatment where they believe their own safety is at risk.
3. Parents are legally obliged to ensure that a sick child has seen a medical professional and therapists may be seen as accomplices if they do not comply with this.
4. Food poisoning is on the list of diseases that have, by law, to be notified to the medical health office via the client's GP.

Research on Reiki

Reiki has been the subject of numerous studies, although these have the limitation of often being small scale and limited in scope. Interestingly, although reiki is viewed as having a holistic effect by practitioners and increasing balance both physically, mentally and spiritually, much of the research in the past has been quantitative rather than qualitative. In their review of reiki, Miles and True (2003) point out that much reported reiki research consists of 'case reports, descriptive studies or randomized controlled studies with a small number of patients'. The review is useful in listing a good number of research trials. In 2007, Miles reviewed reiki's use for 'Mind, body, and spirit support of cancer patients'. In it, she states that reiki has been 'identified as an evidence-based complementary therapy for symptom control and quality of life' by Berenson.

As opposed to the UK, where the authors are not aware of government-funded research into reiki, the USA has funded a number of trials of reiki via the National Center for Complementary and Alternative Medicine. This may demonstrate that there is a different attitude towards complementary therapies in the US healthcare market.

Recent US-government funded studies included looking at reiki's ability to improve wellbeing for patients with advanced AIDS, and evaluate its effects on dimensions of wellbeing and quality of life, the effectiveness of reiki in the treatment of fibromyalgia, the effect of reiki and relaxation response therapy with cognitive restructuring in patients with prostate cancer, a study to determine whether reiki energy healing affects anxiety and disease progression in patients with localized prostate cancer who are candidates for radical prostatectomy, the use of reiki for patients with diabetic neuropathy and the effects of reiki upon stress.

Salach (2006) used her PhD thesis to look into the effects of reiki on depression and anxiety in the Alzheimer's and dementia population. The results were encouraging, both for mitigating depression and anxiety and for suggesting that the results of reiki were cumulative and lasting. The study was small scale and recognized some weaknesses, which could be overcome in future research design.

Researchers at the University of Arizona have taken a different approach to research into reiki. They set about seeing if it was possible to physically measure what, if anything, was emanating from practitioners as they practised reiki using a standard scientific instrument. The instrument picked up an increase in energy in the extra low frequency range when practitioners focused on the flow of reiki (Melinda Connor, 2006, personal communication).

The University of Arizona was careful to recruit highly regarded reiki practitioners for its trials (Melinda Connor, personal communication, 2006). The same university also experimented on giving reiki to rats who had been stressed by noise (as measured by microvascular leakage). Compared with control groups, reiki significantly reduced the leakage in the treated rats (Baldwin and Schwartz, 2006). Later research by the same team on laboratory rats has also confirmed reiki's ability to reduce raised heart rates caused by white noise compared with sham (or fake) reiki (Baldwin et al., 2008). Neither, however, significantly reduced blood pressure.

While there have been a good number of research studies into the effect of distant healing in general, one interesting approach was reported by Achterberg et al. (2005). This team used functional magnetic resonance imaging (fMRI) to show that when senders of various healing modalities had an intention to send healing, the recipients' brains showed levels of activity in the anterior and middle cingulate area, precuneus, and frontal area at a significant level compared to activity when there was no intention to heal.

Research has also been carried in reiki on non-human recipients. Rubik et al.'s (2006) research was carried out on bacterial cultures that had been heat-shocked as a stressor. Controls were used and a contrast of healing and non-healing contexts. The question of placebo can therefore be completely discounted. This would call into question the conclusions that Ernst and Singh (2008: 324) draw that the trials showing beneficial effects of reiki are likely down to a placebo effect. They also state that the 'concepts of Reiki are contrary to our understanding of the laws of nature'. However, just because something is not understandable in the current common scientific paradigm does not mean it is invalid, it simply means that our understanding of the 'laws of nature' may not yet be fully developed. The bacteria receiving reiki were shown to increase significantly more in number than the controls, demonstrating that reiki had the ability to enable them to overcome the effects of heat-shocking. The study also explored the effect of practitioner well-being on healing results and indicated that where social, physical or emotional health was compromised, results were less effective. This implies that the more balanced physically and mentally the practitioner, the more effective the results.

In summary, outside the UK, there has been considerable research into reiki (Table 29.1), much of which has suggested that further research is merited.

Table 29.1 Reiki research findings

Author	Summary
Miles, P. and True, G. (2003) Reiki: review of a biofield therapy history, theory, practice and research, *Alternative Therapies in Health and Medicine*, **9**(2): 62–72	Useful review and discussion of the wide range of research conducted into reiki
Miles, P. (2007) Reiki for mind, body and spirit support cancer patients, *Advances in Mind-Body Medicine*, **22**(2): 20–6	Useful review of reiki's use in local hospitals, cancer centres, community centres and cancer support groups. Lists a number of small studies focused on reiki's usefulness to relieve symptoms
Salach, M.D. (2006) The Effects of Reiki, a Complementary Alternative Medicine, on Depression and Anxiety in the Alzheimer's and Dementia Population, PhD thesis, San Francisco State University	Research carried out with the assistance of the US Institute of Aging. Small study reporting positive benefits, with a significant reduction of depression and anxiety
Achterberg, J., Cooke, K., Richards, T. et al. (2005) Evidence for correlations between distant intentionality and brain function in recipients: a functional magnetic resonance imaging analysis, *Journal of Alternative and Complementary Medicine*, **11**(6): 965–71	While not reiki specific, demonstrated that an intention to send healing distantly to someone can be correlated to brain function changes in that individual. This is supporting evidence for the fact that distant healing can be used in reiki to create physical effects
Rubik, B., Brooks, A. and Schwartz, G. (2006) In vitro effect of reiki treatment on bacterial cultures: role of experimental context and practitioner well-being, *Journal of Alternative and Complementary Medicine*, **12**(1): 7–13	Showed that reiki can improve the 'wellbeing' of shocked bacterial cultures, indicating that its results are not reliant on a placebo effect
Baldwin, A. and Schwartz, G. (2006) Personal interaction with a reiki practitioner decreases noise-induced microvascular damage in an animal model, *Journal of Alternative and Complementary Medicine*, **12**(1): 15–22	Using reiki decreased microvascular damage caused to rats who had been stressed by noise. The results were real and could not be attributable to placebo
Baldwin, A., Wagers, C. and Schwartz, G. (2008) Reiki improves heart rate homeostasis in laboratory rats, *Journal of Alternative and Complementary Medicine*, **14**(4): 417–22	Reiki is shown to reduce stress in rats, supporting its use as a method to reduce stress in humans

Practice Issues

When looking for a reiki practitioner, the public may require answers to a number of questions. These may include: the length of the reiki session, how the reiki is given and how long the practitioner has been working professionally. Probably the most important questions are: are they a member of a professional body, are they insured and are they on a national register? Therefore it is important that those wishing to train ensure that the teachers they select also meet certain criteria.

Health and safety is also important when it comes to giving reiki. Not only should practitioners be fully aware of their responsibilities under the Health and Safety at Work Act, but they should also ensure that they practise according to legal requirements. One area that is sometimes neglected is ensuring that practitioners maintain the highest standards of hygiene themselves; most practitioners think about maintaining a clean and tidy personal appearance, including nails and hair, but some may overlook basic things such as cigarette smells or the smell of spicy food on their breath.

Chapter Summary

Reiki is a safe, low-risk therapy that is simple and easy to learn but requires daily practice and real dedication from its mature practitioners. It has been shown in trials to be of benefit physically, emotionally and spiritually and is being used in hospitals, hospices and drug treatment centres around the world.

REVIEW QUESTIONS

1 What is reiki?
2 Who is the founder of reiki?
3 What is a lineage in reiki?
4 What is its importance for registration?
5 Who can reiki be given to as a therapy?
6 Which three main ways can reiki be given?

CHAPTER LINKS

For further discussion of the healing uses of reiki, see Chapter 30.

FURTHER RESOURCES

Fulton, E. and Prasad, K. (2006) *Animal Reiki: Using Energy to Heal the Animals in Your Life*, Berkeley, CA, Ulysses Press. Clear and concise handbook of holistic reiki practice.

Hall, M. (2000) *Reiki for the Soul: 10 Doorways to Inner Peace*, London, Thorsons. An interactive book by an international authority on reiki.

Lubeck, W., Petter, F.A. and Rand, W.L. (2004) *The Spirit of Reiki*, Varanasi, Pilgrims Publishing. Past and present of reiki, written by three acknowledged masters of the subject.

Quest, P. (2002) *Reiki for Life: The Essential Guide to Reiki Practice*, London, Piatkus. Standard text on reiki.

Stiene, B. and Stiene, F. (2003) *The Reiki Sourcebook*, Winchester, O Books. Good introductory book, covering historical, research and practical aspects.

Stiene, B. and Stiene, F. (2005) *The Japanese Art of Reiki: A Practical Guide to Self-healing*, Winchester, O Books. Good guide to reiki practice.

Web Links

www.reikicouncil.org.uk – The Reiki Council is the lead advisory body for those practising reiki professionally. Contains information on standards for professional reiki practitioners and member associations.

www.grcct.org – The General Regulatory Council for Complementary Therapies is the only independent UK regulator in operation for complementary therapies.

http://nccam.nih.gov/health/reiki/ – The National Center for Complementary and Alternative Medicine is part of the US National Institutes of Health. Includes a list of research being funded by it into reiki.

30 Healing

SALLY CANNING

Learning outcomes

By the end of this chapter, you should be able to:

■ appreciate the significance of the journey towards becoming a healer

■ understand how the healer practises

■ know what healing entails

■ understand what is meant by energy psychology and emotional freedom technique

■ appreciate the relevance of practice examples

This chapter discusses healing through the focus of the author's own practice, rather than examining a range of major physical, mental, spiritual or psychic approaches from a theoretical point of view. The author uses reiki and related approaches, hence the concentration on these here. Healing is a personal act and, as becomes clear later in the chapter, the intention of the practitioner is crucial to this. This makes it important to know where the author is coming from and the chapter begins by placing the author in relation to healing practice.

Becoming a Healer: Elements of Healing

Energy therapies, including reiki, can make a significant contribution to healing. They are noninvasive, totally pure and safe techniques that work on the mind, body and soul and can be transformative and life-changing. I came to energy therapies at a time in my life when I was most open and in need. As a teacher, I wanted to know more about the effects of healing, its history and the possibilities for someone like myself to do the work I felt I was drawn to do. Such was the effect of this information on my life that I gave up a happy and stable career teaching personal development and counselling in adult education, coupled with independent life skills to adults with learning disabilities in social services day centres, in favour of what turned out to be the best job in the world and a quantum leap in quality of life.

I learned that many different cultures throughout history have demonstrated healing arts that used touch to transfer healing energy. Early references can be found in both Eastern and Western writings. Often passed down by oral tradition, energy healing is found around the globe, including China, Japan and other Asian countries, India, Peru, Australia and among Native American tribes. Each has several common elements, including touch, offering caring and using human energy in healing.

Touch is a basic human instinct each of us is born with. Reaching out and touching another person is a universal action that shows love and caring. Traditionally the laying on of hands evokes images of religious ceremonies and church gatherings. However, in recent years, there has been greater acceptance among healthcare professionals of the benefits and effects of energy healing, which utilizes the human capacity to consciously direct the flow of healing, multidimensional energies into the human body and the body's associated physical and spiritual energy system to bring about healing changes.

Nowadays, many people are proactive about their health and wish to learn tools for self-healing. Many want to learn more to deepen their existing practices and many others are on the path of self-discovery and transformation. As we begin to understand that our health is in direct relationship with our mental, emotional and energetic patterning, it becomes apparent that we hold the power of health in our own hands. Even children can do it. Energy healing is an innate human skill. The study of healing techniques, the theories of energy and knowledge of anatomy and physiology assist in refining the work but they are not essential. I discovered that 'we are more than this physical body' and healing is multidimensional – energy healing works on several levels at once – spiritual, emotional, mental and physical.

We are energetic beings whose ailments may be healed not only by modern medicine but also by different forms and frequencies of energy. According to Einstein and quantum physics, the biochemical molecules that make up the physical body are actually a form of vibrating energy. This is where the term 'vibrational medicine' comes from. Vibrational medicine works on the principle that human bodies comprise different, interrelated fields of energy, which may be out of balance and are restored to balance through healing. The natural tendency of blocked energy is to move towards release and the natural tendency of the body is to move towards balance.

Trauma, emotional and mental stress, false belief systems and blocks to our personal growth can be stored in the energy fields of our bodies, affecting our ability to function at our full potential. Ideally, our energy pathways would be free flowing, actively circulating to clear stagnant energies and bring in fresh, healthy energy. However, the pathways can become blocked and healing may be helpful in removing these blockages. These blocks obstruct the vital flow of energy through our body and energy systems that are necessary for our health and wellbeing. Over time, this leads to illness and depleted mental and emotional reserves.

Consciousness, as a form of energy, plays a large part in the maintenance of health. Consciousness resides not only in the brain and central nervous system but is also an integral part of the human heart. Heart-based consciousness acts from a centre of love, compassion and empathy towards others. Our emotions – which may be called 'energy in motion' – are influenced by a spiritual energy field that encompasses and influences the entire physical body and nervous system.

How the Healer Practises

Intention is the key to healing. The practitioner works with 'intention', which means a conscious desire to aid the client in healing. Often something manifested as a physical illness is rooted in deeper emotional or spiritual issues. During energy work, a client may have an emotional release that might be accompanied by specific memories, or may be experienced as pure emotion, which arises for 'no reason'. Release may be dramatic, with tears, sobbing or similar outward signs. If the client and practitioner stay centred and continue energy work, the emotion can be fully released from the energy field.

Energy medicine is an inherently spiritual practice that can lead to spiritual growth for both practitioner and client. It may create a change in consciousness, which allows us to feel a deeper connection with the self.

In distance healing, when people pray for another person to be healed, they usually ask for some kind of 'divine intervention'. Both prayer and hands-on healing may produce healing effects by the same mechanism – the divine energies of the creator/universe. Most healers acknowledge that they are not doing the healing – they are simply a channel or vehicle for a higher healing energy. Even eminent scientific thinkers like Albert Einstein acknowledged the existence of God as an influence in the creation of the universe.

What Healing Entails

I am passionate about empowering and enabling people on all levels of their being – mental, emotional, physical and spiritual – to be the best they can. I recognize a need for healing at a deep level in this fast-paced world for those who cannot and would not wish to commit to longer term programmes of healing, and also for those who wish to take a more cerebral approach to their healing.

I work on the premise that all healing is self-healing. I like the definition of a healer as someone 'who was sick and got well' and the definition of a great healer as someone 'who was very sick and got well quickly'. In truth, you cannot heal any person other than yourself – we practitioners are merely the facilitators in the scenes we play.

The discovery of energy psychology and meridian energy therapies was a real revelation and a joy for me. Meridian energy therapies are amazing techniques for helping people to free themselves from stress and anxiety, traumas, emotional and physical pain, and limiting beliefs to enable them to take responsibility for optimum health and happiness. This remarkable family of self-help and practitioner methods are at the forefront of defining personal development and personal empowerment in the twenty-first century.

Energy Psychology

'Energy psychology' is an umbrella term to convey a range of noninvasive techniques that work with the subtle energies circulating within the body. The field is unified by the underlying principle that every upsetting emotion, disturbing memory, limiting thought, irrational or self-destructive impulse is associated with a corresponding disturbance in the body's subtle energy system.

All energy psychology techniques work by releasing the underlying energy disturbances from the human energy system in order to recognize and deal with the root cause of our particular issues, behaviours or beliefs. Energy psychology allows those wishing to take responsibility for themselves to discover how they might move forward, breaking through their limiting belief systems and emotional blocks that keep them stuck and prevent them from moving forwards in their lives. By resolving disturbances in the subtle energy system, we can produce a sense of balance, calm and clarity in our thoughts, emotions and actions.

The beauty of these techniques is that they put the participant in control. By looking at our own behaviour and feeling the associated feelings, we are able to identify specific areas to be worked on to release energy blocks in order to move forward in our relationships, work and other areas of our lives. This work enables us to have choices about what happens. We cannot change external events; however, we can change the way we respond to them. It raises our own self-awareness – enabling us to view events and situations in a calm, level-headed way. We are able to assess our own expectations and our responses/reactions to the expectations of others. These methods are often rapid – really quick and easy. We are able to look at motivational factors, values and beliefs from our own personal conditioning and to find out where the triggers and blocks occur that create self-sabotage and limiting beliefs.

Emotions

How is it that although many of us may be given the same life experiences, we respond emotionally in very different ways? When you are given a compliment, are you happy and energized by it, or are you embarrassed and uncomfortable? When hearing that you've been made redundant from your job, are you angry and hurt as though you have been hit hard in your body, or do you experience it as life's experiences teaching you some profound lesson?

On all levels of our being, health is about flow. We understand that physically we eat, digest, process the goodness and extract the waste from food, which flows in, through and out of our system. The energy system of the body behaves in the same way. We take in energy from all life's experiences – our surroundings, what we see, hear and sense and what people say and do. We handle it, process it and let it go.

Problems occur when we do not handle this incoming energy in a positive way. Particular types of energy – a look, comment, accident, unexpected news, trauma, or just the sheer volume we have to deal with at any one time – build up until we feel an emotion such as stress, anger, anxiety, frustration, hurt, often accompanied by a physical sensation, or pressure in the body, that is, tightness in the chest, stomach, shoulders or head.

These emotional responses and physical sensations arise from the disturbances in the subtle energy body. Even years later, when you think of a comment made by a particular person, or an incident, you may experience similar feelings. Meridian therapies provide highly effective personal tools to alleviate these often distressing symptoms, to restore the energetic flow and the body's equilibrium.

Other Healing Techniques

Other healing techniques and treatments include thought field therapy, emotional freedom technique, EmoTrance, Be Set Free Fast (Behavioral & Emotional Symptom Elimination Training For Resolving Excess Emotion: Fear, Anger, Sadness & Trauma), Tapas Acupressure Technique and other such therapies. Each of these methods works intentionally with the human energy systems, for example the meridian system. Other deep therapies that access subconscious information may also act energetically, that is, they may cause energetic releases and healing, for example EMDR (eye-movement, desensitization and reprocessing). However, such therapies do not intentionally utilize the body's energetic systems and are not, therefore, called 'energy psychology' therapies.

Traditionally, counselling, psychotherapy and many other 'talking therapies' act deeply to help release emotional blocks, foster healing and change emotional patterns. However, energy psychology techniques add one more unique therapeutic dimension. By correcting a disruption in the energy system, these techniques can bring balance within a disturbed internal pattern, thus promoting inner harmony. Sessions are client oriented and depending on the training of the qualified practitioner, they may choose any one of a number of techniques depending on the client's moment to moment needs. Energy psychology techniques are powerful tools for personal empowerment and development and may be effective in work with a multitude of emotional issues.

Practice example

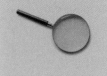

Kristina had a phobia of flying. Over time, her recognizable symptoms of distress, such as a pounding heart, lumps in the throat, distorted perceptions and negative emotions (fear, panic, anger, helplessness and confusion), were replaced by peaceful feelings. This was achieved using the natural resources of the body's energetic system.

The changes Kristina experienced may occur within a single session of treatment, and yet the inner transformation is often profound and enduring. Frequently, the treatment of one issue has the added bonus of eliminating other emotional issues.

Uses of Energy Psychology

Energy psychology can be used effectively for a huge number of physical, mental and spiritual problems, including:

- Painful memories, grief and traumatic experiences
- Anger, rage, resentment, irritability
- Moodiness, sadness, depression, low self-esteem, insecurity, irritable bowel syndrome
- Relationship difficulties, performance issues, and limiting beliefs.

As with all other therapeutic interventions, energy psychology techniques do not work with every single client. However, clinical experience shows that most people can benefit. The techniques are known to produce good results for self-help and supporting clinical treatments. However, because energy psychology is powerful and can cause deep emotional release, it is recommended that long-standing and deep-rooted issues be addressed initially by a trained and licensed practitioner.

Emotional Freedom Technique

Emotional freedom technique (EFT) originates in applied kinesiology (a chiropractic diagnostic method using manual muscle testing for medical diagnosis and a subsequent determination of prescribed therapy) and thought field therapy and is a simple, noninvasive meridian-based technique for releasing the underlying energy that causes negative emotions. It is often the introduction to meridian energy therapies. Gary Craig, a widely respected authority on energy therapies, originated this remarkable technique, basing it on the principle that an upsetting experience or problem is associated with a disturbance in the body's energy system. EFT is a form of psychological acupressure, working with the same energy meridians; however, where acupuncture uses needles to stimulate and unblock the channels, EFT uses a system of tapping with the fingers on 13 specific meridian points on the face, hands and upper body while using statements relating to and directly focusing on the issue being addressed: for example thinking the thought that created the emotion, or focusing on the limiting belief. The process enables clients to work rapidly through layers of emotions, beliefs and memories to locate the root cause of their issues.

EFT has gained a well-deserved reputation for giving rapid, long-lasting relief from anxiety, stress, trauma of all descriptions, fears of flying, spiders or heights, addictions, lack of self-esteem/confidence, and a whole host of other human conditions, including, from my own experience, the control and removal of physical pain, asthma, Ménière's disease (a condition of the inner ear affecting balance and hearing). It is often effective where all else has failed and many therapists, counsellors, trainers and health professionals claim that it has transformed the way they work, often 'leapfrogging' people through their process. For others who come to meridian therapies as a first stop, the effects are often staggeringly effective, as it can remove fears, phobias and disabling beliefs in a short space of time. It is not unusual to hear clients talk of life-changing experiences in a single session.

EFT may be utilized with clients who are willing and able to express their feelings and emotions. However, the beauty of this process is that it may also be used in total confidentiality. It is not strictly necessary for the person to share anything with the therapist. The whole process may be conducted inside the client's own mind while following the protocol, or by substituting keywords for the painful memories or incidents. The results are self-evident in the physiological responses and signals when a session is at a close, by which time the client is usually relieved and relaxed, even when more sessions are required.

EFT does not profess to perform miracles in the way of eradicating negative memories and issues. However, it may remove debilitating feelings such as anguish, guilt, sorrow, anger, fear or resentment, which may have been engulfing a person for years, thereby freeing them to view the original incident with a calm, detached attitude of 'It happened, it's over and I'm OK', enabling them to move on and to experience life from a different, improved, often liberating perspective.

During the first session, clients are taught the technique for self-empowerment, enabling each individual to take charge of their own ongoing wellbeing. This is EFT in its simplest form:

- identifying the issue
- deciding on a suitable 'set-up statement', which is said out loud three times while rubbing 'the sore spot'
- tapping with two or three fingers on specific meridian points.

For the beginner, EFT is as simple as that. There is no need to worry about getting it wrong. Any tapping stimulates the meridians, is relaxing and calming and makes you feel better.

EFT with a qualified practitioner entails more involved preparation. This includes mapping the aspects of the problem, which are then given ratings on a scale of 0–10 to ascertain where to start the process. The highest numbers indicate the greatest disturbance in the energy system.

Practitioners will then often muscle test a series of statements for psychological reversal, or what we might call 'self-sabotage', as, even though we may think we are ready to let go of a certain issue, we may, in fact, have unconscious reasons for holding onto it. Therefore, muscle testing on 'I want to get rid of this problem' may test positive; however, 'I want to get rid of this problem now' may elicit a different response, which would in itself give a new avenue for exploration.

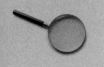

John has a fear of spiders and an intermittent back pain. To direct the tapping to the required area, we focus the mind on the problem by using a statement: for example, 'I am scared of spiders', or in the case of physical ailments and pain: 'My back is killing me.'

The set-up statement must be meaningful to the client, using their own phraseology and words, and is spoken while rubbing the sore spot on the chest, and phrased as: 'Even though I'm scared of spiders, I love and accept myself' (or words to that effect). This is repeated three times while rubbing John's sore spot continuously. Following this, all the points are tapped seven to nine times while John repeats a shortened version of the statement – the reminder phrase, 'I'm scared of spiders.'

The next step, the '9 gamut', often raises a smile and furrowed brow when a sequence of eye movements and humming is introduced. This involves looking up, down, down to the right, down to the left, circling the eyes all the way around like a clock, one way and then again in the opposite direction. John is then asked to hum one bar of a familiar tune, for example 'Happy Birthday to You', perhaps one, two, three, four, five times, quickly, and then to hum the tune again.

The thinking behind this process comes from both kinesiology and neurolinguistic programming, which state that where you place the eye will influence which part of the brain is in use. For example, when looking down to the right, we access the lower left portion of the brain (the kinaesthetic area where we feel emotions). The humming-counting-humming manoeuvre is to switch between hemispheres quite quickly. The humming sequence engages right-brain activity, and counting, left-brain action. Overall this procedure is a useful brain balancing exercise.

Tapping on each of the points is then repeated. This process, which actually only takes about two minutes, is called the 'EFT round'. At the end of the round, the client is again asked how they feel on a scale of 0–10. Usually the number will have reduced. If it has not, it may be that the set-up statement was not precise enough and may need to be reconsidered. However, where the number is lower, another round may be conducted, with the thought held in the mind of how the feelings are in the moment, until the scale has reduced, ideally, to zero.

When the issue is resolved, the client is left with the memory without the associated feelings. At this stage, we refer back to the aspects to re-evaluate the remaining issues. Often previously high scores have reduced and, in some cases, disappeared altogether, highlighting areas that require further consideration.

The important thing is to continue testing: 'So what happens if the spider is still? Now what happens when the spider moves, or runs across the floor? How do you react to the thought of lots of tiny spiders, or the idea of a big one in the corner of the room?' The aim is to remove the irrational fear and resulting associated behaviour.

Some Examples from Practice

These examples are taken from practice in particular aspects of people's lives, where healing skills are used. They provide a flavour of the possible range of settings and areas where healing has applications.

Practice example

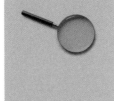

I worked with Frieda for about half an hour on her lifelong fear of wasps. After the treatment, she bemoaned the fact that although she was no longer panic-stricken about the sight or sound of wasps, she still wouldn't like one to come too close to them. 'Who would?' was my response. However, six months later, she helped her partner to remove a wasps' nest from under a tiled roof, with all due caution but absolutely no histrionics.

Practice example

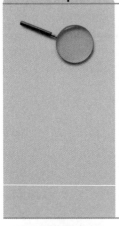

I have worked with people on Jobseeker's Allowance who attend a service provider for various skills training activities. This training is compulsory and if not attended, people lose part or all of their benefits. The skills training entails people gaining communication skills, writing a CV and other basic skills. Some of these people have had jobs in the past, while some have never had a job, do not want one and come from families where the parent/s have never worked. I provided counselling-type skills to help with any emotional barriers to employment, such as confidence and self-esteem issues. This is on a non-compulsory basis and does not affect their benefit entitlement; it is an extra service provided and paid for by a progressive management. The responses of members of this group have been very positive. Anger is a common feeling expressed by them. Some of the young men have criminal records related to their rages erupting in violence.

Practice example

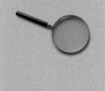

Detlev, aged 23, has a court appearance pending, possibly resulting in prison again, for violence. We worked on his anger feelings, uncovering various aspects relating to his father's rejection of him when he left when he was two. It emerged that he had a fear of loving people, in case they left him. He could not get a job, as he was verbally abusive in interviews, feeling intimidated and threatened by everyone, especially when he was nervous. A 30-minute session led to Detlev changing his attitude from surly to sweet and he left the session with his head high, a large smile and a resolute attitude towards his changed future.

Practice example

During the first encounter, Sadik avoided eye contact and blushed whenever asked a question. It emerged that he was bullied at school for being taken there by his mother, was dyslexic and firmly believed himself to be 'thick, slow and stupid'. He suffered low self-confidence and self-esteem and was unwilling to speak above a whisper. He thought the therapist was having fun at his expense when she showed him 'this silly tapping thing'. He managed to tap along for a couple of rounds before refusing to do any more. The following week he attended again, tapped for the whole session and said that even his dad and best mate had noticed the change in his level of eye contact, confidence and talkativeness.

Chapter Summary

This chapter has examined aspects of healing, but does not claim to be a comprehensive treatment of this vast topic. It focuses on the author's own practice and as such is a personal statement, the illustrations throughout the chapter being intended to demonstrate the positive aspects of energy therapies, EFT and other related healing approaches.

REVIEW QUESTIONS

1 What is energy healing?
2 What is the principle on which vibrational medicine is based?
3 What do the initials EFT stand for and what does this approach entail?

CHAPTER LINKS

For further discussion of reiki, see Chapter 29.

FURTHER RESOURCES

Eden, D. and Feinstein, D. (2000) *Energy Medicine,* Harmondsworth, Penguin. Useful general account of energy approaches to managing and affecting the body's energy systems.

Hartmann, S. (2000) *Adventures in EFT: The Essential Field Guide to Emotional Freedom Techniques,* 6th edn, Eastbourne, DragonRising. Clear, concise, definitive guide for newcomers to EFT.

Quest, P. (2002) *Reiki for Life: The Essential Guide to Reiki Practice,* London, Piatkus. Practical handbook for the beginner as well as for the more advanced practitioner.

Stein, D. (1995) *Essential Reiki: A Complete Guide to an Ancient Healing Art,* Freedom, CA, Crossing Press. An encyclopedic coverage of reiki, yet a personal account, rooted in the author's own views.

Web Link

www.chisuk.org.uk/bodymind/whatis/reiki.php – A useful website offering information on many aspects of complementary healthcare.

Part VI

Resource file

Energy Therapies

This resource file gives supplementary information on energies therapies, over and above the individual areas of practice referred to in the preceding two chapters, and offers suggestions for further reading.

For many people, reiki is central to healing and this book reflects that emphasis, with reiki figuring centrally in Chapter 29. However, reiki and healing are part of the broader field of energy approaches, which include therapeutic touch, pranic healing and spiritual healing.

- **Emotional freedom technique** is a technique based on acupuncture, used in particular for treating emotional problems (see Chapter 30).

Further Resource

Look, C. (2005) *Attracting Abundance with EFT: Emotional Freedom Techniques*, Bloomington, IN, Authorhouse.

- **The Feldenkrais method** was developed by Moshe Feldenkrai (1904–84). It is quite a diffuse approach, in the sense that it is not based on a single statement of theory and application, so much as being a tradition that evolved through its founder's lifetime and continues to evolve. In simple, somewhat oversimplified terms, it uses the notion of energy and a system of exercises to improve the functioning of the body.

Further Resources

Ruthy, A. (1994) *Mindful Spontaneity: Lessons in the Feldenkrais Method*, Berkeley, CA, North Atlantic Books.

Shafarman, S. (1997) *Awareness Heals: The Feldenkrais Method for Dynamic Healing*, Reading, MA, Addison-Wesley.

- **Polarity therapy** was developed by Oliver Stone in the 1940s and uses the notion of energy flows

through the body, which the therapist manipulates with the aim of holistic healing.

Further Resources

Beaulieu, J. (1994) *Polarity Therapy Workbook*, New York, BioSonic Enterprises.

Stone, R. (1986) *Polarity Therapy: The Complete Collected Works*, vols I and II, Sebastopol, CA, CRCS Publications.

- **Pranic healing** is a modern approach drawing on ancient ideas, and developed by Choa Kok Sui (1953–2007). It rests on an understanding of people's auras, shakra and ki, applied to balancing levels of their positive energy.

Further Resources

Sui C. (1990) *Pranic Healing*, Newburyport, MA, Red Wheel Weiser.

Co, S. and Robins, E. (2004) *Your Hands can Heal You*, Tampa, FL, Free Press.

- **Radiesthesia** is a general term used to refer to techniques similar to dowsing, used to detect minerals such as water, or to identify what may be referred to as bodily 'radiation'.

Further Resource

Hartman, J. and Kleiner, E. (1999) *Radionics and Radiethesia*, College Park, MD, Aquarian Systems.

- **Radionics** is the use of bodily substances, such as a hair, to help heal the person from a distance.

Further Resource

Tansley, D., Rae, M. and Westlake, A. (1992) *Dimensions of Radionics*, 2nd edn, Blue Ridge Summit, PA, Brotherhood of Life.

Dance Movement Therapy, Dramatherapy, Art Therapy, Music Therapy and Play Therapy

SUE JENNINGS

Learning outcomes

By the end of this chapter, you should be able to:

- understand the wider context of human development, play and the arts
- grasp the main features that differentiate the arts therapies
- appreciate the similarities and differences between arts therapies and arts activities
- follow the importance of play, games and artistic activities in people's lives

Background

The arts have traditionally been part of children's playing and games, indoors and outdoors, singly and in groups – dancing and skipping, clapping and singing, wood whittling and making mud pies, storytelling and playing make-believe games – all examples of what we might define as 'the arts' and 'play'. We can find references to the social and spiritual functions of music in the Bible:

> Praise him with a bugle blast,
> Praise him with lute and lyre,
> Praise him with the drum and dance,
> Praise him with strings and flute,
> Praise him with resounding cymbals. (Psalm 150)

This is a typical example of a children's game from a traditional undated nursery rhyme:

> Girls and boys come out to play
> The moon doth shine as bright as day
> Leave your supper and leave your sleep

> And join your playfellows in the street
> Come with a whoop, come with a call
> Come with a goodwill or not at all.

If we consider the early development of the child, we can see that healthy attachment development between mother and baby includes creative playing (Jennings, 2006, 2010). There is movement (rocking and bouncing), music and rhythm (lullabies and nursery rhymes, such as pat-a-cake, pat-a-cake), sensory play (blowing bubbles and stroking) and dramatic play (imitation and mimicry).

So the arts and play or the arts within play are an intrinsic part of healthy child development and lead to self-expression, confidence, mastery, coordination, social awareness, adaptability, emotional regulation and sheer enjoyment. The arts and play therapies are now considered 'mainstream' practices that are regulated by professional and governmental bodies, whereas historically they were seen very much as 'fringe medicine':

> If the arts play such an important role in healthy development we can see how they are an important part of the healing process for people who are unwell in mind, body or spirit. (Jennings, 2010)

Equally we can see how over history, the arts are central to both celebration and healing. Whether we look at the Old Testament, the *Mahabharata* (a Sanskrit epic of ancient India), listen to Shakespeare or the Greek Muses, the arts have always been a positive force for maintaining health or dealing with ill health and death:

> And thou didst change my mourning into dancing,
> Stripping my sackcloth, girdling me with joy,
> That my soul might sing thy praises without ceasing. (Psalm 30)

The above extract is a poignant reminder of the importance of the arts in relation to death and bereavement (Schaverien, 2002). All major life events and transitions were traditionally accompanied by artistic performances or rituals and there was always the feeling 'that it works'. However, now we have to demonstrate evidence-based practice and it is far more difficult to prove that the arts and arts therapies make any impact at all. Nevertheless, attempts are being made to create a scientific milieu for the practice of the arts therapies and play therapy – *The Arts in Psychotherapy* journal carries many research papers and the British Association of Dramatherapists has its own newsletter (*The Prompt*) and a research discussion group (http://groups.yahoo.com/group/BADthResearch/).

The following sections will give a short introduction to each of the arts therapies and play therapy. It must be borne in mind, however, that it is very much a Western approach to segregate the arts into separate specialisms, as in Eastern and Asian countries, one is more likely to find an integrated approach (Chabukswar, 2003). Many people believe that since dance needs music and drama needs images, they cannot be divided. There are many movements towards 'arts and healing' or 'the healing arts' or 'arts in hospitals'. These do not suggest that they are therapy initiatives but that their arts programmes are essentially healing. An example of an integrated initiative is the Birmingham Centre for Arts Therapies (BCAT), where all the arts therapies are offered for children and adults. BCAT is the only training and therapy centre to my knowledge that can provide an integrated approach where all the arts and play therapies are provided. Furthermore, there are initiatives there to increase the dialogue between these disciplines. The arts therapies can collectively be referred to as 'creative arts therapies', although historically the term was 'creative therapy' (Jennings, 1975). We will focus on how the arts and play are practised as therapy in the UK and indicate the main pioneers in each of the subjects.

State Regulation and Professional Associations

Art, music and dramatherapy practitioners have been state registered through the Health Professions Council (HPC, www.hpc-uk.org/) since 27 November 1997. Dance movement therapy is about to join and play therapy has applied. The HPC approves training courses and has a list of registered members. You are only allowed to practise as an arts therapist if you are on the state register. You have protection of your title and practice, since only those people who have successfully completed an approved course and maintain their state registration are allowed to call themselves arts therapists. You have to have regular supervision of your practice.

Each of the arts therapies and play therapy has a professional association with full membership criteria and codes of ethics and practice, support research and approve courses for continuing professional development. They publish regular journals and newsletters and maintain up-to-date websites, listed at the end of this chapter. There is some attempt to have conjoint work with conferences and collaborative working parties. However, the only two associations that I know that have one big umbrella for all the art therapies are YAHAT in Israel for all four arts therapies and also psychodrama, and the Irish Association of Creative Arts Therapists, which represents music therapy, art therapy, dramatherapy and dance movement therapy.

Arts therapists work within the NHS, social services and for the Home Office. They also work attached to GP surgeries, bereavement support services and child and adolescent services. Play therapists work within social services, children's hospitals and hospices and in private practice. Arts and play therapists also work in schools and special needs provision.

Dance Movement Therapy

Much of the early influence in dance movement therapy or DMT is from the pioneering work of Rudolf Laban (1879–1958) and his complete movement system and annotation. Laban's work has influenced educators and therapists for decades and he was the inspiration for early movement and dance therapists in the UK such as Marion North and Veronica Sherborne. Sherborne worked primarily with children with learning needs; she has made several films (www.concordmedia.

co.uk/?STitle=M) and wrote a book *Developmental Movement for Children* (1990), which continues to inspire dance movement therapists and dramatherapists.

The Sesame Institute also influenced this development, with the Sesame approach to therapy, which uses drama and movement to promote healing and change. It has done much to move forward the idea of movement in therapy, especially with the work of Marian Lindkvist, Sesame's founder.

Dance movement therapists believe that DMT strengthens the mind-body connections and is able to integrate the whole person through movement and dance. There are several variations in training models in the UK and perhaps the most exciting new initiative is the Integrative Dance Therapy course based at the University of Worcester. It emphasizes cross-cultural and 'eclectic intervention that provides a springboard for the systematic use of imaginative learning processes' (Brathwaite, 2009, personal communication) and gives a historical basis in the cross-fertilization of popular, indigenous and high dance forms.

Another approach is 'dance voice' that develops both the use of movement and voice within the therapeutic process. There is also an approach called medical DMT that focuses its practice on people who are 'medically ill'.

Practice example

Alice had been referred to a DMT group after three months of individual play therapy: she was anxious about her body and whether she could control it. Might it overwhelm her? Might it shame her? The therapist allowed the group of four women to slowly explore their expression of feelings and moods through movement, and then hold a movement 'conversation' of contrasting feelings. In shared discussion, it turned out that all the members had anxiety about loss of control. During the weeks, they moved and danced their anxiety, there was a complete shift in feelings and Alice realized that she could go out socially and dance and she soon joined a recreational class.

Dramatherapy

The first pioneer of dramatherapy in the UK was drama educator Peter Slade (1912–2004) in the 1950s and 60s. Slade paved the way for two later pioneers, Sue Jennings who focused on the developmental model EPR (embodiment-projection-role) for dramatherapy, and Marian Lindkvist who led the Sesame approach, which is also influenced by Jung and Laban. Dramatherapy models have burgeoned to include the 'para-theatre' approach of Steve Mitchell and the 'core process model' of Phil Jones. However it is described, dramatherapy is the application of the creative process of drama and theatre art to physical, mental or social ill health. Some dramatherapists choose a psychotherapeutic approach, others focus on the art form itself.

Dramatherapy builds on the ancient roots of ritual, theatre and storytelling and includes techniques of movement and mime, sand play and sculpting, masks and enactment, ritual, role-play, theatre texts and myths. Dramatherapy allows us to explore our personal stories, and ancient tales are explored as a means of gaining an understanding of our own story. The fact that theatre is 'distanced' from our own experience means that we can stand back and look at things afresh.

Dramatherapy can help us to express those experiences that are difficult to express because it includes verbal and nonverbal methods. Recent research in neuroscience enables us to demonstrate that mental processes are in fact dramatic processes within a theatre structure of the mind (Jennings, 2009).

Dramatherapists work individually and in groups in all spheres of mental ill health, and with people with learning needs. They also work in the prison service and in aftercare. Dramatherapy has been shown to improve thought processes in people with thought disorder, to transform behaviour patterns in children who have been excluded, and to improve communication with children on the autistic spectrum. There is impressive dramatherapy research with people who hear voices by Dr John Casson (2004).

Practice example

A dramatherapy group took place in a psychiatric hospital for people with personality disorders; they had also been sexually abused as children and several of them had an eating disorder. There was a reluctance to engage with the idea of drama and extreme emotions were expressed in all conversations. The dramatherapist developed the idea of 'differentiating feelings' – maybe we feel very angry about some things but only a little bit angry about others. Members of the group brought in pictures from magazines and newspapers that showed feelings and everyone tried to identify them. Interestingly, they got them wrong as often as right. We then role-played without words, just body shape, situations that made us feel angry, sad, scared or happy and 'a lot and a little'. Group members gradually began to experience that their feelings need not be so overwhelming, and that overreacting to everything could be confusing both to themselves and others.

Art Therapy

Art therapy was pioneered in the UK by Edward Adamson (1911–96), who worked for over 30 years at Netherne psychiatric hospital. He collaborated with Adrian Hill, an artist, who taught art to soldiers in sanatoria. Adamson was founder and first chair of the British Association of Art Therapists, and in more recent years, he became critical of art therapy for training people with a background in psychology rather than art, asking in a 1987 interview for the *New York Times*: 'Can't the psychologist remain a psychologist and not try to take over art?' Other art therapy pioneers came from the field of art education, including Edith Kramer, and from the psychoanalytic field, including Margaret Naumberg and Elinor Ulman. More recently, Diana Waller has strongly supported the state registration of art therapists, and, as a pioneer herself, has strongly endorsed the move to 'art psychotherapy' rather than 'art therapy'. There appear to be two main movements – one focusing on the art process and the other focusing on the psychotherapeutic process.

Art therapists use a variety of art media including paints, crayons, pastels, pencils, clay, collage, weaving, papier-mâché and modroc (plaster impregnated bandage), and work in diverse settings including palliative care, all branches of psychiatry, and child and adolescent services.

There is research into art therapy and schizophrenia (Ruddy and Milnes, 2003) and art therapy and eating disorders (Jennings and Minde, 1994; Gilroy, 2006).

Practice example

Ida was an inpatient in a surgical ward for repeated self-harming, having lost a lot of blood the last time. Her wrists had to be stitched and she felt very uncomfortable. The art therapist visited her and Ida shared her starvation, binging and vomiting routine that she had tried to keep hidden. She said that cutting herself was the same as throwing up – getting rid of all the nasty parts of her body. The art therapist asked her what it would feel like for them all to be joined together. Ida used some clay and worked in the enamel dish that was on her bedside table in case she was sick. The sick bowl now contained a beautifully formed young woman that Ida had modelled out of the clay. She looked up and said: 'now that is all joined back together.' This was her first step to overcoming her bulimia and self-harming.

Music Therapy

Music therapy was first pioneered in the UK by French classical cellist Juliette Alvin (1897–1982) in the 1960s and 70s. Mary Priestly, one of her students, developed the model known as 'analytic music therapy'. Nordoff-Robbins music therapy is the other model practiced in the UK, based on the principles of the pioneering music therapy work of Paul Nordoff (1909–77), American pianist and composer, and Clive Robbins (1927–), British educationalist.

Music as a healing art is well documented in traditional literature and religious texts. Early references suggest that people felt better by listening to music, for example Duke Orsino in Shakespeare's *Twelfth Night*, and Saul breathing more freely after David played his lyre in the Old Testament. There is also an association that plays music to people, mainly on the harp, to help them feel better, although it does not purport to be a therapy.

Contemporary music therapy focuses on participation in a musical experience, whether individually or in groups, for therapy to be possible. It may be based on musical improvisation or more formal musical structures, and participants are allowed to choose their own instruments or sing, closely followed by the music therapist.

There is detailed documentation of the effectiveness of music therapy as stroke therapy because it has been shown that music affects parts of the brain, thereby influencing mood and social relations (Aldridge, 2006). Music therapy can reduce depression and anxiety and improve general awareness (Glausiusz, 2001; Sachs, 2002). Music therapy is also effective in therapy for people with schizophrenia (Gold et al., 2005).

Practice example

Jamie was referred to a playgroup for children with special needs where there were both nursery nurses and teachers, and drama and music therapists. Jamie was born with no eyes and a slighted distorted skull. Although nearly three years old, he could not walk, and apparently was passed around family members in the evenings where he was rocked and cuddled. He still used a feeding bottle and the medical view was that he was very severely brain damaged. The music therapist had other ideas, especially after a session when Jamie obviously responded both to rhythm and pitch when she played the piano. After assessment, she announced that he had a musical intelligence of around seven years. She was able to use the music for him to catch up his developmental stages, and as an outlet for his frustrated feelings. Eventually he went to a residential school for children without sight, rather than one for children with learning difficulties.

Play Therapy

Ann Cattanach has done more than anyone else to pioneer the development of play therapy in the UK. She started the first training programme that later moved to the University of Roehampton. She was the first person to train therapists in the co-construction approach to play therapy, and has published many books, especially on working with children who have been sexually abused.

Play therapists in the UK are moving rapidly towards Masters-level training and are hoping to be state registered within the next few years. As with all the arts therapies, there are several strands to the play therapy training and practice, which include co-construction, Rogerian, arts and play, and psychotherapeutic/psychoanalytic models. Play therapy is still an emergent profession and is finding its own identity within the plethora of child-centred practices that include play, for example play worker, therapeutic play worker, paediatric occupational therapist, social worker, special needs teacher, as well as the arts therapists who also use play within their practice. Dramatherapists especially include dramatic play in their work with children and teenagers.

Practice example

Mary was initially referred to play therapy because she was eneuretic. She was 10 years old, wetting her bed on most nights as well as often not 'making it' to the loo at school or when she was out of the house. Her parents put her in nappies and were brusque and controlling in their handling of the situation. In the play therapy, after initial diffidence regarding 'making a mess', she began to play with wet sand. She made puddles and splashed the water, pouring it from on high and seeing it spray over everything. Slowly all her play became focused on mess-making, with the addition of finger paints and clay. It became apparent that her body had been responding to the overbearing control at home, and that she had never really learned to play. She looked relieved that no one was angry with her for making a mess or, as she disclosed, 'for getting it wrong'. Some counselling was arranged for her parents to understand their daughter's needs, where her mother shared her frustration with having to be neat and tidy all the time. Her father acknowledged that mess was difficult for him and suddenly he elected to go into personal therapy to deal with his control needs. The bed-wetting stopped after the messy play and she was then referred for DMT to build up her confidence in her body.

Chapter Summary

In this brief chapter, I have attempted to give an overview of all the arts and play therapies and how they are now practised in UK. All the arts therapies have websites that give more information about professional training. Each training course has an individual philosophy and there is variation in the course content. However, their diversity is their strong point because people can choose a course that feels right for them. Meanwhile, if you enjoy your creativity, you will start to feel better immediately. As C.S. Lewis put it: 'How can we see clearly if our eyes are full of tears?'

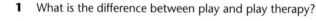

REVIEW QUESTIONS

1   What is the difference between play and play therapy?
2   How can the arts be a therapy?
3   Why is creativity 'good for us'?

FURTHER RESOURCES

Dance movement therapy

Chodorow, J. (1991) *Dance Therapy and Depth Psychology*, London, Routledge. Early definitive and important text.

North, M. (1990) *Personality Assessment through Movement*, London, Northcote House. Accessible and useful for practitioners.

Payne, H.L. (2003) *Creative Movement and Dance in Groupwork*, Milton Keynes, Speechmark. Practical ideas and application.

Stanton Jones, K. (1992) *An Introduction to Dance Movement Therapy in Psychiatry*, London, Tavistock/Routledge. Important text for clinical application.

Dramatherapy

Gersie, A. (1995) *Dramatic Approaches to Brief Therapy*, London, Jessica Kingsley. Excellent contribution to understanding brief therapy in a variety of settings.

Grainger, R. (1990) *Drama and Healing*, London, Jessica Kingsley. First book to evaluate dramatherapy practice.

Jennings, S. (1998) *Introduction to Dramatherapy: Ariadne's Ball of Thread*, London, Jessica Kingsley. Clear foundation to understanding dramatherapy theory and practice.

Pearson, J. (1996) *Discovering the Self through Drama and Movement*, London, Jessica Kingsley. Clear introduction to the Sesame method.

Pitruzella, S. (2004) *Introduction to Dramatherapy*, London, Routledge. Fascinating introduction from a new perspective.

Art therapy

Case, C. and Dally, T. (1990) *Working with Children in Art Therapy*, London Routledge. Early book on the subject but still full of insights.

Liebmann, M. (1994) *Art Therapy with Offenders*, London, Jessica Kingsley. Important book by one of the pioneers of forensic art therapy.

Malchiodi, C. (2006) *The Art Therapy Source Book*, New York, McGraw-Hill. Excellent text with a wide remit.

Shaverien, J. (2002) *The Dying Patient in Psychotherapy*, Basingstoke, Palgrave Macmillan. Unique book by an established art therapist.

Waller, D. (1993) *Group Interactive Art Therapy*, London, Routledge. One of the few books on art therapy with groups.

Music therapy

Aldridge, D. (2000) *Music Therapy in Dementia Care*, London, Jessica Kingsley. Excellent text for working in this difficult area.

Bruscia, K. (1987) *Improvisational Models of Music Therapy*, Springfield, Charles C Thomas. Early text on one approach to music therapy.

Perret, D. (2005) *Roots of Musicality: Music Therapy and Personality Development*, London, Jessica Kingsley. Clear concise understanding of the subject.

Stige, B. (2002) *Culture Centred Music Therapy*, Gilsum NH, Barcelona Publishers. One of the few books to address cross-cultural application.

Whipple, J. (2004) Music in intervention with children and adolescents with autism, *Journal of Music Therapy*, **41**(2): 990–1006. Important paper on application with people on the autistic spectrum.

Play therapy

Carroll, J. (1998) *Introduction to Therapeutic Play*, Oxford, Blackwell Science. Good all-round introduction to the subject.

Cattanach, A. (ed) (2002) *The Story So Far: Play Therapy Narratives*, London, Jessica Kingsley. Definitive text for all therapists.

Cattanach, A. (2008) *Play Therapy with Abused Children*, London, Jessica Kingsley. Excellent book on play therapy and abuse.

Jennings, S. (1999) *Introduction to Developmental Play Therapy*, London, Jessica Kingsley. Solid introduction linking theory to practice.

Stagnitti, K. and Cooper, R. (2009) *Play as Therapy: Assessment and Therapeutic Intervention*, London, Jessica Kingsley. Excellent book on methods and evaluation.

General

Casson, J. (2004) *Drama, Psychotherapy and Psychosis*, London, Routledge. Important book on research and practice.

Part VI

Chabukswar, A. (2003) Birth of a story: story-circles in therapy, *The Prompt*, summer, newsletter of the British Association of Dramatherapists. Clarifies how stories work.

Gersie, A. and King, N. (1990) *Storymaking in Education and Therapy*, London, Jessica Kingsley. Abundant material for therapeutic practice.

Jennings, S. and Minde, A. (1994) *Art Therapy and Dramatherapy: Masks of the Soul*, London, Jessica Kingsley. First book to write about dramatherapy and art therapy.

Jones, P. (1996) *Drama as Therapy, Theatre as Living*, London, Routledge. Sound book on theory and practice.

Karkou, V. and Sanderson, P. (2006) *Arts Therapies: A Research Map of the Field*, Edinburgh, Elsevier. Definitive study – comprehensive and useful.

Web Links

www.admtuk.org.uk – Association for Dance Movement Therapy UK

www.bcat – Birmingham Centre for Arts Therapies

www.badth.org – British Association of Dramatherapists

www.sesame-institute.org – Sesame Institute

www.baat.org – British Association of Art Therapists

www.apmt.org – Association for Professional Music Therapists

www.musictherapy.org – Music as Therapy charity

www.bapt.uk.com – British Association of Play Therapists

www.playtherapy.org.uk – Play Therapy UK

www.actionwork.com – Actionwork

www.psychodrama.org.uk – British Psychodrama Association

www.londoncentreforpsychodrama.org – London Centre for Psychodrama

www.rowancentre.net – Rowan Centre

www.dramatherapy.net – Dramatherapy Network

Resource file

Expressive Therapies

This resource file gives supplementary information on expressive therapies, over and above the individual areas of practice referred to in the preceding chapter, and offers suggestions for further reading.

A wide variety of therapies draw on the expressive arts and people's capacity and motivation to express themselves. Some of these therapies, such as art therapy, dramatherapy, play therapy and music therapy (Chapter 31), are used in close conjunction with conventional health and social work methods. This is particularly the case with children who have been abused and adults experiencing post-traumatic shock. Other less widely known therapies such as writing therapy and photo therapy are also used.

The playing of familiar music and the reading of stories are methods that have been used by relatives and friends to communicate with a child or adult in a coma.

■ *Photo therapy* is a therapeutic approach (Adams, 2007: 401) somewhat overshadowed by other expressive therapies, and may be used on its own or combined with other approaches. Jackson and Jackson (1999: 7–8) illustrate the uses of photographic therapy with disabled people, to help a person gain new skills, reach emotional stability or reduce uncertainties. Also, they show how photography contributes to a sense of achievement, helps a person to grieve and offers a stimulus for memories after a special event or outing (Jackson and Jackson, 1999: 9–10).

Further Resource

Jackson, E. and Jackson, N. (1999) *Learning Disability in Focus: The Use of Photography in the Care of People with a Learning Disability*, London, Jessica Kingsley.

■ *Poetry therapy* has the potential to make a major contribution to therapy, for four reasons:

1. Poems selected can be short
2. They tend to appeal to the emotions
3. They tend to be focused sharply on particular aspects
4. They often possess the power of expression to make a unique contribution to the therapeutic process (Adams, 2007: 401).

Further Resource

Gladding, S. (2003) *Poetry Therapy: Theory and Practice*, London, Routledge.

■ *Sound therapy* is akin to music therapy, in that it relies on the therapist using musical instruments or the human voice in a skilled way, as part of therapy. Repeated instrumental phrases or human chanting may be used either to relax or stimulate the person.

Further Resource

Dewhurst-Maddock, O. (1993) *Sound Therapy: Heal Yourself with Music and Voice*, Englewood Cliffs, NJ, Prentice Hall/IBD.

■ *Visualization therapy* is a form of therapy that encourages the use of the right side of the brain, reportedly more engaged in creative and emotion-laden activity.

Further Resources

Diemer, D. (2000) *The A B C's of Chakra Therapy: A Workbook*, New Delhi, Motilal Banardsidass.

Wills, P. (1994) *Visualisation*, London, Hodder Arnold.

Part VI

Continuing Education and Professional Development

Part VII
Continuing Education and Professional Development

We are reaching the end of the book, but this final part marks a transition rather than an end, that is, the shift to a continuing process of professional and personal development. Chapter 32 explores possible pathways forward, professionally and academically. It does this in conjunction with the resource file that follows. This gives details of how to gain access to continuing education and professional development. The appendix on useful practitioner and professional regulating organizations can also be read in conjunction with this chapter.

Continuing Professional Development

ROBERT ADAMS

Part VII

Learning outcomes

By the end of this chapter, you should be able to:

- clarify what is meant by continuing professional development
- explore what it means to engage in practice development
- identify routes to further education and training
- understand the procedures, costs and other implications
- access relevant professional bodies.

This chapter starts where Chapter 2 left off. Chapter 2 set the scene for the rest of the book, by examining the realities of developing ourselves as critically reflective practitioners. Here, at the end of the book, we acknowledge that in one sense, although we have finished this book, we are only at the start of another process – the process of practice development – to which there is no ending.

This chapter discusses the opportunities that exist for further study and/or work experience and provides relevant information on how to access these. The three main routes to further professional development are through:

1. being supervised by a more qualified and experienced practitioner
2. membership of a practitioner organization
3. joining a course or practice development programme based in a college or university.

Continuing Professional Development

Continuing professional development is the systematic process by which the complementary practitioner maintains and updates expertise, that is, knowledge,

375

understanding and skills, thereby improving performance in practice. It is possible to engage in this in a structured way, by enlisting the help of an experienced colleague, or group of colleagues. You may be lucky enough to be able to ask an experienced colleague to act as a regular reflector, while you talk through your work with particular patients or clients (Figure 32.1).

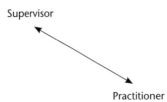

Supervisor

Practitioner

Figure 32.1 Supervision

This reflective process is part of what a professional supervisor would do, if appointed by your employer. There is a hierarchical element in most of these supervisory relationships, represented in Figure 32.1 by the downhill slope from the supervisor to the practitioner. Another possibility is that you engage in what is called 'co-supervision', which is where you exchange roles back and forth and supervise each other in turn (Figure 32.2).

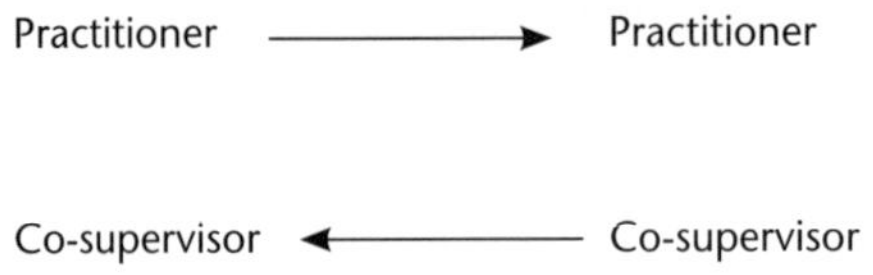

Practitioner ⟶ Practitioner

Co-supervisor ⟵ Co-supervisor

Figure 32.2 Co-supervision

Or it may be that you can join a group of practitioners and discuss your cases as a group (Figure 32.3). It is clear from Figure 32.3 that this opens up more possibilities, but is also more complex, from the point of view of supervisory and co-supervisory relationships.

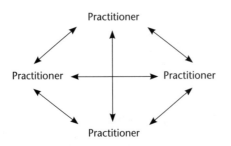

Practitioner

Practitioner   Practitioner

Practitioner

Figure 32.3 Group supervision

Integrative Practice Development

Spend a few minutes considering what the term 'integrative' means to you in relation to the development of practice.

Practice is an ongoing integrative activity, rather than one which ever achieves integration, in a final sense. If you accept this idea, it means that our professional development never finishes, and inseparable from this, of course, is the reality that our personal development never finishes.

'Practice development' is the term I use to refer to the continuing challenge of developing as a critically reflective practitioner. It integrates what you are learning from experience with your continually developing understanding and expanding the knowledge you gain about the research that feeds the evidence base for practice. These ingredients interact with each other and also contribute to integrative practice (Figure 32.4).

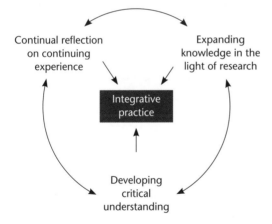

Figure 32.4 Integrative practice development

Further Education and Training

There are training and career opportunities in complementary health practice, but hard work is necessary in order to manage the business side as well as the practice. It is necessary to overcome the fact that some people believe that complementary and alternative practitioners are not adequately qualified and deliver inferior services. To achieve this, the new practitioner needs to work to establish a reputation as being credible and reliable.

Part VII

Continuing Education

Qualifications are available at different levels. The more creditable courses are assessed and validated by external professional and/or academic bodies such as professional councils, colleges or universities. On the whole, a course that only has academic validation is not likely to lead to a professional qualification, without involvement by the relevant professional body. The person intending to practise should seek a course accredited by the professional body. When choosing a course, it is advisable to find out how much practice the programme entails. A reasonable balance between the academic/classroom sessions and practice sessions is necessary. The balance considered reasonable will vary according to the area of practice. It is necessary to distinguish between work experience and practice learning, which entails supervision and the development of expertise through being taught, or observed and given critical feedback, while practising. Another aspect to consider is the content of the programme. It is worth asking a practitioner to consider the content of the course and comment on its relevance.

As mentioned in Chapter 12, an active approach to research is part of lifelong personal and professional development.

Regulation

It is important to consider what area or areas of practice in which one wishes to develop expertise. It is wise to consult the relevant bodies that regulate the respective areas of practice. The field of complementary therapies is becoming more regulated. The regulatory situation varies in different countries. At present, only a small number of professional areas, such as chiropractic and osteopathy, are subject to statutory regulation. Other practitioners come under the umbrella of the self-regulating Complementary and Natural Healthcare Council.

Costs

Grants are available in the UK to some categories of students in further and higher education. The rules for eligibility for grants are complex. Broadly speaking, students up to about age 18 or 19 in sixth form colleges and further education colleges are entitled to free full-time education and most A level or equivalent courses can be taken on this basis. There are some courses where equipment is required and this is normally an additional cost incurred by the student, unless the student is eligible for an additional grant or bursary. It is necessary to bear in mind that equipment can be costly. For example, a folding chair for reflexology treatment can cost up to £200, while oils and herbal preparations for aromatherapy and herbal medicines can be expensive.

Some complementary therapy courses are run in further education colleges, while an increasing number are developing in higher education as part of undergraduate degree provision. This means that the professional qualification may be awarded alongside an honours degree. In this case, the normal regulations governing eligibility for higher education grants apply to students. These vary in different countries of the UK. Details of the application process can be obtained from UCAS (www.ucas.ac.uk). Career development loans are also available in some circumstances for a proportion (usually up to 80%) of the cost of course fees for job-related courses. Under certain circumstances, living expenses can be added to the loan. Some courses, such as foundation degrees, are designed for students to take while continuing to work and this makes it possible to earn money to offset against course fees and other expenses.

Chapter Summary

This chapter has considered pathways forward for the future professional development of practitioners in complementary therapy and alternative medicine. A number of aspects need considering, notably different pathways to continuing professional development, the matter of regulation and the costs of relevant educational and qualification programmes.

CHAPTER LINKS

For further discussion of legal registration and regulation, see Chapter 5.

For further discussion on running a small business in complementary therapies and/or alternative medicine, see Chapter 7.

For further information about professional organizations and links, see Appendix 1 and the resource file below.

FURTHER RESOURCES

Alexander, L. (2001) *Getting into Complementary Therapies*, Richmond, Trotman; Brown, L. (1994) *Working in Complementary and Alternative Medicine*, London, Kogan Page; Fulder, S. (1996) *Handbook of Alternative and Complementary Medicine*, Oxford, Oxford University Press; Wilson, L. (2000) *Becoming a Complementary Therapist*, Oxford, How to Books; *Complete Guide to Healthcare Professions Courses*, UCAS/Trotman guide series. All books on moving into complementary practice.

Higgins, N. (2002) *Careers in Complementary Medicine: Your Questions and Answers*, Richmond, Trotman. Slim book containing a straightforward sequence of commonly asked questions, with answers.

Maher, G. (1992) *Start a Career in Complementary Medicine: A Manual/Directory of Courses in Alternative and Complementary Medicine*, Harrow, Tackmart Publishing. Practical guidance on routes to qualification in different areas of complementary practice.

Resource file

Further Study

This resource file contains basic information about further study, in two categories:

- gaining access to courses
- identifying relevant journals and similar sources of information.

Gaining Access to College and University-based Courses

There are courses in complementary therapies and alternative medicine in colleges and universities. Courses can be found that are uncertificated, as well as at foundation degree, undergraduate and postgraduate levels. The nature and number of courses offered changes constantly. In 2009, there were approximately 70 foundation degrees in aspects of complementary therapies, about 30 honours undergraduate degree programmes and a handful of postgraduate degrees.

Foundation Degree Forward (FDF) is the higher education organization that promotes employer-led courses in the UK. Foundation degrees are intended to be work-based courses, so they offer the opportunity for students at work to study at the same time. The FDF website (www.fdf.ac.uk) contains details of the different foundation degrees available at any time.

Access to undergraduate and, since 2007 with the introduction of the UKPASS information system for intending postgraduate students (www.ukpass.ac.uk), postgraduate courses in higher education in the UK (degrees, foundation degrees, higher national diplomas and other courses) is through UCAS. UCAS (www.ucas.ac.uk) manages the process of application on behalf of students and the institutions offering the courses for which they apply.

Prospects (www.prospects.ac.uk) also gives information about postgraduate study, including masters and doctorate degrees and offers careers advice, including information on jobs and CV, applications and interview guidance.

Identifying Relevant Journals and Similar Sources of Information

The detailed information and guidance given in the resource file at the end of Chapter 2 should make it straightforward to gain access to journals, databases and other relevant sources of information.

The following are some relevant journals:

Acupuncture in Medicine
Acupuncture Today
Alternative & Complementary Therapies
Alternative Medicine
Alternative Medicine Review
Alternative Therapies in Health and Medicine
Alternative Therapies in Women's Health
American Journal of Chinese Medicine
American Journal of Homeopathic Medicine
Aromatic News
Australian Journal of Medical Herbalism
Australian Journal of Music Therapy
Better Nutrition
BMC Complementary and Alternative Medicine
Body Sense
California Chiropractic Association Journal
California Journal of Oriental Medicine
Canadian Journal of Herbalism
Chinese Journal of Integrative Medicine
Chiropractic Journal
Chiropractic Journal of Australia
Clinical Chiropractic
Complementary and Alternative Medicine (eCAM)
Complementary Health Practice Review
Complementary Therapies in Clinical Practice
Complementary Therapies in Medicine
Dragons Tale
Dynamic Chiropractic
Focus on Alternative and Complementary Therapies
Health and Homeopathy
Healthy Way
Herb Quarterly

Integrative Cancer Therapies
Integrative Medicine: A Clinician's Journal
International Journal of Applied Kinesiology and
    Kinesiologic Medicine
International Journal of Aromatherapy
International Journal of Clinical and Experimental
    Hypnosis
Journal of Alternative and Complementary Medicine
Journal of Bodywork and Movement Therapies
Journal of Chinese Medicine
Journal of Chiropractic Education
Journal of Chiropractic Humanities
Journal of Chiropractic Medicine
Journal of Complementary and Integrative Medicine
Journal of Complementary Medicine (Australia)
Journal of Ethnopharmacology
Journal of Herbal Pharmacotherapy
Journal of Herbs, Spices & Medicinal Plants
Journal of Manipulative and Physiological Therapeutics
Journal of Medicinal Food
Journal of the American Chiropractic Association
Journal of the Australian Traditional-Medicine Society
Journal of the Canadian Chiropractic Association
Macrobiotics Today
Massage & Bodywork
Massage Therapy Journal
Massage Today

Massage World
National Journal of Homoeopathy
Positive Health Magazine
Scientific Review of Alternative Medicine

The following are examples of a few other sources of useful information and publications:

http://bmj.com/cgi/collection/complementary_medi-
    cine – *British Medical Journal* articles since January
    1998 on complementary medicine
www.chisuk.org.uk – Complementary Healthcare
    Information Service, UK
www.elsevier.com/wps/find/journaldescription.cws_
    home/704176/description#description – *Comple-
    mentary Therapies in Clinical Practice*
www.elsevier.com/wps/find/journaldescription.cws_
    home/623020/description#description – *Comple-
    mentary Therapies in Medicine*
www.pharmpress.com/shop/journals.asp?a=1&cid=27
    – *Focus on Alternative and Complementary Therapies*
www.internethealthlibrary.com – Internet Health Library
www.liebertpub.com/products/product.aspx?pid=26 –
    Journal of Alternative and Complementary Medicine
www.bepress.com/jcim/ – *Journal of Complementary
    and Integrative Medicine*
www.noah-health.org – New York Online Access to
    Health (NOAH)

Appendices

Professional Organizations and Related Contacts

The following is not a complete list but it does give entry to the websites of some of the more established complementary professions. The list is a starting point only, in the sense that it only indicates possible sources, since within each area of practice, a search using a search engine such as Google, with either the heading of UK, international or country, will produce many opportunities for further links.

UK

Aromatherapy and Allied Practitioners Association
www.aromatherapyuk.net

Aromatherapy Council
www.aromatherapycouncil.co.uk

Aromatherapy Organizations Council
www.dunromin.demon.co.uk

Aromatherapy Trade Council
www.candleliteliving.co.uk

Association of Master Herbalists
www.associationofmasterherbalists.co.uk

Association of Natural Medicine
www.associationnaturalmedicine.co.uk

Association of Traditional Chinese Medicine
www.atcm.co.uk

Ayurveda Institute
www.ayurveda.com

British Acupuncture Council
www.acupuncture.org.uk

British Association for Nutritional Therapy
www.bant.org.uk

British Chiropractic Association
www.chiropractic-uk.co.uk

British Complementary Medicine Association
www.bcma.co.uk

British Herbal Medicine Association
www.bhma.info

British Homeopathic Association
www.trusthomeopathy.org/faculty

British International Spa Association
www.spaassociation.org.uk

British Osteopathic Association
www.osteopathy.org

College of Ayurveda
www.ayurvedacollege.org.uk

College of Practitioners of Phytotherapy
www.phytotherapists.org

Complementary Medical Association
www.the-cma.org.uk

Complementary and Natural Healthcare Council
www.cnhc.org.uk

Complementary Therapists Association
www.complementary.assoc.org.uk

Dr Edward Bach Centre
www.bachcentre.com

Federation of Holistic Therapists
www.fht.org.uk

Foundation for Traditional Chinese Medicine
www.ftcm.org.uk

General Chiropractic Council
www.gcc-uk.org

General Osteopathic Council
www.osteopathy.org.uk

General Regulatory Council for Complementary
Therapists
www.grcct.org

Holistic Local (social networking and business
directory)
www.holisticlocal.co.uk

Institute for Complementary and Natural Medicine (also administers the Register of Complementary Practitioners)
www.i-c-m.org.uk

National Institute of Medical Herbalists
www.nimh.org.uk

Northern Ireland Association of Traditional
Chinese Medicine
www.niatcm.com

Prince's Foundation for Integrated Health
www.fih.org.uk

The Nutri Centre (based at the Hale Clinic,
London, leading dispensary and centre for
complementary medicine)
www.nutricentre.com

The Reiki Association
www.reikiassociation.org.uk

Society of Homeopaths
www.homeopathy-soh.org

Society of Teachers of the Alexander Technique
www.stat.org.uk

Unified Register of Herbal Practitioners
www.urhp.com

WITNESS (organization working with people
abused by health and social care workers)
www.popan.org.uk

International

Alternative Medicines College of Canada
www.alternativemedicinecollege.com

American Alternative Medicine Association
www.joinaama.com

American Chinese Medicine Association
www.americanchinesemedicineassociation.org

American Herbalists Guild
www.americanherbalistsguild.com

American Holistic Medicine Association
www.holisticmedicine.org

Asia Pacific Traditional Medicine and Herbal
Technology Network
www.apctt-tm.net

Australian Traditional Medicine Society
www.atms.com.au

Ayurveda Medical Association of India
www.ayurveda-amai.org

Bach flower remedies
www.edwardbach.org

Canadian College of Naturopathic Medicine
www.ccnm.edu

Canadian Natural Health Association
http://toronto.ibegin.com/misc/
canadian-natural-health-association

Canadian Society of Chinese Medicine and
Acupuncture
www.tcmcanada.org

Centre for Traditional Medicine (USA)
www.centerfortraditionalmedicine.org

European Herbal and Traditional Medicine
Practitioners' Association
www.ehtpa.eu

International Aromatherapy Association
www.internationalaromatherapyassociation.com

International Association of Crystal Healing
Therapists
www.iacht.co.uk

International Association of Reiki Professionals
www.iarp.org

International Association for the Study of
Traditional Asian Medicine
www.iastam.org

International Center for Reiki Training
www.reiki.org

International Chiropractors Association
www.chiropractic.org

International Council of Reflexologists
www.icr-reflexology.org

International Expressive Arts Therapy Association
www.ieata.org

International Federation of Professional
Aromatherapists
www.aromatherapy-studies.com

International Healing and Professional Spiritual
Professionals Association
www.onlinehealers.org

International Natural Healers Association
www.internationalhealers.com

International Reflexology Association
www.holisticbenefits.com

International Register of Consultant Herbalists
and Homeopaths
www.irch.org

International Reiki Association
www.internationalreikiassociation.com

International Self-realization Healing Association
www.novelguide.com

National Ayurvedic Medical Association (USA)
www.ayurveda-nama.org

Osteopathic International Alliance
www.oialliance.org

Prometra International (advocates traditional medicine in Africa)
www.prometra.org

Reflexology Association of America
www.reflexology-usa.org

Reiki Alliance Worldwide
www.reikialliance.com

Traditional Medicine Association (South Africa)
www.botany.uwc.ac.za

World Federation of Chinese Medicine Societies
www.wfcms.org

APPENDIX

2 Key Concepts

(Meanings of Chinese terms contributed by Fanyi Meng)

aetiology   the study of the causes of diseases and medical conditions

allopathic medicine   orthodox or conventional medicine, which treats illnesses, diseases or conditions with remedies that aim to manage, change, modify or eliminate these

alternative medicine   holistic approaches to healing, health or wellbeing that are alternatives to conventional medicine

artery   a blood vessel that carries blood away from the heart to the peripheral capillaries

asymptomatic   (of a disease or suspected disease) without sumptoms

balanced resting state   'unwinding' by lying on one's back, knees up and head on a comfortable amount of books, just high enough for the head to be a continuation of the direction of the back, without it being pulled back or pushed into the throat

biochemical processes   processes involving chemical activity

biomedical approaches   approaches to explaining illnesses in terms of their natural scientific, for example physiological, biologically based causes rather than the complexity of their individual and social origins

biopsychosocial   an alternative to the biomedical approach to ill health, which emphasizes not just the social context of the patient but also the role of the system of healthcare in creating and relieving conditions and illnesses

capillary   a minute blood vessel, connecting an arteriole (small artery) and a venule

cleaning   the process of physically removing contaminants, which does not necessarily entail eliminating them

clinical waste	waste that has been in contact with bodily fluids
code of ethics	the set of rules and standards of conduct that professionals should follow
cognition	referring to ways in which we are aware of, experience and know the world around us
critical analysis	the set of describing and analytic skills on which we draw when we engage in the process of reflecting on practice in the light of our existing knowledge and understanding, and posing questions about how well we have done and whether we could do differently and better next time
disinfection	the process of reducing contaminants, but will not eliminate microbial infection
dissection	cutting up and separating parts, for example in the study of anatomy
dosha	term used in Ayurvedic medicine for the healthy functioning of the body
evaluation of practice	the term used to refer to how we judge our practice and the practice of others
evidence-based practice	approach not based on custom and practice but following research evidence
experiential learning	different ways in which people draw on their previous and current primary (from direct experience) and secondary (from experience gained through formally acquired learning) learning from experience
hazard	the manner in which a situation or an object may cause harm
herbal decoction	the extraction of substances by boiling plants
holism	derived from the Greek *holos* meaning a whole or complete
holistic approaches	approaches to health and healing that take into account the needs of the whole person and body
homeostasis	the maintenance of balance in the healthy functioning of the cells, tissues, organs and systems of the body
infection	the process of invasion of the body by organisms that produce disease – whether bacteria or viruses
informed consent	the practitioner has to explain the consequences of a particular decision, treatment or intervention, so that the person understands the nature of the consequences – possible, probable or certain – of anything that is or is not done
interstitial fluid	the fluid in the tissues that fills the spaces between cells
meridians (经络)	pathways through which the qi (chi) flows
MRSA	methicillin resistant *Staphylococcus aureus* – a dangerous and potentially fatal form of the common bacterium *Staphylococcus aureus*,

	which is resistant to methicillin, a form of antibiotic drug similar to penicillin, and so cannot easily be treated when it invades the body
oral tradition	handed down by word of mouth rather than through printed words
palpation	a method of clinical examination that uses gentle pressure of the fingers to feel the condition of organs beneath the skin, detect growths, changes in the size of underlying organs, and unusual tissue reactions to pressure
pathogenesis	the origin, development and resultant effects of a disease
pathology	the study and diagnosis of diseases and conditions through examination of the body
pathophysiology	the study of abnormalities in the body brought about by a disease or condition
physiomedicalism	the integration of holistic ideas of natural therapeutic healing, modern medical understandings and the botanic healing system
placebo	a false or 'dummy' treatment or drug, which looks just like the real treatment but has no effect
practice	the integrative process of gathering knowledge and understanding and incorporating this into actions, on which the practitioner continually reflects
qi (**chi**, 气, 氣)	Chinese term for vital materials bearing energy in the body, which is also considered to be the internal healing power
reductionist approach	approach that understands happenings, illnesses or conditions not with reference to their complexity but through simplifying this
reflective practice	the systematic process of describing practice, identifying its main features, highlighting its significance, exploring its complexity, evaluating its strengths and weaknesses and clarifying what would be done differently next time
reflexivity	how we bring to bear on our reflections on another person's situation our emotions and thoughts in relation to our own experience and learning
research	the term used to refer to systematic attempts to focus on particular aspects of a subject and, rather than relying on opinions, establish patterns, processes, outcomes or effectiveness
risk	the calculated chance that harm will occur
self-awareness	the knowledge and understanding we have of our own values, beliefs and actions
showing expertise	using appropriate knowledge, understanding and skills in practice and taking responsibility for continuing professional development
sterilization	the process of eliminating viable microorganisms from an object

Taoism (道) ancient Chinese philosophy based on the teachings of Lao Tzu from the 6th century BC

values beliefs, standards and ideals about what is considered desirable or worthwhile

vein a blood vessel that carries blood from the capillaries back to the heart

venule a minute vein that receives oxygen-depleted blood from the capillaries and returns it to the heart via the veins

wellbeing state of good health of mind, body and spirit

yin and yang (陰陽) terms in Chinese philosophy referring to the opposite and complementary qualities of many phenomena in the world. They do not refer to conflicts or tensions but do refer to dual relationships, which in some circumstances may counterbalance each other

Bibliography

Acheson, Sir Donald (1998) *Independent Inquiry into Inequalities in Health*, London, TSO.

Achterberg, J., Cooke, K., Richards, T. et al. (2005) Evidence for correlations between distant intentionality and brain function in recipients: a functional magnetic resonance imaging analysis, *Journal of Alternative and Complementary Medicine*, **11**(6): 965–71.

Adams, R. (1990) *Self-help, Social Work and Empowerment*, Basingstoke, Macmillan – now Palgrave Macmillan.

Adams, R. (ed.) (2007) *Foundations of Health and Social Care*, Basingstoke, Palgrave Macmillan.

Adams, R. (2008) *Empowerment, Participation and Social Work*, Basingstoke, Palgrave Macmillan.

Albright, P. (1997) *Complementary Therapies: A Marshall Health Guide*, London, Marshall.

Aldridge, D. (2006) *Music Therapy Research and Practice in Medicine: From Out of the Silence*, London, Jessica Kingsley.

Ali, M. (2001) *The Integrated Health Bible*, London, Vermilion/Random House.

Andrews, M., Angone, K., Cray, J. et al. (eds) (1999) *Nurse's Handbook of Alternative and Complementary Therapies*, Springhouse, PA, Springhouse.

Argyle, M. (1988) *Bodily Communication*, London, Methuen.

Arnett, F., Edworthy, S., Bloch, D. et al. (1988) The American Rheumatism Association 1987 revised criteria for the classification of rheumatoid arthritis, *Arthritis & Rheumatism*, **31**(1): 315–24.

Austin, D., Bower, H., Creswell, J. et al. (1998) *Total Health: The Essential Family Guide to Conventional and Complementary Medicine*, London, Marshall Publishing

Azaizeh, H., Saad, B., Khalil, K. and Said. O. (2006) The state of the art of traditional Arab herbal medicine region of the Mediterranean: a review, *Evidence Based Complementary Alternative* Medicine, **3**(2): 229–35.

Baerlein, E. (1978) Hand healing, in M. Hulke (ed.) *The Encyclopedia of Alternative Medicine and Self-help*, London, Rider.

Bajaj, S. and Vohora, S.B. (2000) Anti-cataleptic, anti-anxiety and anti-depressant activity of gold: preparations used in Indian systems of medicine, *Indian Journal of Pharmacology*, **32**: 339–46.

Bakx, K. (1991) The 'eclipse' of folk medicine in western society, *Sociology of Health and Illness*, **13**: 20–8.

Baldwin, A. and Schwartz, G. (2006) Personal interaction with a reiki practitioner decreases noise-induced microvascular damage in an animal model, *Journal of Alternative and Complementary Medicine*, **12**(1): 15–22.

Baldwin, A., Wagers, C. and Schwartz, G. (2008) Reiki improves heart rate homeostasis in laboratory rats, *Journal of Alternative and Complementary Medicine*, **14**(4): 417–22.

Bandler, R. and Grindler, J. (1982) *Reframing: Neuro-linguistic Programming and the Transformation of Meaning*, Boulder, CO, Real People Press.

Bannerman, R.H., Burton, J. and Ch'en W.-C. (eds) (1983) *Traditional Medicine and Health Care Coverage: A Reader for Health Administrators and Practitioners*, Geneva, WHO.

Barnett, L. and Chambers, M. (1996) *Reiki Energy Medicine: Bringing Healing Touch into Home, Hospital, and Hospice*, Rochester, VT, Healing Arts Press.

Bratman, S. (2007) *Complementary and Alternative Health: The Scientific Verdict on What Really Works*, London, Collins.

BMA (British Medical Association) (1993) *Complementary Medicine: New Approaches to Good Practice*, Oxford, Oxford University Press.

Bronfort, G., Haas, M., Evans, R. et al. (2008) Evidence-informed management of chronic low back pain with spinal manipulation and mobilisation, *The Spine Journal*, **8**: 213–25.

Brown, G.W. and Harris, T. (1978) *Social Origins of Depression: A Study of Psychiatric Disorder in Women*, Abingdon, Taylor & Francis.

Burton, R. (1932) *The Anatomy of Melancholy*, orig. published 1621, London, Everyman.

Buxton, P. (2002) The principles of osteopathy, *The Osteopath*, March, 23–5.

Caldicott, F. (1997) *Caldicott Committee Report on the Review of Patient-identifiable Information*, London, DH.

Caldicott Standards (2002) *Implementing the Caldicott Standard into Social Care*, Health Service Circular/LAC circular, HSC2002/003/LAC 2.

Cant, S. and Sharma, U. (1999) *A New Medical Pluralism? Alternative Medicine, Doctors, Patients and the State*, London, UCL Press.

Cash, M. (1996) *Sports and Remedial Massage Therapy*, London, Ebury Press.

Cash, M. and Ylinen, J. (1992) *Sports Massage*, London, Hutchinson.

Cassidy, J.D., Boyle, E. and Côté, P. et al. (2008) Risk of vertebrobasilar stroke and chiropractic care, *Spine*, **33**(4S): 176–83.

Casson, J. (2004) *Drama, Psychotherapy and Psychosis: Dramatherapy and Psychodrama with People who Hear Voices*, Hove, Routledge.

Chabukswar, A. (2003) Birth of a story: story-circles for healing and change, *The Prompt*, summer, newsletter of the British Association of Dramatherapists.

Chief Executives' Group (2007) *Common Values Statement by the Chief Executives' Group of the Health Care Regulators on Professional Values*, www.health.ac.uk/media/docs/advisory-board/meetings/2007.

Chishti, H.G.M. (1991) *The Traditional Healer's Handbook: A Classic Guide to the Medicine of Avicenna*, Rochester, VT, Healing Arts Press.

Conable, B. and Conable, B. (2000) *What Every Musician Needs to Know About the Body: The Practical Application of Body Mapping and the Alexander Technique to Making Music*, Portland, OR, Andover Press.

COT (College of Occupational Therapists) (2005a) *Occupational Therapists in Independent Practice (OTIP): Code of Business Practice*, London, College of Occupational Therapists.

COT (College of Occupational Therapists) (2005b) *College of Occupational Therapists Code of Ethics and Professional Conduct*, London, College of Occupational Therapists, www.cot.co.uk/.

Cottrell, D. (1993) In defence of multidisciplinary teams in child and adolescent psychiatry, *Psychiatric Bulletin*, **17**: 733–5.

Credit, L.P., Hartunian, S.G. and Nowak, M.J. (2003) *Your Guide to Alternative Medicine*, New York, Square One Publishers.

Crellin, J. and Ania, F. (2002) *Professionalism and Ethics in Complementary and Alternative Medicine*, Binghampton, NY, Haworth.

Davies, C. (ed.) (1981) *Rewriting Nursing History*, New York, Barnes & Noble.

DH (Department of Health) (2004) *Choosing Health: Making Healthy Choices Easier*, White Paper, Cm 6374, London, TSO.

DH (Department of Health) (2007) *Trust, Assurance and Safety: The Regulation of Health Professionals in the 21st Century*, White Paper, Cmnd 7013, London, TSO.

DH/DfES (Department of Health/Department for Education and Skills) (2004) *National Service Framework for Children, Young People and Maternity Services*, London, TSO.

DiGiovana, E.L. (2001) *An Encyclopaedia of Osteopathy*, Indianapolis, American Academy of Osteopathy.

Eisenberg, D.M., Kessler, R.C., Foster, C. et al. (1993) Unconventional medicine in the United States, *New England Journal of Medicine*, **328**: 246–52.

Eisenberg, D.M., Davis, R.B., Ettnes, S.L. et al. (1998) Trends in alternative medicine use in the United States, 1990-1997, *Journal of American Medical Association*, **280**: 1569–75.

Ernst, E. and Singh, S. (2008) *Trick or Treatment: Alternative Medicine on Trial,* London, Bantam Press.

European Society of Cardiology (2005) Guidelines for the diagnosis and treatment of chronic heart failure: executive summary, the Task Force for the Diagnosis and Treatment of Chronic Heart Failure of the European Society of Cardiology, *European Heart Journal*, **22**: 247–3.

Frawley, D. (2003) *Ayurvedic Healing: A Comprehensive Guide*, 2nd edn, Delhi, Motilal Banarsidass.

Friedson, E. (1970) *Profession of Medicine: A Study of the Sociology of Applied Knowledge*, New York, Dodd Mead.

Fulder, S. (1997) *The Handbook of Alternative and Complementary Medicine: The Essential Health Companion*, 3rd edn, London, Vermilion.

Gascoigne, S. (1997) *The Chinese Way to Health: A Self-help Guide to Traditional Medicine*, London, Hodder & Stoughton.

Gilroy, A. (2006) *Art Therapy, Research and Evidence-based Practice*, London, Sage.

Glausiusz, J. (2001) The genetic mystery of music, *Discover Magazine*, August.

Glover, C.A. (2002) *Glossary of Osteopathic Terminology*, Chevy Chase, MD, American Association of Colleges of Osteopathic Medicine.

Godogama, S. (2001) *The Handbook of Ayurveda*, Edinburgh, Kyle Cathie.

Gold, C., Heldal, T.O., Dahle, T. and Wigram, T. (2005) Music therapy with schizophrenia and schizophrenia type illnesses, *Cochrane Database Syst. Rev.* (2) CD004025.

Gordon, S. (2005) *Integrated Health Care in Europe*, Kenninghall, Norfolk, European Council for Classical Homeopathy, www.epha.org/a/516.

GOsC (General Osteopathic Council) (2005) *Code of Practice*, London, GOsC.

GOsC (General Osteopathic Council) (2008) *The Statutory Register of Osteopaths*, London, GOsC.

Hahnemann, S. (1995) *Organon of the Medical Art*, 6th edn, trans. S. Decker, ed. and annotated by W. Brewster O'Reilly, Washington, Birdcage Books.

Hamonet, C. (2003) Andrew Taylor Still and the birth of osteopathy, *Joint Bone Spine*, **70**(1): 80–4.

Han, S., Hur, M., Buckle, J. et al. (2006) Effect of aromatherapy on symptoms of dysmenorrhea in college students: a randomized placebo-controlled clinical trial, *Journal of Alternative and Complementary Medicine*, **12**(6): 535–41.

Haralambos, M. and Holborn, M. (2008) *Sociology: Themes and Perspectives*, 7th edn, London, Collins Educational.

Haug, M. (1973) Deprofessionalisation: an alternative hypothesis for the future, *Sociological Review Monograph*, **20**: 195–211.

Hayden, C. (1999) Infantile colic and cranial osteopathy, *The Tide*, autumn: 14–17.

Healthwork UK (2002) *National Occupational Standards for Reflexology*, London, Healthwork UK.

HM Treasury (2003) *Every Child Matters*, Green Paper, Cm 5860, London, TSO.

House of Lords (2000) *Complementary and Alternative Medicine*, Sixth Report, Select Committee on Science and Technology, London, TSO, www.parliament.the-stationery-office.co.uk/.

Hulke, M. (ed.) (1978) *The Encyclopedia of Alternative Medicine and Self-help*, London, Rider.

Illich, I. (1975a) *Tools for Conviviality*, London, Fontana.

Illich, I. (1975b) *Medical Nemesis: The Expropriation of Health*, London, Marion Boyars.

Illich, I., Zola, I.K., McKnight, J. et al. (1977) *Disabling Professions*, London, Marion Boyars.

InterSurvey (2000) *Survey of Alternative Medicine*, www.intersurvey.com.

Izhar, N. (1989) The Unani traditional medical system in India: a case study in health behaviour, *Geographica Medica*, **19**: 163–85.

Jackson, E. and Jackson, N. (1997) *Learning Disability in Focus: The Use of Photography in the Care of People with a Learning Disability*, London, Jessica Kingsley.

Jennings, S. (1975) *Creative Therapy*, London, Pitman.

Jennings, S. (2006) *Creative Play with Children at Risk*, Milton Keynes, Speechmark.

Jennings, S. (2010) *Neuro-Dramatic-Play and Attachment*, London, Jessica Kingsley.

Jennings, S. and Minde, A. (1994) *Art Therapy and Dramatherapy: Masks of the Soul*, London, Jessica Kingsley.

Jessup, R.L. (2007) Interdisciplinary versus multidisciplinary care teams: do we understand the difference?, *Australian Health Review*, August: 3–5, http://findarticles.com/p/articles/mi_6800/is_/ai_n28446050.

Jones, F.P. (1997) *Freedom to Change: The Development and Science of the Alexander Technique*, 3rd edn, London, Mourits.

Kemm, J. and Close, A. (1995) *Health Promotion: Theory and Practice*, Basingstoke, Macmillan – now Palgrave Macmillan.

Kolb, D.A. (1984) *Experiential Learning: Experience as the Source of Learning and Development*, London, Prentice Hall.

Kowalski, L. (2002) Use of aromatherapy with hospice patients to decrease pain, anxiety and depression and to promote an increased sense of well-being, *American Journal of Hospice and Palliative Care*, **19**(6): 381–6.

Lad, V. (2001) *Textbook of Ayurveda: Fundamental Principles*, vol. 1, Albuquerque, NM, Ayurvedic Press.

Lad, V. (2006) *The Complete Book of Ayurvedic Home Remedies*, London, Piatkus Books.

Lee, R.P. (2001) The primary respiratory mechanism beyond the craniospinal axis, *American Academy of Osteopathy Journal*, spring: 24–34.

Lewith, G. (2002) *Understanding Complementary Medicine*, London, BMA.

Little, P., Lewith, G., Webley, F. et al. (2008) Randomised controlled trial of Alexander technique lessons, exercise and massage (ATEAM) for chronic and recurrent back pain, *British Medical Journal*, 337: 438.

McCarter, D.F., Courtney, A.U. and Pollart, S.M. (2007) Cerumen impaction, *American Family Physician*, 75: 1523–8.

Macdonald, P. (1989) *The Alexander Technique as I see It*, Eastbourne, Alpha Press.

McKinlay, J. and Arches, J. (1985) Towards proletarianization of physicians, *International Journal of Health Sciences*, **15**: 161–95.

Maddalena, S. (1999) *The Legal Status of Complementary Medicines in Europe: A Comparative Analysis*, Bern, Stämpfli.

Maher, G. (1992) *Start a Career in Complementary Medicine: A Manual/Directory of Courses in Alternative and Complementary Medicine*, Harrow, Tackmart Publishing.

Manga, P., Angus, D., Papadopoulos, C. and Swan, W. (1993) *The Manga Report Summary: The Effectiveness and Cost-effectiveness of Chiropractic Management of Low Back Pain*, University of Ottawa.

Manga, P., Angus, D.E. and Swan, W.R. (1993) Effective management of low back pain: it's time to accept the evidence, *Journal of Canadian Chiropractic Association*, **37**(4): 221–9.

Maury, M. (2004) *Marguerite Maury's Guide to Aromatherapy: The Secret of Life and Youth*, London, Random House.

Miles, P. (2007) Reiki for mind, body and spirit support cancer patients, *Advances in Mind-body Medicine*, **22**(2): 20–6.

Miles, P. and True, G. (2003) Reiki: review of a biofield therapy history, theory, practice and research, *Alternative Therapies in Health and Medicine*, **9**(2): 62–72.

Millerson, G. (1964) *The Qualifying Association*, London, Routledge.

Mills, S. (1997) *Professional Organisation of Complementary and Alternative Medicine in the United Kingdom 1997*, Centre for Complementary Health Studies, University of Exeter.

Mills, S. and Budd, S. (2000) *Professional Organisation of Complementary and Alternative Medicine in the United Kingdom 2000*, Centre for Complementary Health Studies, University of Exeter.

NASW (National Association of Social Workers) (1999) *Code of Ethics of the National Association of Social Workers*, Washington, NASW.

National Institutes of Health (1994) *Alternative Medicine: Expanding Medical Horizons*, Washington, DC, US Government Printing Office.

Navarro, V. (1978) *Class, Struggle, the State and Medicine*, London, Martin Robertson.

NCB (National Children's Bureau) (2005) *Healthy Care Programme Handbook*, London, NCB.

NMC (Nursing and Midwifery Council) (2007) *The Code: Standards of Conduct, Performance and Ethics for Nurses and Midwives*, London, NMC, www.nmc-uk.org/aArticle.aspx?ArticleID=3056.

Nutbeam, D. (1998) *Health Promotion Glossary*, Geneva, WHO.

Oschman, J. (2000) *Energy Medicine: The Scientific Basis*, 8th edn, Edinburgh, Churchill Livingstone.

Ovretveit, J. (1986) *Organising Multidisciplinary Community Teams*, Uxbridge, Brunel Institute of Organisational and Social Studies, Brunel University.

Ovretveit, J. (1997) Planning and managing interprofessional working and teams, in J. Ovretveit, P. Mathias and T. Thompson (eds) *Interprofessional Working for Health*, Basingstoke, Macmillan – now Palgrave Macmillan.

Parsons, T. (1959) The social structure of the family, in R.N. Anshen (ed.) *The Family: Its Functions and Destiny*, New York, Harper & Row.

Parsons, T. (1965) The normal American family, in S.M. Farber (ed.) *Man and Civilization: The Family's Search for Survival*, New York, McGraw-Hill.

Patwardhan, B., Warude, D., Pushpangadan, P. and Bhatt, N. (2005) Ayurveda and traditional Chinese medicine: a comparative overview, *Evidence-based Complementary and Alternative Medicine*, 2(4): 465–73.

Payne, M. (2000) *Teamwork in Multiprofessional Care*, Basingstoke, Palgrave – now Palgrave Macmillan.

Peters, D. (ed.) (2008) *Family Guide to Complementary and Conventional Medicine*, London, Dorling Kindersley.

Peterson, D.H. and Bergmann, T.F. (2002) *Chiropractic Technique: Principles and Procedures*, 2nd edn, St Louis, Mosby.

Pietroni, P. (1991) *The Greening of Medicine*, London, Victor Gollancz.

Pike, S. and Forster, D. (eds) (1997) *Health Promotion for All*, Edinburgh, Churchill Livingstone.

Pittilo, M. (2008) *Report to Ministers from the Department of Health Steering Group on the Statutory Regulation of Practitioners of Acupuncture, Herbal Medicine, Traditional Chinese Medicine and Other Traditional Medicine Systems Practised in the UK*, Aberdeen.

Pole, S. (2006) *Ayurvedic Medicine: The Principles of Traditional Practice*, Edinburgh, Churchill Livingstone.

Quest, P. (2003) *Self-healing with Reiki*, London, Piatkus Books.

Rafferty, J. and Tsikovdas, A. (2007) Ear candling: should general practitioners recommend it?, *Canadian Family Physician*, 12: 2121–2.

Reflexology Forum (2006) *Core Curriculum for Reflexology in the United Kingdom*, London, Douglas Barry.

Reich, C. (1971) *The Greening of America*, Harmondsworth, Penguin.

Robinson, L. and Thomson, G. (2004) *The Complete Classic Pilates Method*, London, Pan.

Roter, D.L. and Hall, J.A. (2006) *Doctors Talking with Patients/Patients Talking with Doctors*, 2nd edn, Westport, CT, Praeger.

Rubik, B., Brooks, A. and Schwartz, G. (2006) *In vitro* effect of reiki treatment on bacterial cultures: role of experimental context and practitioner well-being, *Journal of Alternative and Complementary Medicine*, **12**(1): 7–13.

Ruddy, R. and Milnes, D. (2003) Art therapy for schizophrenia or schizophrenia like illnesses, *Cochrane Database Syst. Rev.* (2) CD003728.

Ryan, T. and Pritchard, J. (eds) (2004) *Good Practice in Adult Mental Health*, London, Jessica Kingsley.

Saad, B., Azaizeh, H. and Said, O. (2005) Tradition and perspectives of Arab herbal medicine: a review, *eCAM*, **2**(4): 475–9.

Saad, B., Azaizeh, H., Abu-Hijleh, G. and Said, O. (2006) Safety of traditional Arab herbal medicine, *cCAM*, **3**(4): 433–9.

Sachs, O. (2002) When music heals body and soul, *Parada Magazine*, 31 March.

Saks, M. (1998) Medicine and complementary medicine, in G. Scambler and P. Higgs (eds) *Modernity, Medicine and Health: Medical Sociology Towards 2000*, London, Routledge.

Salach, M.D. (2006) The Effects of Reiki, a Complementary Alternative Medicine, on Depression and Anxiety in the Alzheimer's and Dementia Population, PhD thesis, San Francisco State University.

Schaverien, J. (2008) *The Revealing Image: Analytical Art Psychotherapy in Theory and Practice*, London, Jessica Kingsley.

Schön, D.A. (1983) *The Reflective Practitioner: How Professionals Think in Action*, New York, Basic Books.

Shapiro, R. (2008) *Suckers: How Alternative Medicine Makes Fools of Us All*, London, Harvill Secker.

Shealy, C.N. (2000) *The Directory of Complementary Therapies*, Lewes, Time Life Books.

Sherborne, V. (1990) *Developmental Movement for Children*, Cambridge, Cambridge University Press.

Smith, A. (1997) *Practical Ayurveda*, York Beach, ME, Samuel Welser.

Smith, M.C., Reeder, F., Daniel, L. et al. (2003) Outcomes of touch therapies during bone marrow transplant, *Alternative Therapies in Health and Medicine*, **9**(1): 40–9.

Spencer, J.W. and Jacobs, J.J. (1999) *Complementary Alternative Medicine: An Evidence-based Approach*, St Louis, MI, Mosby.

Stevens, C. (1987) *The Alexander Technique*, London, Macdonald.

Still, A.T. (1899) *Philosophy of Osteopathy*, Kirksville, MO, AT Still.

Still, A.T. (1908) *Autobiography of AT Still*, Kirksville, MO, AT Still.

Stone, J. (2005) *Development of Proposals for a Future Voluntary Regulatory Structure for Complementary Healthcare Professions* (the Stone Report), London, The Prince of Wales' Foundation for Integrated Health.

Stone, J. and Lee-Treweek, G. (2005) Regulation and control, in G. Lee-Treweek, T. Heller, H. MacQueen et al. (eds) *Complementary and Alternative Medicine: Structures and Safeguards*, Abingdon, Routledge.

Stone, J. and Matthews, J. (1996) *Complementary Medicine and the Law*, Oxford, Oxford University Press.

Stuart-Cole, E. (2007) General infection prevention and control, in R. Adams (ed.) *Foundations of Health and Social Care*, Basingstoke, Palgrave Macmillan.

Sullivan, C. (1997) Introducing the cranial approach in osteopathy and the treatment of infants and mothers, *Complementary Therapies in Nursing and Midwifery*, **3**(7): 2–26.

Sullivan, H. and Skelcher, C. (2002) *Working Across Boundaries: Collaboration in Public Services*, Basingstoke, Palgrave Macmillan.

Thiel, H.W., Bolton, J.E., Docherty, S. and Portlock, J.C. (2007) Safety of chiropractic manipulation of the cervical spine, *Spine*, **32**(21): 2375–8.

Thompson, N. (2003) *Communication and Language: A Handbook of Theory and Practice*, Basingstoke, Palgrave Macmillan.

Tisserand, R. and Balacs, T. (1995) *Essential Oil Safety: A Guide for Health Professionals*, Edinburgh, Churchill Livingstone.

Tones, K. and Tilford, S. (2001) *Health Promotion: Effectiveness, Efficiency and Equity*, 3rd edn, Cheltenham, Nelson Thornes.

Totman, R. (1979) *Social Causes of Illness*, London, Souvenir Press.

Turner, B.S. (1995) *Medical Power and Social Knowledge*, London, Sage.

UK BEAM Trial Team (2004) United Kingdom back pain exercise and manipulation (UK BEAM) randomised trial: effectiveness of physical treatments for back pain in primary care, *British Medical Journal*, www.bmj.com/cgi/content/abstract/329/7479/1377.

UKCC (United Kingdom Central Council for Nursing, Midwifery and Health Visiting) (2002) *Standards for the Administration of Medicines*, London, UKCC.

UN (United Nations) (1948) *Universal Declaration of Human Rights*, Geneva, UN.

Van der Velde, G., Hogg-Johnson, S., Bayoumi, A. et al. (2008) Identifying the best treatment among common nonsurgical neck pain treatments, *Spine*, 33(4S): 184–91.

Vick, D.A., McKay, C. and Zengerle, C.R. (1996) The safety of manipulative treatment: review of the literature from 1925 to 1993, *Journal of American Osteopathic Association*, **96**(2): 113–15.

Vickers, A. (1996) *Massage and Aromatherapy: A Guide for Health Professionals*, London, Chapman & Hall.

Vickers, A. and Zolman, C. (1999) Clinical review. ABC of complementary therapies. The manipulative therapies: osteopathy and chiropractic, *British Medical Journal*, **319**: 1176–9.

Visser, G.J. and Peters, L. (1990) Alternative medicine and general practitioners in the Netherlands: towards acceptance and integration, *Family Practice*, **7**(3): 227–32.

Votsmeier, A. (1996) Kurt Goldstein and Holism, lecture held at GTILA Summer Residential Program, Barcelona, www.gestaltpsychologie.de/Lago1_ho.pdf.

Webb, E.C. (1977) *Report of the Committee of Inquiry into Chiropractic, Osteopathy, Homeopathy and Naturopathy* (Webb Report), Canberra, Australian Government Publishers.

WHO (World Health Organization) (2001) *Regulatory Situation of Herbal Medicines: A Worldwide Review*, Geneva, WHO.

WHO (World Health Organization) (2002) *Key Points: WHO Traditional Medicine Strategy 2002–2005*, Geneva, WHO.

Witz, A. (1992) *Professions and Patriarchy*, London, Routledge.

Woodham, A. (1994) *HEA Guide to Complementary Medicine and Therapies*, London, Health Education Authority.

Young, M. (2002) *Women and Pain: Why It Hurts and What You Can Do*, New York, Hyperion.

Name Index

A

Acheson, D. 42
Adams, R. 47, 48, 86, 123
Adamson, E. 365
Albright, P. 33
Aldred, E.M. 79
Aldridge, D. 366
Alexander, F.M. 217, 325, 326–7, 333
Alexander, L. 379
Ali, M. 47
Ali al-Rahawi 92
Al-Khafaji, H. 241
Alvin, J. 366
Andrews, M. 37
Ania, F. 54
Arches, J. 138
Argyle, M. 105
Arnett, F. 198–9
Aromatherapy Trade Council 53
Austin, D. 33
Avicenna 52, 129, 217
Azaizeh, H. 127, 134

B

Baerlein, E. 52
Bajaj, S. 132
Baker, K. 241
Bakx, K. 136
Balacs, T. 53, 289
Baldwin, A. 346
Banks, S. 98
Bannerman, R.H. 56
Bartram, R. 280
Bayly, D.E. 317, 323
Beck, E.R. 215
Beers, M.H. 171, 186, 202, 215
Bergmann, T.F. 300, 301
Bickley, L.S. 171, 186, 202, 215
Bikkhu, T. 267
Birch, S.J. 241, 255
Birmingham Centre for Arts
    Therapies 362–3
Black, D. 42
Bodeker, G. 72
Bonamin, V. 228
Bone, K. 280
Boyd, H. 228
Bratman, S. 33, 115, 116, 117, 119
Brayne, H. 87
Brechin, A. 20
British Association of Art Therapists
    365
British Association of
    Dramatherapists 362
British Complementary Medicine
    Association 22, 55
British Medical Association 31, 33,
    34, 37, 55

British Osteopathic Council 310, 311
British Osteopathic Journal 311
British Reflexology Association 322
British School of Osteopathy 304
Bronfort, G. 298
Brown, G.W. 137
Buckle, J. 289
Budd, S. 55
Buhner, S.H. 280
Bulman, C. 20
Burkholder, P. 79
Burton, R. 133
Buxton, P. 305

C

Caldicott, F. 100
Cant, S. 134
Care Quality Commission 87
Carr, H. 87
Cash, M. 30
Cassidy, C. 241
Cassidy, J.D. 300
Casson, J. 365
Cattanach, A. 367
Centre for Complementary Health
    Studies 55
Cheng, X. 241
Chishti, H.G.M. 132, 139
Christensen, P.J. 112
Citizens Advice Bureau 88
Clark, M. 171, 186, 202
Close, A. 44, 47, 48
Cohen, M. 72
College of Occupational Therapists
    75, 77, 78, 79, 93, 98
Collins, M. 314
Commission for Social Care
    Inspection 87
Committee on the Environment,
    Public Health and Consumer
    Protection 54
Complementary and Natural
    Healthcare Council 55, 318, 378
Compton Burnett, J. 217
Conable, B.H. 328
Conable, B.J. 328
Cottrell, D. 67
Craig, G. 355
Credit, L.P. 33
Crellin, J. 54
Culpeper, N. 217

D

Davies, C. 137
Davies, H. 106
Deadman, P. 241
De Alacantara 235
Department for Education and Skills
    43, 60, 61

Department of Communities and
    Local Government 60, 61
Department of Health 42, 43, 48,
    55, 60, 61, 279, 311
Derrickson, B. 171, 186, 202
Dewey, J. 333
Dimond, B. 59
Drake, R.L. 151

E

Eden, D. 359
Einstein, A. 352
Eisenberg, D.M. 33, 34
Ellis, A. 151
Ernst, E. 346
European Commission 56
European Parliament 54, 56, 57
European Society of Cardiology 156
European Union 55, 279

F

Fallowfield, L. 106
Fauci, A.S. 186
Federal Regulatory Council 55
Fédération des Professionnels 54
Feinstein, D. 359
Felt, R.L. 241
Field, B. 151
Fitter, M.A. 255
Fitzgerald, W. 316–17
Flaws, B. 242
Forster, D. 48, 49, 62
Foundation for Holistic Spirituality 43
Foundation for Integrated Health 318
Foundation for Integrated Medicine 55
Foundation for Paediatric
    Osteopathy 309
Friedson, E. 137
Fulder, S. 33, 35
Fulton, E. 348

G

Galen 216
Gascoigne, S. 137
Gattefosse 283
Gelb, M. 334
General Chiropractic Council 53,
    294
General Council and Register of
    Osteopaths 304
General Medical Council 55
General Osteopathic Council 53, 56,
    59, 93, 304, 310
General Regulatory Council for
    Complementary Therapies 55
Gilling, C. 112
Gilroy, A. 366
Glausiusz, J. 366
Glover, C.A. 307

Subject Index